Exercise Physiology

Physiologie de l'effort

FITNESS AND PERFORMANCE CAPACITY STUDIES

ÉTUDES PHYSIOLOGIQUES DE LA CONDITION PHYSIQUE ET DE L'APTITUDE À LA PERFORMANCE

A collection of the formal papers presented at the *International Congress of Physical Activity Sciences* held in Quebec City, July 11-16, 1976, under the auspices of the CISAP-1976-ICPAS Corporation.

Recueil des communications présentées dans le cadre du *Congrès international des sciences de l'activité physique* qui eut lieu à Québec, du 11 au 16 juillet 1976, sous les auspices de la Corporation du CISAP-1976-ICPAS.

Compiled and edited by

Recueilli et édité par

FERNAND LANDRY, Ph.D.
WILLIAM A. R. ORBAN, Ph.D.

Published by

Publié par

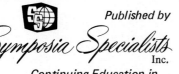
Inc.
Continuing Education in Sports Sciences

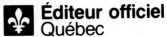
Éditeur officiel
Québec

Released through
SYMPOSIA SPECIALISTS, INC. · 1460 N.E. 129th Street
Miami, Florida 33161, U.S.A.

JOINT PUBLICATION / COPRODUCTION

L'Editeur officiel du Québec

Le Haut-commissariat à la jeunesse,
aux loisirs et aux sports du Québec

Symposia Specialists Incorporated

Associate producers/Producteurs délégués
Michel Marquis
Miriam Hochberg

WORLDWIDE DISTRIBUTION / DISTRIBUTION MONDIALE

Symposia Specialists Incorporated
Miami, Florida 33161 U.S.A.

SOLE DISTRIBUTOR FOR QUEBEC
DISTRIBUTEUR UNIQUE AU QUÉBEC

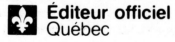

Éditeur officiel
Québec

Library of Congress Catalog
Card No. 78-55934
ISBN 0-88372-107-4

Table of Contents

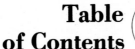

Table des matières

PREDICTION OF OUTSTANDING ATHLETIC ABILITY
La prédiction de l'aptitude à la haute performance

8th INTERNATIONAL SCIENTIFIC AQUATIC SYMPOSIUM
AQUATICS AND HUMAN PERFORMANCE
8e Symposium scientifique international sur les activités aquatiques
Activités aquatiques et performance humaine

iii

ACUTE AND CHRONIC EFFECTS OF EXERCISE AND TRAINING
Effets aigus et chroniques de l'exercice et de l'entraînement physiques

INDIVIDUAL SCIENTIFIC CONTRIBUTIONS
Communications scientifiques individuelles

Neurological—Neuromuscular and Muscular Aspects
Aspects neurologiques, neuromusculaires et musculaires

Kunio Kikuchi and Minoru Wada
Department of Health and Physical Education,
Faculty of Integrated Arts and Sciences, Hiroshima
University, Hiroshima, Japan

Biochemical Aspects
Aspects biochimiques

Fitness and Performance Capacity
Condition physique et aptitude à la performance

LA COMMISSION SCIENTIFIQUE
THE SCIENTIFIC COMMISSION

L'Exécutif — The Executive

Fernand Landry *Québec*
Président — President
William A.R. Orban *Ottawa*
Vice-président — Vice-president
Paul Godbout *Québec*
Secrétaire — Secretary

Membres — Members

Gerald Kenyon *Waterloo*
Arthur Sheedy *Montréal*
Roy J. Shephard *Toronto*
Yves Bélanger *Québec*
Gouvernement du Québec
Quebec Government

Paul S. Woodstock *Ottawa*
Gouvernement du Canada
Government of Canada
Jean Loiselle *Montréal*
COJO
Laurent Bélanger *Montréal*
APAPQ
Gordon R. Cumming *Winnipeg*
CASS — ACSS
Gregg McKelvey *Ottawa*
CAHPER
Gilles Houde *Ville de Laval*
Le Secrétaire exécutif et trésorier
The Executive Secretary and Treasurer
Gilbert Michaud *Québec*

CONSEILLERS INTERNATIONAUX
INTERNATIONAL ADVISERS

Tr Hon. — Rt. Hon.
Philip Noel-Baker *Grande-Bretagne*
Président — President *Great Britain*
CIEPS — ICSPE
Raudol Ruiz Aguilera *Cuba*
Jean Borotra *France*
Günter Erbach *Rép. démocr. allemande*
German Democratic Republic

Julien Falize *Belgique—Belgium*
Vladimir Roditchenko *URSS—USSR*
Franz Lotz *Rép. fédér. d'Allemagne*
Federal Republic of Germany
Tetsuo Meshizuka *Japon—Japan*
Leona Holbrook *EU—USA*
Nadir M. Souelem *Egypte—Egypt*

Le Congrès international des sciences de l'activité physique, 1976
a été placé sous le distingué patronage de L'UNESCO, Organisation
des Nations Unies pour l'éducation, la science et la culture.

The International Congress of Physical Activity Sciences, 1976
has been placed under the distinguished sponsorship of UNESCO,
United Nations Educational, Scientific and Cultural Organization.

Acknowledgements

The *Scientific Commission* wishes to express its deepest appreciation to the Director General of UNESCO, Mr. AMADOU MAHTAR M'BOW. for having granted the official sponsorship of his organization to the *International Congress of Physical Activity Sciences — 1976.*

The *Scientific Commission* also wishes to express its sincere appreciation and thanks to the governments, as well as to the associations, committees and groups which have provided the financial, scientific and professional assistance necessary for the planning, organization and conduct of the *International Congress of Physical Activity Sciences — 1976.*

FINANCIAL AND ADMINISTRATIVE ASSISTANCE
— THE GOVERNMENT OF CANADA
  · Health and Welfare Canada
    Fitness and Amateur Sport Branch
  · Secretary of State
— THE QUEBEC GOVERNMENT
  · Haut-commissariat à la jeunesse, aux loisirs et aux sports
  · Le ministère des Affaires intergouvernementales
  · Le ministère des Affaires culturelles
  · Le ministère du Tourisme, de la chasse et de la pêche

— THE ORGANIZING COMMITTEE OF THE OLYMPIC GAMES OF MONTREAL

SCIENTIFIC AND PROFESSIONAL COOPERATION AND ASSISTANCE
— International Council for Sport and Physical Education
  · International Committee for Sociology of Sport
  · International Committee of History of Sport and Physical Education
  · International Work Group for the Construction of Sport and Leisure Facilities (IAKS)
  · Research Group on Biochemistry of Exercise
  · Working Group on Sport and Leisure
— International Council for Health, Physical Education and Recreation
— International Society for Sports Psychology
— International Society of Cardiology
— International Sports Press Association
— Association internationale des écoles supérieures d'éducation physique et de sport (AIESEP)
— International Society of Biomechanics
— American Alliance for Health, Physical Education and Recreation (AAHPER)
— American Academy of Physical Education
— American College of Sports Medicine
— National College Physical Education Association for Men (USA)
— Council for National Cooperation in Aquatics (USA)
— Canadian Association for Health, Physical Education and Recreation (CAHPER)
  · History of Sport and Physical Activity Committee
  · Sociology of Sport Committee
  · Philosophy Committee

Remerciements

La *Commission scientifique* exprime sa haute appréciation au Directeur général de l'UNESCO, M. AMADOU MAHTAR M'BOW, pour avoir bien voulu accorder le patronage de son organisme au *Congrès international des sciences de l'activité physique — 1976.*

La *Commission scientifique* tient aussi à exprimer ses remerciements les plus sincères aux institutions gouvernementales, ainsi qu'aux organismes, associations et comités qui lui ont procuré les appuis financiers, scientifiques et professionnels nécessaires à la planification et au déroulement du congrès.

L'ASSISTANCE ADMINISTRATIVE ET FINANCIERE

— LE GOUVERNEMENT DU CANADA
  · Santé et bien-être social Canada
    Direction générale de la santé et du sport amateur
  · Secrétariat d'Etat

— LE GOUVERNEMENT DU QUEBEC
  · Haut-commissariat à la jeunesse, aux loisirs et aux sports
  · Le ministère des Affaires intergouvernementales
  · Le ministère des Affaires culturelles
  · Le ministère du Tourisme, de la chasse et de la pêche

— LE COMITE ORGANISATEUR DES JEUX OLYMPIQUES DE MONTREAL

COLLABORATION SCIENTIFIQUE ET PROFESSIONNELLE

— Le Conseil international pour l'éducation physique et le sport (CIEPS)
  · Le Comité international pour la sociologie du sport
  · Le Comité international de l'histoire de l'éducation physique et du sport
  · Le Groupe international de travail pour les équipements de sport et de loisir (IAKS)
  · Le Groupe de recherche sur la biochimie de l'effort
  · Le Groupe de travail Sport et loisirs

— Le Conseil international sur l'hygiène, l'éducation physique et la récréation (ICHPER)
— La Société internationale de psychologie du sport (ISSP)
— La Société internationale de cardiologie
— L'Association internationale de la presse sportive
— L'Association internationale des écoles supérieures d'éducation physique et de sport
— La Société internationale de biomécanique
— American Alliance for Health, Physical Education and Recreation (AAHPER)
— American Academy of Physical Education
— American College of Sports Medicine
— National College Physical Education Association for Men (USA)
— Council for National Cooperation in Aquatics (USA)
— Canadian Association for Health, Physical Education and Recreation (CAHPER)

  · History of Sport and Physical Activity Committee
  · Sociology of Sport Committee
  · Philosophy Committee

ACKNOWLEDGEMENTS

- · Exercise Physiology Committee
- · Psycho-motor Learning and Sports Psychology Committee
- · Biomechanics Committee
- · Administrative Theory and Practice Committee

— Canadian Council for Cooperation in Aquatics
— Association des professionnels de l'activité physique du Québec (APAPQ)
— Canadian Association for Sports Sciences (CASS-ACSS)
— La Ville de Québec
— L'Université Laval

The Scientific Commission extends its deepest gratitude to all the individuals who, in the last three years, have worked behind the scenes in a most efficient and generous manner.

By formal resolution of the Scientific Commission at its meeting of April 28, 1977, Messrs. Fernand Landry and William A.R. Orban, respectively President and Vice-President of the Corporation were mandated to carry out the production of the official proceedings of the CISAP-1976-ICPAS (resolution CS 77-01-11).

NOTICE

By decision of the Scientific Commission, *French* and *English* were adopted as the two official languages of the International Congress of Physical Activity Sciences – 1976.

In these Proceedings, the communications appear *in the language in which they were presented* for French and English and *in English* as concerns the papers which were delivered in either German, Russian or Spanish. Abstracts in the two official languages accompany each paper included in Books 1 and 2 and the seminar presentations in the other books of the series.

REMERCIEMENTS

- · Exercise Physiology Committee
- · Psycho-motor Learning and Sports Psychology Committee
- · Biomechanics Committee
- · Administrative Theory and Practice Committee
- — Le Conseil canadien de coopération en activités aquatiques
- — L'Association des professionnels de l'activité physique du Québec
- — L'Association canadienne des sciences du sport (CASS-ACSS)
- — La Ville de Québec
- — L'Université Laval

La gratitude de la Commission scientifique s'étend à toutes les personnes qui, au cours des trois dernières années, et trop souvent dans l'ombre, ont apporté leur efficace et généreuse collaboration.

Par résolution de la Commission scientifique à sa réunion du 28 avril 1977, MM. Fernand Landry et William A.R. Orban, respectivement président et vice-président de la Corporation, ont été mandatés pour effectuer la production des actes du CISAP-1976-ICPAS (résolution CS 77-01-11).

AVERTISSEMENT

Les langues *anglaise* et *française* furent adoptées par la Commission scientifique commes langues officielles du Congrès international des sciences de l'activité physique – 1976. De ce fait, les communications apparaissent au présent rapport officiel *dans la langue où elles ont été présentées* pour ce qui est de l'anglais et du français, et dans la langue *anglaise* pour ce qui est des communications qui furent faites dans les langues allemande, russe et espagnole.

Des résumés dans chacune des deux langues officielles accompagnent chacune des communications qui paraissent aux Volumes 1 et 2 ainsi que les présentations faites par les conférenciers invités dans les autres volumes de la série.

Preface

The staging of international scientific sessions on the occasion of the Olympic Games has become a well-established tradition.

The themes of the congresses held at the times of the Games celebrating the last five olympiads illustrate that the movement has indeed become multidisciplinary and international.

In choosing *Physical activity and human well-being* as the central theme of the Québec Congress, the Scientific Commission endeavored to offer to the eventual delegates from the entire world, on the eve of the Olympic Games of Montreal, a large and democratic platform for the sharing of knowledge and the exchange of viewpoints on the problems now confronting sport internationally. For each one of the *subthemes* retained in the program, four speakers of different disciplines and of international reputation were invited by the Scientific Commission to give their viewpoint or that of their discipline on the proposed subjects. Additionally, the Scientific Commission offered a series of twenty (20) seminars of monodisciplinary character, in which at least three specialists of international reknown were invited to express themselves on selected topics. One hundred and twenty-seven (127) speakers from all corners of the world thus accepted the invitation of the Scientific Commission and were present at the Québec Congress.

Over and above the thematic and disciplinary seminars which constituted the heart of its program, the Scientific Commission also reserved a large portion of the time to the presentation of individual scientific contributions in sixteen (16) different disciplines and in six (6) special events.

The work sessions, numbering more than eighty (80), made it possible for more than three hundred (300) authors from all corners of the world to present the results on their research and scholarly work.

The central objective of the whole Congress was to bring frontier knowledge pertaining to sport and physical activity in general to the attention of the maximum number of persons. To that effect, the invited speakers were urged to present — the results of the latest research or scholarly work on the subjects proposed — the most convincing facts or ideas — the disciplinary practices, questions or issues which were in greater debate or contention — whenever

Préface

La tenue de sessions scientifiques internationales à l'occasion des Jeux olympiques est une tradition maintenant bien établie. Les thèmes des congrès qui ont effectivement eu lieu aux temps de célébration des cinq dernières olympiades confirment certes la multidisciplinarité et l'internationalisme du mouvement.

En choisissant pour thème du Congrès *L'activité physique et le bien-être de l'homme*, la Commission scientifique canadienne souhaitait donner aux délégués éventuels du monde entier, à l'occasion des Jeux olympiques de Montréal, une plate-forme large et démocratique permettant un libre échange des points de vue sur les problèmes qui confrontent le sport partout. Pour chaque *sous-thème* retenu, quatre conférenciers de disciplines différentes et de réputation internationale furent invités par la Commission scientifique canadienne à venir donner leur point de vue ou celui de leur discipline d'appartenance sur le sujet proposé. En plus, la Commission scientifique avait prévu la tenue de séminaires à caractère monodisciplinaire, donnant l'occasion à au moins trois spécialistes, dans chacune des vingt (20) disciplines impliquées, de faire état des connaissances sur des sujets choisis. Un total de cent vingt-sept (127) conférenciers de tous les coins du monde répondirent ainsi à l'invitation de la Commission scientifique canadienne et furent présents à Québec.

Au delà des séminaires thématiques et disciplinaires constituant le coeur du programme, la Commission scientifique a voulu réserver une place importante du programme à la présentation de communications scientifiques individuelles dans l'éventail des disciplines impliquées.

Les sessions de travail, au nombre de plus de quatre-vingt (80), permirent à plus de trois cents (300) auteurs de livrer à leurs pairs de tous les coins du monde les résultats de leurs réflexions et de leurs recherches.

Le rapport scientifique que constitue la présente série de publications se veut donc un bilan général de ce que dit la recherche et de ce que sont les réalités de la pensée et de la pratique courante, à travers le monde, sur des sujets précis touchant l'activité physique en général. Notre Commission scientifique canadienne avait à cet effet incité tous les auteurs à faire ressortir — l'état des connaissances, des

possible, the various implications relative to the education, health, or well-being of the people.

It was judged acceptable at the Québec Congress that speakers addressing themselves to the same topics present complementary, differing or even opposed viewpoints on the subjects, questions or issues at stake. It was in the discussion periods, which were made an essential and integral part of all work sessions, that the data and the viewpoints were exposed to questions, commentaries and criticisms from the audience, in the full respect of democratic principles and of the basic regards due to each person.

The reports which constitute the present series of publications are in reality the responsibility of their authors; consequently, they should not be interpreted as necessarily reflecting the opinion of the editors or those of the members of the Canadian Scientific Commission.

We believe that in actual fact, the body of knowledge relative to the potential contribution of physical activity to human well-being will have progressed significantly at the time and as a result of the Québec session.

The series of volumes constituting the present scientific report illustrates, in our opinion, the fact that the Canadian Scientific Commission has endeavored to build a program which was consistent with the highest contemporary international standards. To that effect, the Scientific Commission had chosen to function on a democratic basis which it believes unprecedented in this type of international effort; both the quality and the representativity of the professional and scientific organizations which were invited to contribute to the total endeavor do indeed illustrate this fact.

The members of the Canadian Scientific Commission believe that they were correct in assuring that there would be place, within the framework of the CISAP-1976-ICPAS program, for contributions stemming from all the branches and sectors of human knowledge which may be interested, from one angle or the other, in physical activity and sports as contemporary phenomena.

The success of the Québec Congress is owed outright to the efforts of the members of the Scientific Commission, the International Advisors, the members of the Executive, the Executive Secretary and Treasurer as well as to those of the numerous collaborators who have in fact consecrated so much energy to the pursuit of the objectives. At the critical stages of our collective endeavor, the professional and scientific contributions of a large

travaux de recherche et des réflexions de pointe sur le sujet, — les faits et/ou les idées les plus convaincants, — les pratiques ou les questions en discussion et en contention, — le cas échéant, les implications diverses qui touchent l'éducation, le bien-être, la santé ou la qualité de vie des citoyens.

Il était bien sûr accepté au Congrès de Québec que des conférenciers différents présentent, sur un même sujet, des vues personnelles, complémentaires, divergentes, ou même carrément opposées. Ce fut à ce sujet dans les périodes de discussions, parties intégrantes de toutes les sessions de travail, que les données et les points de vue ont été exposés aux questions, aux commentaires et aux critiques, dans le plus grand respect cependant des principes démocratiques et des égards dus à la personne.

Les travaux qui paraissent à la présente série n'engagent donc en fait que leurs auteurs; ils ne doivent pas être interprétés comme reflétant nécessairement les opinions des éditeurs ou celles des membres de la Commission scientifique.

Nous croyons cependant que l'ensemble des connaissances relatives à la contribution potentielle de l'activité physique au bien-être de l'homme aura progressé de façon significative, au moment, et comme résultant de notre session de Québec.

Les divers volumes du présent rapport scientifique illustrent bien, croyons-nous, le fait que la Commission scientifique canadienne s'est appliquée à édifier un programme qui soit conforme aux standards les plus élevés de l'heure et a de plus choisi de fonctionner sur des bases démocratiques sans précédent dans ce genre d'effort international. Les qualités et la représentativité des organismes scientifiques et professionnels qui ont été mis à contribution dans l'ensemble du projet témoignent, entre autres, de cet état de choses.

Nous croyons avoir eu raison d'avoir voulu et d'avoir fait qu'il y ait place, dans le cadre des débats du CISAP-1976-ICPAS, pour des apports en provenance de toutes les branches du savoir humain qui s'intéressent à l'activité physique sous l'une ou l'autre de ses formes.

Le succès remporté par le Congrès de Québec ne saurait cependant que revenir de plein droit aux membres de la Commission scientifique, aux Conseillers internationaux, aux membres de l'Exécutif, au Secrétaire exécutif et trésorier, ainsi qu'aux nombreux autres collaborateurs, bref à tous ceux et celles qui, effectivement, ont mis la main à la pâte. Aux moments les plus importants de notre cheminement critique, les apports professionnels et scientifiques en

number of persons, foreigners as well as Canadians, have indeed been generous, efficient and noteworthy.

The co-editors

William A.R. Orban, Ph.D.
Vice-president of the
Scientific Commission

Fernand Landry, Ph.D.
President of the
Scientific Commission

PREFACE

provenance d'un grand nombre de personnes, étrangers et canadiens, ont été en effet on ne peut plus généreux, efficaces et marquants.

Les co-éditeurs

William A.R. Orban, Ph.D.
Vice-président de la
Commission scientifique

Fernand Landry, Ph.D.
Président de la
Commission scientifique

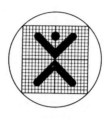

Prediction of Outstanding Athletic Ability

La prédiction de l'aptitude à la haute performance

Prediction of Athletic Performance: Genetic Considerations

Vassilis Klissouras

Data from twin studies show that discriminating biological factors in outstanding performance are genetically determined. However, appropriate training stimuli can profoundly affect the expression of their genetic potential within the fixed limits of heredity. The genetic factors are decisive in the attainment and prediction of outstanding athletic performance. The basic biophysical disposition must be present for the possibility of being an outstanding athlete to arise. The psychological and other factors nevertheless determine how close the athlete approaches his absolute limits of performance.

Introduction

The degree to which we can predict potential athletic performance depends to a large extent upon our knowledge of the relative importance of heredity in human diversity. In this connection an attempt is made in this paper to unravel the following questions:

1. To what extent do genetic differences account for existing individual differences in physiological capacities?

2. Does maximal exposure of an individual to environmental influences, such as physical training, increase his functional capacity, and to what extent? And further, does the ontological time factor during exposure affect the magnitude of change?

3. Is there a genotype-environment interaction? In other words, does the same training stimulus produce a change of different magnitude in different genotypes?

Genetic Influences

From comparison of intrapair differences between identical and nonidentical twins, it is possible to answer the first question since, in

---

Vassilis Klissouras, Department of Physiology and Physical Education, McGill University, Montreal, Quebec, Canada.

Our studies on twins were supported by grants from the Medical Research Council of Canada and the Quebec Ministry of Education.

effect, phenotypic variability in identical twins is due solely to environmental agents, whereas that in nonidentical twins is due to both genetic fluctuations and extragenetic influences.

In an early study based on the variance of such intrapair twin differences we found that the contribution of heredity to the interindividual differences in maximal oxygen uptakes, which is used as a performance criterion of functional capacity, is relatively high [5]. Figure 1 depicts the data obtained in this study from 25 (15 monozygous [MZ] and 10 dizygous [DZ]) pairs of twin boys. It may be seen that the intrapair difference tends to be smaller between identical than nonidentical twins. In fact, the experimental error could account for all intrapair differences in identical twins.

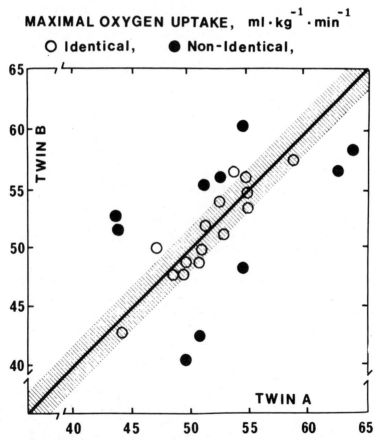

FIG. 1. Intrapair values of maximal oxygen uptake for identical and nonidentical twin boys between 7 and 13 years of age. (Data from Klissouras [5].)

Statistical treatment revealed that the difference in intrapair variance between MZ and DZ twins was significant well beyond the 0.01 probability level. It should be noted that young twins were used as subjects in this study to insure that environmental influences were comparable for MZ and DZ twins. It could be argued, however, that DZ pairs would be under more diverse environmental influences than MZ pairs during the developmental period. Thus, a follow-up study was conducted to determine whether the small intrapair differences observed between identical twins and the marked differences between nonidentical twins persist throughout life [7]. Thirty-nine pairs of twins (23 MZ and 16 DZ) of both sexes, ranging in age from 9 to 52 years, were used as subjects. In twins exposed to similar environments at different stages in their lives, any demonstrable differences between DZ as compared with MZ twins must be an expression of the relative strength of the genotype. In those exposed to contrasting environments, the resulting differences may provide a measure of this responsiveness to environmental forces. The obtained results shown in Figure 2 confirmed our earlier conclusion that heredity alone accounts almost entirely for existing differences in maximal oxygen uptake.

One may still wonder whether intrapair differences in maximal oxygen uptake could possibly be related to differences in mode of life. Reference may be made to some case studies [7]. In one case of nonidentical twins, aged 21 years who lived apart since 16, one twin had trained strenuously for competitive middle distance running, whereas his brother had never participated in sports of any kind. Therefore, it was surprising to find that the untrained twin had a maximal oxygen uptake of 56.0 $ml \cdot kg^{-1} \cdot min^{-1}$ as compared with a value of 52.8 for his trained counterpart. One cannot escape the inference that if it were not for the physical training the intrapair difference between this twin pair would have been greater. Further, the implicit postulate of this observation is that some individuals with a weak genotype have to use a greater amount of physical activity to attain an average adaptive value, whereas those with generous native endowment may not need more than a threshold exposure to maintain their already high adaptive value.

Another two cases are also intriguing. Two identical brothers, 40 years of age, had been separated at age 12 and had had different life styles. More important, one twin had engaged in vigorous training for competitive basketball (12 to 30 years, 18 to 30 on the national level), whereas his brother was only moderately active during the same period. For the last ten years neither of them had been involved in regular physical exertion. When tested, their maximal oxygen

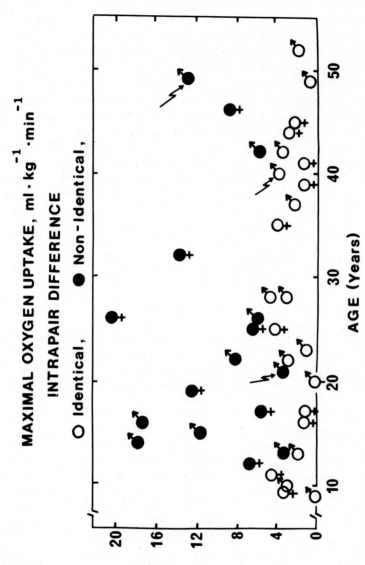

FIG. 2. Intrapair difference in maximal oxygen uptake in identical and nonidentical twins of different age. Arrows indicate three case studies discussed in the text. (Data from Klissouras et al [7].)

uptake was closely similar — the absolute values being 37.8 and 41.7 $ml \cdot kg^{-1} \cdot min^{-1}$ for the trained and untrained twin, respectively. In another case, nonidentical twins had a maximal oxygen uptake of 31.9 and 45.0 $ml \cdot kg^{-1} \cdot min^{-1}$ at age 49. They had lived together all their lives, had the same profession and both played competitive soccer from early childhood until they were 22 years of age. These observations support the notion that "natural tendency inevitably asserts itself."

However, it is necessary to resort to statistical analysis in order to determine to what extent individual differences are attributable to genetic variation and to what extent to environmental conditions. This is done with the computation of heritability indices which are based on a comparison of intrapair variances observed in MZ and DZ twins. In DZ twins the variance of the differences in a given attribute between partners is partly dependent upon hereditary variance $(\sigma^2 H)$, partly due to environmental effects $(\sigma^2 E)$ and partly affected by the error of measurement $(\sigma^2 e)$.

$$\sigma^2 DZ = \sigma^2 H + \sigma^2 E + \sigma^2 e \qquad (1)$$

MZ twins share a common heredity and any intrapair difference is attributed solely to monogenetic influences, namely, environment and error of measurement:

$$\sigma^2 MZ = \sigma^2 E + \sigma^2 e \qquad (2)$$

Equations 1 and 2 may be combined and by eliminating the environmental effect $(\sigma^2 E)$ which is assumed to be equal for MZ and DZ twins, we derive the following equation which denotes the variance in DZ twins due to genetic differences:

$$\sigma^2 H = (\sigma^2 DZ - \sigma^2 e) - (\sigma^2 MZ - \sigma^2 e) \qquad (3)$$

Further, if we arrange the above equation in a ratio form and refer to the term $\sigma^2 H$ as heritability estimate (Hest) we have:

$$Hest = \sigma^2 DZ - \sigma^2 MZ / \sigma^2 DZ - \sigma^2 e \times 100 \qquad (4)$$

This heritability index contrived by Holzinger and elaborated by others [5] may then be applied to the population from which the twin sample was drawn, to signify to what extent genetic differences account for existing individual differences in a given variable. If the heritability index is unity, then the heredity may be considered the cause of the variation observed. If the coefficient is zero, the variation may be attributed solely to environmental influences. If the variation is partly affected by environment and partly conditioned by heredity, the index will fall between and its proximity to unity is taken as an indication of the relative strength of the genotype.

Heritability indices are presented in Figure 3 for some metabolic, cardiorespiratory, pulmonary and neuromuscular attributes. It must be noted that Hest were calculated only if the variance ratio (F = $\sigma^2 DZ/\sigma^2 MZ$) was significant in a statistical sense, for otherwise any inference drawn from these estimates would have little meaning. Several workers have conducted extensive investigations in this area and have disclosed similar results for a number of physiological, biochemical and morphological variables. Mention should be made in particular of the work of Schwarz and Cergienko in the Soviet Union, Komi in Finland, Howald in Switzerland, Kovar in Czechoslovakia, Gedda, Venerando and Milani-Comparetti in Italy and Pirnay and Petit in Belgium.

In Soviet literature Schwarz has reported Hest for some 35 different measurements and found, for example, a Hest of 0.79 for $\dot{V}O_2$max, 0.88 for PWC_{170}, 0.86 for lean body weight, 0.91 for sprint running (60 to 100 meters) and 0.79 for 2 to 3 km country skiing [13]. Venerando and Milani-Comparetti have reported Hest for over 70 variables. Their Hest for maximal oxygen uptake (0.94), maximal heart rate (0.91) and vital capacity (0.91) are comparable to our findings [16]. Kovar found a Hest of 0.83 and 0.85 for vertical jump and throw of a medicine ball, both of which are tests for maximal muscular power [10].

Komi and co-workers have computed in two different studies a Hest not different from unity (0.99 and 0.98) for maximal muscular power measured by running on a staircase [8, 9]. A similar value (0.97) was found for the maximal power of forearm flexor muscles, calculated from force-velocity data (B. Jones, unpublished observations at the author's laboratory).

The introduction of the muscle biopsy technique has made it possible in recent years to analyze the structure of the human skeletal muscle and its bioenergetic systems. In fact, it has revolutionized our experimental approach in exercise physiology. Howald and associates took biopsies from the vastus lateralis of 17 twin pairs (11 MZ and 6 DZ) and studied the ultrastructural components and the activities of some energy-transforming enzymes in the muscle cells [1]. They observed no significant intrapair difference between MZ and DZ for (a) morphometric parameters volume density of myofibrils, of mitochondria, and of cytoplasm, surface density of inner and outer mitochondrial membranes and ratio of mitochondrial to myofibril volume), (b) the activities of mitochondrial enzymes (succinate dehydrogenase, malate dehydroge-

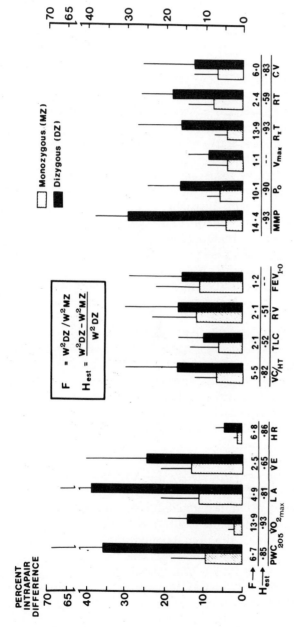

FIG. 3. Percent intrapair differences, their standard deviation, F-ratios and heritability estimates (Hest) of physical work capacity at a heart rate of 205, maximal oxygen uptake ($\dot{V}O_2$ max), maximal work ventilation (VE), maximal heart rate (HR), maximal blood lactate concentration (LA), total lung capacity (TLC), residual volume (RV), vital capacity to body height ratio (VC/Ht), forced expiratory volume at one second (FEV 1.0 sec), maximal muscular power (MMP) of the forearm flexors, maximal isometric force (Po) of the forearm flexors, maximal speed (Vmax) of forearm flexors, reflex time (R × T), reaction time (RT) and conduction velocity (CV). Hest were computed only when the F-ratio was significant at a level higher than 0.05. (Data from Baeriswyl [1], Klissouras [6, 7], Komi [8] and Kovar [10].)

nase and (c) the activities of extramitochondrial enzymes (hexokinase and glyceraldehyde-3P-dehydrogenase [1]. On the basis of
this evidence, the authors concluded that interindividual variability
observed in the cellular metabolic equipment is conditioned primarily by extragenetic influences.

Komi and co-workers reached the same conclusion regarding the
activity of enzymes involved either in ATP turnover during muscle
contraction or in glucose residue metabolism [9]. However, the
striking observation of their study, with profound implications for
prediction of potential performance and sports selection, is the
almost identical percent distribution of the slow twitch fibers (ST%)
in the vastus lateralis muscle of MZ twin brothers in contrast to DZ
twin pairs of both sexes. The respective Hest values of ST% for males
and females were 99.6% and 92.2% [9]. In view of the fact that a
motoneuron innervates a both histochemically and physiologically
uniform type of muscle fiber, the authors suggested that the motor
unit composition in human skeletal muscle is genetically fixed and
they inferred that the genetic factors are decisive in human potential
performance and its prediction.

Finally, mention should be made of the high heritability
estimates for morphological dimensions [15] and motor behavior [6].

The validity of any heritability estimate depends upon the
acceptability of the underlying assumptions. Four basic assumptions
are usually made in the derivation of a Hest. It is assured (1) that
environmental influences are comparable for identical and nonidentical twins; (2) that hereditary variance shows no dominance or
interaction effects; (3) that no correlation exists between parents
due to assortative mating, and (4) that hereditary and environmental
influences are not correlated.

In regard to the first assumption, one has to consider both
prenatal and postnatal environment. It has been argued that
differences in intrauterine position and blood supply to the embryo
and accidental differences in the make-up of the cytoplasm may
result in structural and biochemical differences between MZ twins.
Although such differences in the prenatal environment may exist, no
phenotypical differences that could be ascribed to their effect were
observed in the identical twins studied. These observations strongly
suggest either the quality of prenatal environment or that existing
prenatal differences are not enduring, but are progressively equaled
under the influence of a genetic maturational pacemaker. This, of
course, would only apply to prenatal differences which do not result

in injury of a vital organ, which in turn may cause some developmental anomaly or malformations. In any event, prenatal inequalities would only lead to an underestimation of the share of heredity in the discordance of nonidentical twins. As far as the postnatal environment is concerned, it is believed that no differentiating influences can be operant if both MZ and DZ twins have similar life styles and if they are of a young age, for as children grow older the assumption of a shared environment becomes less certain. All of our Hest are based on twins of young age to insure the environmental comparability. This does not mean that the environment did not vary, but that it varied approximately in the same direction and to the same degree for all individuals under study. However, it must be noted that in some studies no special control is made of the age, socioeconomic, health and physical activity status within or between pairs and thus the comparability assumption is not tenable.

In regard to the tenability of the second assumption, it is conceivable that the interaction between heredity and environment is a source of variation in some variables. It is quite probable that the simple model of heredity plus environment may not be adequate to explain the observed within pair variance of the DZ twins and that it should be modified to include an additional term signifying the mutual interaction between heredity and environment. However, the inclusion of this multiplicative component requires experimental confirmation and can be obtained by "split-twin" experiments, in which one twin trains while his genotypically identical partner acts as a control. With data obtained in this manner it is possible to distinguish three sources of variation: intrapair variation (training effect), interpair variation (genetic disposition), and interaction between the two. We have observed no such interaction for $\dot{V}O_2$ max.

If there is an assortative mating effect (third assumption) and not included in the computation of Hest, the relative strength of the genotype will be underestimated, since such an effect will increase the between families variance and will decrease the within families variance. Although it is doubtful whether biological criteria are used to any appreciable extent in mating (e.g., correlation coefficient between mates is 0.30 for height), a trend for marriages between outstanding athletes should be noted.

The final assumption, that hereditary and environmental influences are not correlated, may be only partially true, since, on the one hand, gifted children are most likely given special opportunity to practice, and on the other, family studies on high performance athletes seem to indicate that sports activity participation is conditioned by genotypic factors [2].

Finally, it must be noted that a high heritability index should not necessarily be interpreted to mean that the genetic factor has an etiologic role in the expressivity of the biological responses under study, nor has it sensible meaning with reference to measurement in an individual. It is erroneous, for example, to interpret a 93% heritability index found for maximal aerobic power variance as meaning that 93% of an individual's $\dot{V}O_2$ is genetically determined and 7% susceptible to environmental modification. As Komi and co-workers put it, "The Hest is only an estimate of the extent to which heredity affects the variation of a given organic attribute, in a given population exposed to common environmental influences at a given time" [8]. Knowledge acquired from Hest should be complemented with information obtained from co-twin analysis on the potency of physical training and only then can the nature-nurture problem be placed in perspective and the environmental forces upon heredity predisposition be evaluated.

Environmental Influences

The potency of environmental forces upon hereditary predisposition can be fully evaluated only if they are given a chance to act maximally. In this context, it is important to know the limits set by the genotype, the relative potency of training at different developmental ages and the extent to which genotype and training stimulus interact. These questions, posed at the beginning of this paper, can be elucidated with the co-twin analysis, where each subject is accompanied by a genotypically identical control.

"Ceiling" of Performance

All functional capacities and physiological processes in man as in all species have a genetically determined ceiling. For example, the upper limit of oxygen uptake is a little over 7 liters/min and that of cardiac output close to 40 liters/min. Additionally, we find that ceilings characteristic of individual genotypes must exist at different levels and the question then arises as to what extent environmental influences such as physical training can raise an individual's capacity above a certain level toward the species maximum value.

To obtain some insight into this question, a pair of identical twins, a trained athlete and his untrained brother, were tested over a period of 1½ years. The untrained twin had a $\dot{V}O_2$ max of 35.9 ml·kg^{-1}·min^{-1} whereas the trained twin had a peak value of only

49.2 ml·kg^{-1}·min^{-1}. This latter value is comparable to an average maximum value of about 50 ml·kg^{-1}·min^{-1} for untrained college men of the same age, well below values reported for top athletes. So despite hard and prolonged training, the trained twin was unable to surpass an average level of adaptive capacity. The reason for this seems to hinge on his low pretraining functional adaptability as judged from that of his identical brother. This observation strongly suggests that rigorous athletic training cannot contribute to functional development beyond a limit set by the genotype. In this connection, the age-old question — "Is an athlete born or made" — is meaningless as phrased. It is not a matter of predetermination versus plasticity, since heredity cannot operate in a vacuum and there must be an appropriate environment where the heredity factor attains full expression. What the question really endeavors to ask is: "Does everybody possess the constellation of genes or the genetic potential which, with appropriate training, can find a phenotypic expression in superior athletic achievement?" In view of the empirical evidence obtained the answer to this latter question is unequivocally negative [4].

Early Training

There is much speculation but little evidence regarding the relative potency of training at different developmental ages. In a recent study [17] we split 12 pairs of identical twin boys (4 sets aged 10 years, 4 sets aged 13 years and 4 sets aged 16 years), so that one twin trained, while his identical brother served as a control and continued in his normal day-to-day activity pattern. The training program was of ten-week duration and was designed to improve primarily the subject's endurance by both interval and continuous exercise. The individual differences for maximal oxygen uptake before and after training are shown in Figure 4. The mean intrapair difference was 11.5% and 13.9% for the 10- and 16-year-old groups, but it was not changed (1.8%) in the 13-year-olds. Since the type, intensity, duration and frequency of exercise were the same for all groups, the reason for this difference in response should be sought for in factors other than training. The most likely explanation for the commensurate increase in $\dot{V}O_2$ in both trained and untrained 13-year-old twins seems to hinge on the influences associated with the adolescent growth spurt that occurs at this age and is assessed by the height velocity. It is possible that hormonal activity is optimum during this age and any additional stimuli such as training cannot override its influence. In this connection one thinks of the anabolic

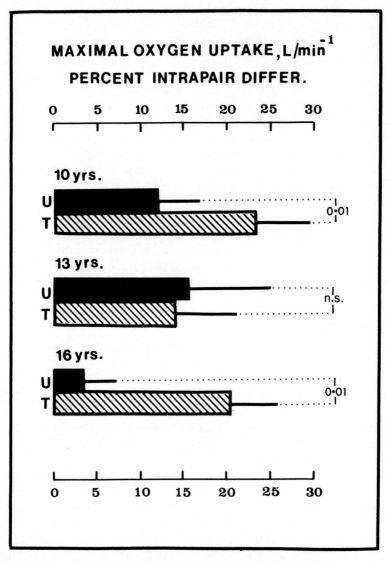

FIG. 4. Mean percent differences, standard deviations and significant levels of maximal oxygen uptake for untrained (U) twins and their trained (T) brothers of three age groups. (Data from Venerando and Milani-Comparetti [16].)

activity of the growth hormone, which stimulates the transport of amino acids across cell membranes and the synthesis of protein. However, some other factors must play an essential role, since the blood growth hormone levels in children and adolescents are not different from that observed in adults during rest and in response to muscular work.

Most likely the ontological time factor is decisive in development of functionally important structures. However, it still remains uncertain at which developmental period the growth-promoting stimuli which act upon the tissues should be applied. The old hypothesis that more might be gained by introducing extra exercise at the time when the growth impulse is the strongest is not tenable anymore in view of the present evidence.

Genotype-Training Interaction

A question of considerable theoretical and practical importance is whether different genotypes respond to a given training stimulus with a change of different magnitude. Split-twin experiments, in which one twin trains and his identical partner acts as a control, make it possible to separate the observed intrapair variance into its three components: that due to heredity, that due to training and that due to the interaction between heredity and training. Eight twin boys underwent a ten-week training program of the same amount and intensity, while their identical brothers restricted their activities to normal daily routines. The $\dot{V}O_2$ max of all twins was measured before and at the end of the ten-week period. The mean $\dot{V}O_2$ max for all experimental and control twins was 51.9 ml·kg^{-1}·min^{-1}, with nonsignificant intrapair differences. The interpair variability ranged from 41.1 to 58.6 ml·kg^{-1}·min^{-1}, so that the interaction hypothesis could be tested. The mean $\dot{V}O_2$ max after training was 59.4 ml·kg^{-1}·min^{-1}, with adjustments for changes observed in the nontrained twins, and the range was 45.2 to 69.3 ml·kg^{-1}·min^{-1}. Treatment of the results with the analysis of variance revealed that the interaction between genotype and training does not contribute significantly to the total variance (Table I). These findings do not support the notion that the magnitude of improvement in $\dot{V}O_2$ max

Table I. Analysis of Variance in $\dot{V}O_2$ max
Figures Based on Eight Twin Pairs*

Sources of Variation	Mean Squares	Variance in Percent of Total Variance
Training	221.72	42
Heredity	69.04	51
Interaction	4.39	7

*From Weber et al [17].

depends upon the relative strength of the genotype. Thus, the inverse relationship occasionally observed between initial level of $\dot{V}O_2$ max and relative improvement should be attributed to the amount and intensity of physical activity which presumably modifies the initial level of $\dot{V}O_2$ max. Further, it is surprising to find that despite strenuous training, the main cause of the total variance in $\dot{V}O_2$ max is still the genetic predisposition. In this context, it should be pointed out that the partitioning of $\dot{V}O_2$ max does not refer to the individual values but to the variation in a population. In view of the available evidence, it is concluded that variability in $\dot{V}O_2$ max observed in a population that has been exposed to common environmental forces may be almost entirely determined by heredity, but its relative contribution to the total variance may be reduced to about 50% with the operation of extreme environmental conditions.

Concluding Remarks

Twin findings make it possible to ascertain the relative strength of the genetic control of individual differences in biophysical variables. From such twin data we now know for example that such discriminating factors in outstanding athletic performance as maximal aerobic power, maximal anaerobic power and capacity, maximal muscular power and percent distribution of slow twitch fibers are genetically determined. Further, we know, at least for some adaptive responses, that appropriate training stimuli can profoundly affect the expression of their genetic potential, but this can occur only within the fixed limits of heredity. The implicit postulate of all these observations is that genetic factors are decisive in the attainment and prediction of outstanding athletic performance. It is clear that the basic biophysical disposition must be present for the possibility of being an outstanding athlete to arise.

Yet, the difference between athletes lies not entirely in physiological functions, histochemical quantities, biochemical activities and morphological dimensions. It lies rather "in their capacity," as Bannister put it, "for mental excitement, which brings with it an ability to overcome or ignore the discomfort, even pain in muscle and brain." Though physiology may indicate biophysical limits, to athletic performance "psychological and other factors beyond the ken of physiology set the razor's edge of defeat or victory and determine how closely an athlete approached the absolute limits of performance."

References

1. Baeriswyl, C., Luthi, Y., Claasen, H. et al: Ultrastructure and biochemical function of skeletal muscle in twins: Genetic and environmental influences. J. Appl. Physiol. (to be published).
2. Gedda, L.: Sports and genetics. A study on twins (351 pairs). Acta Genet. Med. Gemellol. 9:387-408, 1960.
3. Klissouras, V.: Erblichkeit und Training-Studien Mit Zwillingen. Leistungsport 5:357-368, 1973.
4. Klissouras, V.: Genetic limit of functional adaptability. Int. Z. Angew. Physiol. 30:85-94, 1972.
5. Klissouras, V.: Heritability of adaptive variation. J. Appl. Physiol. 31:338-344, 1971.
6. Klissouras, V. and Marisi, D.Q.: Genetic basis of individual differences in physical performance. McGill J. Educ. 11:15-28, 1976.
7. Klissouras, V., Pirnay, F. and Petit, J.M.: Adaptation to maximal effort: Genetics and age. J. Appl. Physiol. 35:288-293, 1973.
8. Komi, P., Klissouras, V., and Karvinen, E.: Genetic variation in neuromuscular performance. Int. Z. Angew. Physiol. 31:289-304, 1973.
9. Komi, P.V., Viitasalo, J.H.T., Havu, M. et al: Physical performance, skeletal muscle enzyme activities and fiber types in monozygous and dizygous twins of both sexes. Acta Physiol. Scand. Suppl. 1976 (In press.)
10. Kovar, R.: Contribution to investigations in genetically condition to human motor behaviour (in Cech). Thesis, University Karlovy, Praha, 1974.
11. Pirnay, J., Klissouras, V. and Petit, J.M.: Fonction pumonaire et génétique. Acta Tuberc. Pneumol. Belg. 63:477-483, 1972.
12. Price, B.: Primary biases of twin studies. Am. J. Human Genet. 2:293-352, 1950.
13. Schwarz, V.: On the relative role of genetic and environmental factors in development of physical work capacity in children: A twin-study (in Russian). Thesis, State University of Tartu, Soviet Union, 1972.
14. Tanner, J.M.: The Physique of the Olympic Athlete. London:L. Allen & Unnin, 1964.
15. Vandenberg, S.G.: How stable are heritability estimates? A comparison of six anthropometric studies. Am. J. Phys. Anthropol. n.s. 20:331-338, 1962.
16. Venerando, A. and Milani-Comparetti: Influenza dell-eredita sull attitudine ai vari Sport. Med. Dello Sport 26:347-352, 1973.
17. Weber, G., Kartodiharjio and Klissouras, V.: Growth and physical training with reference to heredity. J. Appl. Physiol. 40:211-215, 1976.

Prédiction de la performance des athlètes: considérations génétiques

Les études effectuées sur des jumeaux indiquent que les facteurs biologiques distinctifs dans la haute performance sont déterminés génétiquement. Toutefois, des stimuli appropriés d'entraînement peuvent affecter profondément la manifestation du potentiel génétique dans les limites fixées par l'hérédité. Les facteurs génétiques sont décisifs quant à la réalisation et la prédiction d'exploits athlétiques. La présence de la disposition biophysique fondamentale est nécessaire pour que se réalise la possibilité de devenir un athlète extraordinaire. Néanmoins, des facteurs psychologiques et d'autres déterminent jusqu'à quel point un athlète s'approche de la limite absolue de son potentiel.

Prediction of Outstanding Athletic Ability

V. Seliger

Energy metabolism of the organism measured by indirect calorimetry reflects the processes in the active tissue and thus is a good general index of functional capacity. The rate of energy expenditure and the ratio of aerobic and anaerobic energy utilization in specific and nonspecific tests of work performance are examples of such indices. Different substrata for releasing energy according to the different types of activity are discussed as well as the feasibility of biochemical tests. The basis of this discussion is the reseach on hockey players in a game situation.

When assessing a sports performance all athletes, coaches and physicians intensively consider how far the athlete's abilities may be predicted in order to continue the process of increasing his performance and to select him for representative teams, important competitions, etc. We will attempt to discuss this problem and that only from the point of view of physical possibilities of the athlete.

It is well known that different mechanisms and different physiological functions are of deciding importance for different kinds of motor activities and that the athlete can hardly achieve a superior physical performance without possessing a high level of these functions. Hill in 1926, investigating the speed of athletic runs in very short and very long distances, disclosed that the speed expressively decreased with the duration of time required for the performance. There are in the main four phases of changes: The highest speed is attained in athletic sprints (100 and 200 meters), then a rapid fall comes in middle distance runs (400 through 1500 meters), then a gradual decrease follows in long distance events (3 through 15 km) and finally only a very slow decrease succeeds in very long runs (25 through 42 km). The changes in speed of runs, i.e., the changes in physical performance, indicate indirectly that also

V. Seliger, Department of Physiology, Faculty of Physical Education and Sports, Charles University, Prague, Czechoslovakia.

different mechanisms exist that enable achievement of different speeds at different distances.

It is possible to regard the changes in metabolism, reinforcing the performance, as the main mechanism that is involved in a particular kind of motor activity. The studies on metabolism in muscle cells [9] and on the function of organs transporting materials required to insure the metabolism [10] are the most important. It becomes clear that physical performance raises metabolism at the cellular level and that in the training important adaptation changes are induced which enable the athlete to attain a higher specific performance [7, 8]. Energy metabolism of the organism, which may be relatively accurately measured by means of indirect calorimetry, becomes a global index of processes in the active tissues.

From this point of view interest is paid above all to the intensity of the energy expenditures. This decreases very rapidly with the length of the duration of motor activities. In performances of *maximal* intensity metabolism attains energy expenditure of an intensity of 30,000% BMR (20,000% to 35,000%); however, it is possible to achieve performances of that intensity only for several seconds. These types of motor activities include the following: athletic sprints, shot put, throws, jumps, weightlifting, etc. In performances of *submaximal* intensity the energy expenditure achieves around 10,000% BMR (5,000% to 15,000%). Performances of that intensity may last several minutes and include events like 400 and 800 meter running, 100 meter swimming, kayak paddling, etc. The performances of *medium* intensity of metabolism increase the energy expenditure on the average to 2,000% BMR (1,000% to 5,000%), but they may last several tens of minutes, or even one to three hours. These are athletic runs for 5 to 42 km, road cycling competitions, football, basketball, etc. Finally, the performances of *moderate* intensity of metabolism raise the average intensity of energy metabolism to 500% BMR (300% to 1,000%) and they may last several hours. Tourism, climbing, etc., may serve as examples of these performances. If we examine the ratio of the intensity of metabolism in percent BMR to the duration of activity an initial rapid fall of energy expenditure becomes apparent in very intensive activities. In the later stages of longer lasting activities the intensity of energy output decreases very little with the duration of activity. These findings correspond to the results presented by Yamaoka [16]. On the basis of our measurements of 1,114 persons with a medium physical efficiency and in 86 different motor activities, lasting from 0.02 to 21.1 minutes, it was possible to express the curve in a mathematical equation as follows:

% BMR = 1890.4 + 362.1 × t   *duration of activity*

where the intensity of metabolism is expressed in percentage of BMR and the duration of activity (t) in minutes. This equation may be used for predicting the intensity of metabolism for persons at medium performances, if the duration of the particular motor activity is known.

The ratio of aerobic and anaerobic energy output in the total metabolism [13] is a most interesting index. In the very short lasting performances of maximum intensity the energy expenditure is realized anaerobically practically from 100%. There is then a relation between the duration of motor activity and the type of energy metabolism. In performances lasting about 2.5 minutes the share of aerobic and anaerobic metabolism makes 50%; in short lasting performances the share of anaerobic metabolism increases. In longer lasting performances, on the contrary, the proportion of aerobic metabolism is greater. The dependency may be well expressed in an equation that is calculated on the basis of results obtained with the above described sample of persons of medium efficiency:

aerobic metabolism (%) = 32.1 + 46.9 × log t,

where the amount of aerobic metabolism is expressed in percentage of total energy expenditure and the duration (t) in minutes. This relationship enables calculation for practical use of the ratio of aerobic and anaerobic metabolism for the duration of a particular motor activity, assuming a high intensity performance. The findings are on the whole in accordance with currently known data [1, 9].

These are the theoretical bases of mechanisms supporting the performance from the point of view of energy metabolism. The release of chemical energy and its transformation into mechanical energy is realized in a complex process of metabolism. From the preceding statements it would be possible to consider that there are different substrata for releasing energy according to the character of the activity. In principle the energy required for performance is released in muscle cells where the macroergic phosphates and macroergic substrata are utilized and catalyzed by enzymes. The volume of energy capacity remains however relatively small at cell level. Macroergic phosphates release energy in a quite simple and very fast manner, but the total magnitude of energy obtained in this way is relatively small. Therefore, the organism begins immediately with an energy release from the macroergic substrata. First, it is the glycogen depletion, primarily on an anaerobic and then aerobic basis, and then the lipid depletion follows, or even also protein depletion.

Keul et al [9] registered the dynamics of these processes in a well-known graph. If the energy potential in cells is very rapidly consumed, then the regulative mechanism secures some additional amounts of energy, first from the resources stored in the circulating blood, and then from specific stores. This is of fundamental importance from the point of view of energy needs of muscle tissues. The need for energy potentials evokes considerable responses in the activity of the cardiopulmonary system. In our research we have examined different functions. From the point of view of utilization in practice, e.g., the activity index of blood circulation is quite interesting, as measured by heart rate. We registered heart rate telemetrically during all activities and we calculated the average values of heart rate during the performance. It is possible to express mathematically the ascertained heart rate by means of two equations: one in a ratio to the duration of the particular performance and the other to the intensity of the metabolism:

$$HR = 77.2 + 172.5 \times \sqrt{t} - 145.6 \times t + 54.3 \times t^{1.5} - 7.3 \times t^2$$

$$HR = 3.50989 + 7.609918 \times \sqrt{\%BMR} - 0.112076 \times (\%BMR) + \\ + 0.00058 \times (\%BMR)^{1.5} - 0.000001 \times (\%BMR)$$

where the heart rate (HR) is in relation to the duration of motor activity (t) in minutes or in relation to the intensity of the metabolism in percent of BMR. It appears that the highest values of heart rate are attained during performances of submaximal and medium intensity of metabolism, when the transportation system becomes taxed very strongly.

In concluding these theoretical considerations it is necessary to point out that the performance itself depends not only upon metabolism and neuromuscular functions, but that it has also its psychic, tactical and other components. All these are inseparable factors of a physical performance and, of course, a particular performance may be modified in consequence of the influence of these components toward a better as well as lower performance. Also, other factors such as hypoxia, smoking, alcoholism, different diseases, etc., may play an important role on the external and internal environment of the organism.

A question raised very frequently is how to ascertain the abilities and physical capacity of the organism for a performance. The basic known instruments for this purpose are the test of physical efficiency. The *specific tests* employed for this purpose are those which are performance tests identical or at least very close to the competitive activity of the athlete. The *nonspecific tests* use especially exercise on a bicycle ergometer to a maximum workload. This instrument is very advantageous, since it permits adjusting the workload fairly well; also, the results obtained are not influenced by the individual's body weight. The treadmill is also frequently used. This device has a disadvantage in that the units of work must be stated arbitrarily and the workload can be adjusted only in changing the spread or the gradient of the treadmill.

However, should the demand on physical capacity be general, then the functional testing must be very manifold and thorough. The biochemical methods are used more and more frequently, even at a cellular or molecular level [9, 11, 12, 15]. Nevertheless, it remains questionable whether the information on energy potential in cells on the activity of enzymatic systems, subcellular structures, etc., may be utilized widely in practice beyond the basic research. We are of the opinion that the investigation of functional reactions of the organism to physical work may help considerably, be it in a global view of the changes of principal functional systems or in a biochemical examination of blood or urine.

At the Faculty of Physical Education and Sports we work on the theoretical and practical problems of the structure of sports performance in concrete types of sport disciplines [3, 4]. We try to show various demands of sport disciplines on motor, functional and social aspects of the athlete's performance. From the physiological point of view we try to establish the actual demands on particular functional systems as well as on the energy metabolism. Our experiences show that up to the present time the following system seems to be the most suitable:

1. By means of indirect calorimetry to ascertain the average energy expenditure for a particular performance. In case of long-duration performances we take a sample measurement, in a situationally typical performance (which is suggested by the coach) as a model of the actual activity and may last as a rule 15 to 20 minutes, with a longer recovery measured in a sitting rest position for about 30 to 45 minutes. This helps to answer the question of the intensity of metabolism in percent of BMR, in kilocalories per minute or in kilocalories per minute per kilogram, and to calculate the magnitude of energy expenditure during the entire motor activity in kilocalories and the percentual proportion of aerobic and anaerobic metabolism.

2. In laboratory conditions to test physical efficiency of the athlete on bicycle ergometer to a maximum workload. Attention is paid to rest values of functional indices, to values obtained during submaximal workload and maximal workload. We are interested also

in oxygen debt, which is taken for 25 minutes after the work has finished. In addition to functional indices, some other selected biochemical indices are also investigated.

3. In this way the basic metabolic characteristics required by the sports event and the basic functional capacities of individual athletes are observed. From a comparison of demands of functional level required for the particular sport and functional indices of the athlete we are then able to present to the coach or athlete, e.g., the deficiencies of his functional capacities and to recommend ways to improve them by purposeful training. An example of this is in ice hockey.

In a group of players of the Czechoslovak representative team we examined energy expenditure (13 players, age 24.4 years) during one playing period [14]. The measurements were made in an actual game situation during the last change of players and was followed by recovery in a sitting position. The data of energy expenditure and functiorial changes occurring in the progress of the game are presented in Table I. It demonstrates a relatively high energy output realized on an aerobic basis of 66%, while the functional response remained at a submaximal level. With respect to the range of results it is questionable whether the functional response of the organism

Table I. Various Indices of Energy Metabolism and Related
Cardiopulmonary Functions During One Playing
Period in Ice Hockey Players

	$\overline{X}$	SD
A. *Indices of Energy Metabolism*		
Working time (min)	1.17	0.17
Recovery period (min)	21.00	0.00
Energy expenditure (netto):		
kcal	45.6	10.2
kcal/min	39.6	10.8
kcal/min/kg	0.48	0.11
% BMR	3137	774
Percent of metabolism:		
aerobic	31.1	5.6
anaerobic	68.9	5.6
Oxygen debt (1)	6.3	1.7
B. *Changes of the Followed Functional Indices*		
Heart rate (beats/min)	152.2	15.9
Pulmonary ventilation (1/min)	92.0	16.2
Oxygen uptake (1/min)	2.62	0.41
Oxygen uptake (ml/min/kg)	32.1	4.5
Pulse oxygen (ml)	17.2	3.0

reaches maximal values even in a very intensive part of the game. For this reason — and examining also other research findings [2, 5, 6] — we made an effort to estimate the functional indices that a successful ice hockey player should possess at a maximal physical workload (Table II). Individual players were then tested on bicycle ergometer to a maximal workload in order to evaluate the ascertained indices. A comparison with the required norm then makes it possible to draw conclusions for the coach that may help him to improve a required function of the player by rational training. The example in Table III presents players relatively equal at the technical and tactical level, but with explicit functional differences. Player No. 1 has a relatively good capacity to release energy on the anaerobic basis, but very little aerobically. He is able to master short duration speed performances, but he has difficulty with speed endurance work and his performance decreases when he has to stay longer on the ice. Player No. 3 has a

Table II. Expected Level of Main Functional Indices of One Successful Ice Hockey Player Working on the Bicycle Ergometer to Maximal Load

Functional Indices	Values
Heart rate (beats/min)	174-192
W 170 (W)	350
Pulmonary ventilation (1/min)	160
Oxygen uptake (1/min)	4.9
Oxygen uptake (ml/min/kg)	58
Pulse oxygen (ml)	24
Oxygen debt (1)	12

Table III. Examples of Selected Functional Indices Obtained From Three Subjects Exposed to a Maximal Load on Bicycle Ergometer

	Subject 1	2	3
Heart rate (beats/min)	193	185	197
Pulmonary ventilation (1/min)	114	152	169
Oxygen uptake (1/min)	3.9	4.2	4.6
Oxygen uptake (ml/min/kg)	44.8	49.5	58.5
Pulse oxygen (ml)	20.2	22.7	23.4
Oxygen debt (1)	11.2	9.5	9.6
W 170 (W)	215	267	209
Blood lactate (mg%)	117	150	151
pH	7.15	7.18	7.12

high capacity to utilize energy aerobically. He is able to achieve both speed and speed endurance performances and to keep his performance for a longer time. Player No. 2 has capacity for average energy utilization, but the level of his technical and tactical experience is very high, which compensates his lower functional capacity.

In conclusion it may be said — and follows from the above examples — that a certain level of physical condition of the athlete constitutes an essential prerequisite for a good performance in the relevant sports events, and the prescription of a rational training program necessarily requires knowing the athlete's condition on the basis of testing. To a certain extent it may of course be supplemented by other components of the performance, such as technical and tactical preparation, volitional and psychic preparation.

References

1. Astrand, P.O. and Rodahl, K.: Textbook of Work Physiology. New York: McGraw-Hill, 1970.
2. Bouchard, C., Landry, F., Leblanc, C. and Mondr, J.C.: Quelques-unes des caractéristiques physiques et physiologiques des joueurs de hockey et leurs relations avec la performance. Hockey World 9:95, 1974.
3. Choutka, M.: Essai d'analyse de la practique sportive en football. Kinanthropologie 1:251, 1969.
4. Choutka, M.: Studies of the structure of sport performance (in Czech.) Prague:Charles University, 1976.
5. Ferguson, R.J., Marcotte, G.G. and Montpatit, R.R.: A maximal oxygen uptake test during ice skating. Med. Sci. Sports 1:207, 1969.
6. Guminskij, A.A., Tarasov, A.V., Jelizarova, O.S. et al: Following of aerobic and anaerobic indices in ice-hockey player (in Russian). Teor. Prakt. fiz. Kult. 34 (11):39, 1971.
7. Howald, H. and Poortmans, J.R.: Metabolic adaptation to prolonged physical exercise. Basel:Birkhäuser, 1975.
8. Keul, J.: Limiting Factors of Physical Performance. Stuttgart:G. Thieme, 1973.
9. Keul, J., Doll, E. and Keppler, D.: Muskelstoffwechsel. Wiss. Schriftenreihe Dtsch. Sportbundes Bd. 9, München:J. A. Barth, 1969.
10. Pernow, B. and Saltin, B.: Muscle Metabolism During Exercise. New York-London:Plenum Press, 1971.
11. Saltin, B.: Fiber composition and enzyme activity in human skeletal muscle and the importance for work performance. In Hansen, G. and Mellerowicz, H. (eds.): Third Internationales Seminar für Ergometrie. Berlin:Ergon, 1973, p. 15.
12. Saltin, B. and Karlsson, J.: Muscle glykogen utilisation during work of different intensities. In Pernow, B. and Saltin, B. (eds.): Muscle Metabolism During Exercise. New York:Plenum Press, 1971, p. 289.
13. Seliger, V.: The aerobic and anaerobic metabolic rates in physical exercises. In Seliger, V. (ed.): Physical Fitness. Praha:Universita Karlova, 1973, p. 351.

14. Seliger, V., Kostka, V., Grusová, D. et al: Energy expenditure and physical fitness of ice-hockey players. Int. Z. Angew. Physiol. 30:283, 1972.
15. Syrový, I., Gutmann, E. and Melichna, J.: Effect of exercise on skeletal muscle myosin ATP-ase activity. Physiol. Bohemoslov 21:633, 1972.
16. Yamaoka, S.: Studies on energy metabolism in athletic sports. Res. J. Physiol. Educ. 9:28, 1965.

Prédiction de dispositions athlétiques remarquables

Le métabolisme énergétique de l'organisme, mesuré par calorimétrie indirecte, montre les développements dans le tissu actif et constitue, de ce fait, un bon indice de la capacité fonctionnelle. Le taux de dépense énergétique et la proportion d'utilisation d'énergie aérobie et anaérobie au cours d'épreuves précises et générales de rendement au travail sont des exemples de ces indices. L'auteur commente les différents mécanismes pour la libération de l'énergie, selon les différents genres d'activités, ainsi que les possibilités d'épreuves biochimiques. Le texte se fonde sur la recherche effectuée auprès de hockeyeurs au cours de matchs.

Prediction of Outstanding Athletic Ability: The Structural Perspective

J. E. Lindsay Carter

A discussion of the three kinds of predictions and limitations of each is followed by a review of present knowledge regarding anthropometry and prediction of outstanding athletic ability. It is concluded that in terms of absolute somatotype, absolute and relative body dimensions, and body composition clear prototypes exist for outstanding performances requiring strength, speed and stamina. A suitable physique at the outset permits concentration on other qualities for top performance. The prediction of adult athlete physique and performance from the physique of the young athlete can only be done within broad categories.

Introduction

The use of anthropometry to describe the size, shape and composition of athletes has had increasingly wide application during the past 70 years. These descriptions have established that there are differences among sport groups when at least moderate to outstanding levels of performance in these sports have been used as criteria. The causes of these differences have been variously attributed to such influences as genetic endowment, physical training, nutrition and socio-cultural factors. The relative contributions of such influences to the resulting structure are unclear, as is their relationship to performance in a given sport. This leads to the following question: Can we predict outstanding athletic ability from body structure? It is the purpose of this paper to attempt to answer this question and in the process to point out some of the problems associated with such an apparently simple question.

There are three kinds of prediction which are of interest: (1) Does the athlete have the requisite physique to do well in his or her sport? (2) Can we predict the performance of a given athlete in his or her sport or event from physique? (3) Can we predict the

J. E. Lindsay Carter, Department of Physical Education, San Diego State University, San Diego, California, U.S.A.

29

adult athlete's physique from measurements taken on the young athlete? As will be shown, the first question can be more easily answered than the next two. The usual, although limited approach, to these questions is through measuring samples of athletes of known ability levels. The resulting physique profiles potentially represent both any influence of physique on the choice of sport and any effect of practice of a sport on development of physique. From such studies we can derive little about how the physique was achieved. However, they do provide anthropometric prototypes of successful athletes which may be utilized in two ways; physical training programs may be prescribed which will mold given athletes toward the anthropometric prototype, or athletes can be selected for a certain sport based on how closely their anthropometric profiles approximate the prototype for that sport. Biomechanical and physiological prototypes could also be defined for the same purposes, and ideally all approaches could be used. Nevertheless, the influence of physical training upon physique appears small compared with the range of genetically determined variations. Moreover, even at moderate levels of performance, structure alone does not determine performance and that certain performance criteria (e.g., specific motor skills) will be more important than the structure. On the other hand, if these other factors of performance are equated, then physical differences may explain differences in performance to a large extent.

Predicting performance (place, time, distance) of outstanding athletes within a given event on the basis of body structure is difficult, if not impossible, for several reasons. First, the physique is but one aspect of performance. Second, variation in performance criteria of elite athletes is very small, thus the correlation with other criteria (e.g., body measurements), whose variability for the athlete's sport group is also small, is usually low. Elite athletes by definition are the upper 1% of the population in terms of ability and their performances in a given competition may be within 1% of each other. Physiologists might argue that such small differences have no biological significance, but athletes and coaches are seldom impressed by such statements. Finally, much of the analysis in the past has been with single measurements and performance. Recent multivariate studies appear more promising, but they still appear to be most successful in defining groups rather than ordering performance. Furthermore, among athletes, there may be compensating anthropometric attributes, so that individual prediction becomes less reliable. Occasionally, a unique structure will be the reason for success of an individual compared to others.

The possibility of predicting the physique of athletes from pre-adult ages is perhaps the most interesting and at the same time the most dangerous question. It is of practical interest for coaches to select young athletes who will have the most potential to become outstanding, but it is also dangerous from an educational and skill development point of view in that the young athlete may spend years in training for one sport to finally discover that alterations in physique preclude further development. This aspect of the question must be seriously considered by those working with and responsible for the young athlete.

Having posed the questions and the limitations in seeking their solutions, attention must now be turned to a review of present knowledge regarding anthropometry and prediction of outstanding athletic ability. Aspects of anthropometry which will be examined are somatotype, absolute and relative size, and body composition.

Somatotype

The concept of somatotyping is appealing because it is a classification of total body form which can be expressed as a simple three-digit number. The many separate dimensions of human physique are reduced to the somatotype rating which has continuous scales, thereby allowing for many different ratings [4, 20]. In the Heath-Carter method the somatotype is defined as a description of present morphological conformation. It is expressed in a three-digit rating (on open-ended scales) representing evaluation of each of three components of the physique; relative fatness (endomorphy), relative musculoskeletal development (mesomorphy), relative linearity (ecto-morphy). The present somatotype is rated and no assumptions are made regarding permanence. Because this method differs from other methods [8] only studies using the Heath-Carter method will be cited in illustrating this paper.

Three groups of somatotype studies provide us with extensive data on 3189 subjects (approximately 25% ♀) from 53 sport groups. Carter [6, 7] (Carter et al, unpublished studies, 1976) reported on the somatotypes of 792 ♂ and 302 ♀ athletes from 22 sport groups from club through Olympic levels of competition. Stepnicka [28, 29] studied 654 ♂ and 198 ♀ outstanding CSSR athletes in 13 sport groups. De Garay, Levine and Carter [16] presented data on 1102 ♂ and 141 ♀ Olympic athletes from 18 sport groups who competed in Mexico in 1968. According to the authors cited, athletes in general (both ♂ and ♀) are more mesomorphic and less endomorphic than nonathletes of the same age. Some athletes in throwing events (track and field, ♂ and ♀) and in the heavier weight classes for boxing, weightlifting and wrestling are relatively high on endomorphy. These male athlete groups, as well as body builders and gymnasts, are clearly the most mesomorphic athletes. For males, the average mesomorphy is approximately 5½, but some groups have means close to 4 and some as high as 7½. Individual ratings as high as 10 are found in some athletes. Some distance runners and basketball players have mesomorphy ratings lower than 4, but these are usually accompanied by low endomorphy and high ectomorphy ratings. For most athletes in vigorous sports, the average endomorphy is 2 to 2½, and the lowest values possible (1 and 1½) are common in some events (e.g., ♂ distance runners).

The means for most female athlete groups on mesomorphy is 4½, while the least mesomorphic athletes are around 2½ and the most mesomorphic about 6. In contrast to men some successful female athletes have higher endomorphy than mesomorphy; however, most are endomesomorphs or ectomesomorphs. The greatest variation for the somatotype mean values for different sports is in the ectomorphic component.

The somatoplots of each sport group show that there are characteristic somatotype distributions for some sports which show little or no overlap with other sports (e.g., ♂ gymnasts and distance runners). On the other hand, there are some distributions which are similar and overlap considerably, such as track sprinters and sprint cyclists (♂). Other groups such as male soccer and volleyball players have a wide range of somatotypes across the mesomorphic sector of the somatochart [28]. There are differences among events in such sports as track and field, but no differences in others such as rowing and cycling. Athletes with similar somatotypes excel at specific events regardless of race. Variations among the means of selected male and female athlete groups are illustrated in Figures 1 and 2. Just as there is sexual dimorphism in reference populations, it is also present in athletic populations. Furthermore, there are somatotype differences among general populations from different parts of the world [5]. Obviously, countries with large proportions of somatotypes which are similar to the prototypes of outstanding athletes in certain events will have a greater likelihood of providing athletes suited for excelling in these events, while countries which do not have certain somatotypes in their populations will have little likelihood of international success in these events.

The prediction of athletic ability from somatotype (and other physique measures) is determined in part by the contributions of growth and training to somatotype. Present indications are that

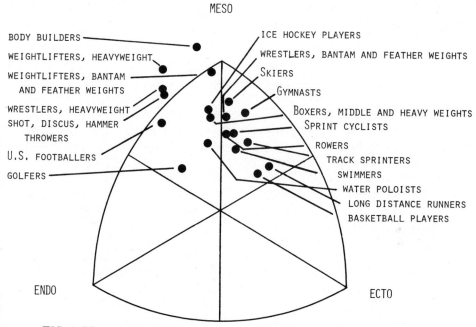

FIG. 1. Mean somatoplots of selected groups of outstanding male athletes.

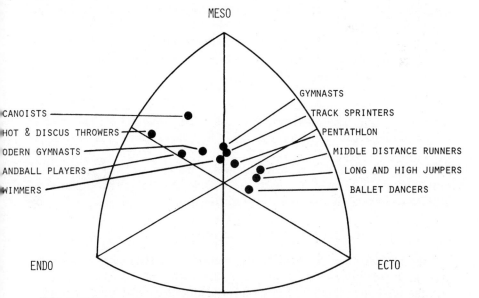

FIG. 2. Mean somatoplots of selected groups of outstanding female athletes.

somatotype changes during growth [13, 19, 24] and that physical training changes the somatotype of young and old men [10, 11]. These changes undoubtedly take place within certain genetic limits, but the relative contributions of all factors are as yet unknown. In the absence of longitudinal somatotype studies on outstanding athletes we can only estimate the prediction of athletic ability from the somatotypes of groups of athletes at different ages and levels of competition. Previous studies on male distance runners, gymnasts, rowers and U.S. football players at different levels of competition and performance show similar somatotype patterns but that the patterns become narrower at higher levels [6, 7, 12]. Figures 3 and 4 present mean somatoplots of sprinters (♂ and ♀), gymnasts (♂ and ♀), distance runners (♂) and bodybuilders (♂). Comparisons of the means show large differences among sports and small differences within sports according to age and level of competition. The means for the male sprinters are clustered near somatotypes 2-5-2, 2-6-3, and 2-5-3, with no clear trend for age and level of competition; although three U.S. samples show a trend toward higher mesomorphy and lower ectomorphy with increasing age. For female sprinters, the two older and higher level athlete groups have higher mesomorphy and lower ectomorphy than the younger U.S. sprinters. The male Olympic distance runners are slightly more mesomorphic and less endomorphic than the younger distance runners. Among the male gymnasts the CSSR group are more mesomorphic and the Mexico Olympic gymnasts more ectomorphic than the others. The AAU placers are more mesomorphic than the nonplacers. Within AIAW female gymnasts, placers were found to be more mesomorphic and less endomorphic than the nonplacers. The youngest gymnasts (14.8 years) were lower on mesomorphy and higher on ectomorphy than the other three groups. Among the bodybuilders, the Novice class were one unit less mesomorphic than the Open class and CSSR athletes, but the Masters class (44.2 years) were the same on mesomorphy as the Novices and were more endomorphic than any of the other groups. These data suggest that the somatotype of the younger athlete must at least approach that of the outstanding athlete to have a chance at success in the sport.

Absolute and Relative Size

While there have been literally hundreds of studies reporting the size and proportion of athletes from different sports, very few studies have described and compared groups of outstanding athletes using anthropometry. The problem of reviewing the literature

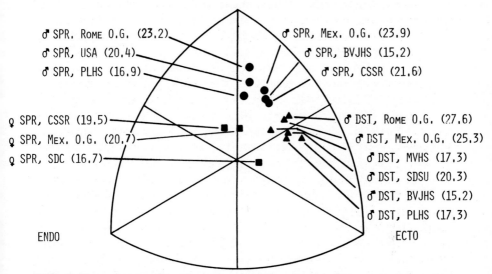

FIG. 3. Mean somatoplots of sprinters (SPR) and long distance runners (DST). The value in parenthesis is the mean age of the group.

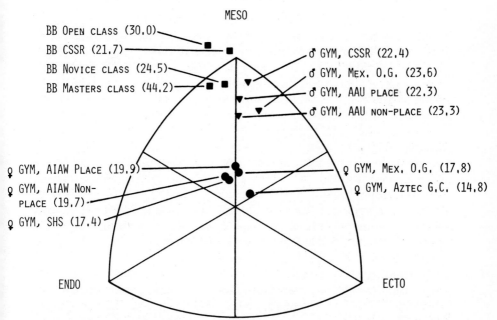

FIG. 4. Mean somatoplots of bodybuilders (BB) and gymnasts (GYM). The value in parenthesis is the mean age of the group.

becomes one of deciding which sports and which of approximately
100 dimensions and proportions should be summarized. To simplify
matters, only selected studies on Olympic and international athletes
which have examined and compared athletes from different sports
and events will be utilized in this paper. Studies on Olympic athletes
have been reported by Kohlrausch [23], Cureton [15], Correnti and
Zauli [14], Tanner [30], Azuma [1] and de Garay, Levine and
Carter [16]. Other studies on international athletes using anthropometry and/or somatotype are those of Tittel [31], Tittel and
Wutscherk [32], Eiben [17], Carter [7] and Stepnicka [29]. Among
these studies most have concentrated on track and field athletes and
only some contain data on female athletes. By far the most extensive
study is that of de Garay et al [16], who studied 1265 athletes from
92 countries who participated in 13 sports at the Mexico Olympics in
1968. Further analyses of these data have been reported by
Hebbelinck, Carter and de Garay [21], Carter [3] and Carter,
Hebbelinck, and de Garay [9]. The major findings from the above
studies are synthesized below. Most statements apply to both male
and female athletes.

Absolute Sizes

Height, weight, segmental lengths, breadths and girths have been
used to describe body size. In general, there are major differences in
body size between competitors in different events within the same
sport and between sports. However, there are examples of similar size
among events such as in rowing and in cycling and also similarity
among sports such as between track sprinters and cyclists. Tittel and
Wutscherk [32] observed differences in body size within and
between strokes for swimmers, but these differences were not as
pronounced in the Mexico Olympic data [16]. Athletes range from
very small (e.g., gymnasts, lowest weight classes in boxing, wrestling
and weightlifting) to very large, e.g., field events (shot, discus,
hammer), upper weight classes in boxing, wrestling and weightlifting,
as well as rowers and some basketball players. Increased height and
weight in some events were related to better performance [32].
Apparently, when other factors are equal, slightly taller and heavier
individuals have an advantage in some events.

In running events, there is a trend toward decreasing height from
400 meters through the marathon. However, some very short and tall
individuals seem to compete with equal success at the longer
distances, suggesting that proportions may be more important than
the absolute height. Kohlrausch [23] observed that the size of the

athletes was related to the stature of the country of the people of origin. De Garay et al [16] found that racial differences within events were similar in pattern to differences among races in general. They also found that in almost all comparisons blacks had narrower pelves than whites. In addition, blacks had longer arms and legs in some events. Tanner [30] showed differences between these two groups within events, but pointed out that the groups were closer to each other within events than they were to athletes in other events. This finding was also supported by de Garay et al [16]. Based on the differences between countries in regard to the body size of their people, Hirata [22] suggested that countries with people whose general size and physique was limited to the characteristics of champions in certain events should concentrate on those events in order to have international success.

There appears to be a secular trend toward increasing body size in some events, but not in others, at the Olympic games [14, 30]. Because of the different proportions of athletes from different ethnic backgrounds participating at recent Games, these trends should be interpreted with caution. Whether single or combined measurements are used, the most successful athletes, male or female, showed inconsistency in their values compared to the means of their groups. Some were near the mean and some were at the extreme of the distributions. De Garay et al [16] showed that in terms of absolute size, female athletes are generally smaller than male athletes except for skinfolds and biiliocristal breadth. Female shot and discus throwers are larger than many male athletes, especially gymnasts and long distance runners.

Relative Size

Proportions allow us to compare athletes of different body size as well as providing another method of looking at biomechanical aspects of performance. However, they also pose statistical and interpretational problems. As with absolute dimensions, proportions have been shown to distinguish between athletes in different sports or events. In some sports this differentiation is in the segmental lengths, while in others it is the breadths or the ratios of bulk to length.

The nature of the differences between black and white athletes is highlighted by proportional analysis. Although there are wide individual variations, black athletes in most sports and events have a relatively narrower pelvis, have longer arms and legs and shorter trunks than white athletes. These differences are also consistent with population findings. Although there have been increases in size in athletes, the proportions have remained the same [14]. Perhaps this emphasizes the biomechanical requirements of the specific event. Again, it should be pointed out that although there are proportional differences among races, the differences between some sports are greater.

Because of statistical difficulties in dealing with proportions, a new approach has been tried with promising results [3]. Recently, Ross and Wilson [26] developed a stratagem for proportionality analysis called the phantom stratagem. Methodologically this approach has the advantages that all individuals are adjusted to the same stature, and the separate variables are all converted to Z-scores, thus facilitating between group, between sex and among variable comparisons. In applying this stratagem to black and white runners and jumpers Carter [3] found through use of stepwise discriminant analysis for each event that approximately 90% of both races could be correctly classified on the basis of three lengths and two breadths. The greatest contributions to the differences between races were due to biiliac breadth, which was narrower in the blacks, and arm length which was longer in the blacks. The only group for which this analysis failed to discriminate was the long distance runners. When this same analysis was applied across the five events for each race separately, the discrimination was very poor (from 0% to 52%) except for black sprinters who were correctly assigned to their event 82% of the time. These results indicate that the skeletal proportions are somewhat similar for all runners and jumpers when race is equated. Recently Sprague [27] used similar techniques to predict swimming times in young male swimmers from skeletal proportions. He found some variables were related but no single physical attribute was found consistently across all strokes. He concluded that prediction of swimming success was poor for young males.

Body Composition

Of great concern to the athlete is the amount of body fat which can be carried without hindering performance. Techniques such as densitometry, hydrometry, x-ray, anthropometric measurements including skinfolds and isotope detection have been used to assess the body fat of athletes. Unfortunately, no universal constants have been found which apply equally well to all groups, including male and female athletes. Because the different methodologies produce differences of 5% or more in an individual's body fatness, quantification of percent body fat in athletes from the many different studies creates serious interpretational problems. Nevertheless, if an attempt is made to take these differences into account, the leanest male athletes appear to be about 3% (which is the approximate value of essential fat) to 7% fat, and the leanest female athletes about 7% (which is essential fat plus sex-specific fat) to 10% fat [2]. With few exceptions, the upper level of fatness for males is about 15% and for females about 22% in outstanding athletes. Even at a relatively high level of competition for female gymnasts the placers are less fat than the nonplacers [18]. Parizkova and Poupa [24] have shown that body fat dynamically fluctuates as a function of the state of physical training.

Correnti and Zauli [14] measured skinfolds on both sides of the upper and lower limbs of track and field athletes and swimmers at Rome in 1960. There appeared to be no differences in skinfold thickness between right and left sides of those participating in unilateral sports. They also found the distance runners had smaller skinfolds than other athletes and that swimmers had larger skinfolds than the runners and stated that skinfolds are an excellent indicator of the state of training. In Tanner's [30] study of Olympic athletes, he examined the widths of fat, muscle and bone on x-rays and found differences in all three tissues among events and some differences between blacks and whites within events. Tittel and Wutscherk [32] found surprisingly high percent fat (13.4%) in middle distance female runners compared to 80 meter hurdlers (7.8%). They also noted higher relative fat (13.3%) in male waterpolo players compared to handball, basketball and volleyball players (10%). The lowest values of fat (7.5%) tended to be in the male distance runners.

Figure 5 shows the sum of three skinfolds for 17 groups of male and female Olympic athletes at Mexico in 1968 [16]. In general, the males have smaller values than the females, but the male water-poloists have higher values than do female divers, sprinters and gymnasts. The smallest skinfolds are found in the male long distance runners and gymnasts. The highest values for females are in the shot and discus throwers. Although not shown in the graph, the highest values for males are found in shot, discus and hammer throwers, as well as some athletes in the heaviest classes of boxing, wrestling and weightlifting [16]. We would expect that the lowest values in body fat (and on endomorphy) might be found in endurance-type athletes whose training and competition involve high energy cost for long periods of time. The fact that, in addition to distance runners, we find gymnasts, wrestlers and weightlifters (below middle weight class) all sharing the lowest levels of fatness indicates the importance of other factors. In gymnastics, wrestling and weightlifting it is

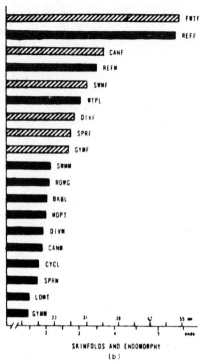

SKINFOLDS AND ENDOMORPHY
(b)

FIG. 5. Means of sum of three skinfolds and endomorphy for selected groups of male and female athlete groups at the Mexico games in 1968. (From de Garay, Levine and Carter [16].)

desirable to be as strong as possible, yet as light as possible, while distance runners should have excellent cardiovascular endurance, yet be as light as possible. In practice, both training and diet are used to control excess fat [5].

References

1. Azuma, T. (ed.): Olympic Medical Archives, Report, Tokyo 1964. The Japanese Olympic Medical Archives Committee, Tokyo, Japan, 1964.
2. Behnke, A.R. and Wilmore, J.H.: Evaluation and Regulation of Body Build and Composition. Englewood Cliffs:Prentice-Hall, Inc., 1974.
3. Carter, J.E.L.: Proportionality characteristics of black and white Olympic runners and jumpers. Paper presented at 23rd Annual Meeting, Amer. College of Sports Med., Anaheim, May 6, 1976.
4. Carter, J.E.L.: The Heath-Carter Somatotype Method. San Diego, California:San Diego State University, Revised edition, 1975.
5. Carter, J.E.L.: Somatotype, growth and physical performance. In Vague, J. and Boyer, J. (eds.): The Regulation of the Adipose Tissue Mass. Amsterdam:Excerpta Medica, 1974.

6. Carter, J.E.L.: Somatotype characteristics of champion athletes. *In* Novotny, V.V. (ed.): Anthropological Congress Dedicated to Ales Hrdlicka. Academia, Czechoslovak Academy of Sciences, Prague, 1971.
7. Carter, J.E.L.: The somatotypes of athletes — A Review. Hum. Biol. 42:535-569, 1970.
8. Carter, J.E.L. and Heath, B.H.: Somatotype methodology and kinesiology research. Kinesiology Rev., 1971, pp. 10-19.
9. Carter, J.E.L., Hebbelinck, M. and de Garay, A.L.: Anthropometric profiles of Olympic athletes at Mexico City. Paper presented at the International Congress of Physical Activity Sciences, Quebec City, July 13, 1976.
10. Carter, J.E.L. and Phillips, W.H.: Structural changes in exercising middle-aged males during a 2-year period. J. Appl. Physiol. 27:787-794, 1969.
11. Carter, J.E.L. and Rahe, R.H.: Effects of stressful underwater demolition training on body structure. Med. Sci. Sports 7:304-308, 1975.
12. Carter, J.E.L., Sleet, D.A. and Martin, G.N.: Somatotypes of male gymnasts. J. Sports Med. Phys. Fitness 11:2-11, 1971.
13. Clarke, H.E.: Physical and Motor Tests in the Medford Boy's Growth Study. Englewood Cliffs:Prentice-Hall, 1971.
14. Correnti, V. and Zauli, B.: Olimpionici 1960. Rome:Marves, 1964.
15. Cureton, T.K.: Physical Fitness of Champion Athletes. Urbana, Ill.: University of Illinois Press, 1951.
16. De Garay, A.L., Levine, L., Carter, J.E.L. (eds.): Genetic and Anthropological Studies of Olympic Athletes. New York:Academic Press, 1974.
17. Eiben, O.E.: The Physique of Women Athletes. Budapest:The Hungarian Scientific Council for Physical Education, 1972.
18. Falls, H.B. and Humphrey, L.D.: Comparison on somatotype and body composition between place winners and non place winners in an AIAW gymnastics meet. Paper presented at the Annual Meeting of A.A.H.P.E.R., Milwaukee, April 4, 1976.
19. Heath, B.H. and Carter, J.E.L.: Growth and somatotype patterns of Manus children, Territory of Papua and New Guinea: Application of a modified somatotype method to the study of growth patterns. Am. J. Phys. Anthrop. 35:49-67, 1971.
20. Heath, B.H. and Carter, J.E.L.: A modified somatotype method. Am. J. Phys. Anthrop. 27:57-74, 1967.
21. Hebbelinck, M., Carter, L. and de Garay, A.: Body build and somatotype of Olympic swimmers, divers, and water polo players. *In* Lewillie, L. and Clarys, J.P. (eds.): Swimming II. Baltimore:University Park Press, 1975.
22. Hirata, K.: Physique and age of Tokyo Olympic champions. J. Sports Med. Phys. Fitness 6:207-222, 1966.
23. Kohlrausch, W. Zuzammenhange von Korperform und Leistung: Ergebnisse der anthropometrischen Messungen und der Athleten der Amsterdamer Olympiade. Arbeitphysiol. 2:187-204, 1929.
24. Parizkova, J. and Carter, J.E.L.: Influence of physical activity on stability of somatotypes in boys. Am. J. Phys. Anthrop. 44:327-340, 1976.
25. Parizkova, J. and Poupa, O.: Some metabolic consequences of adaptation to muscular work. Br. J. Nutr. 17:341-345, 1963.
26. Ross, W.D. and Wilson, N.C.: A strategem [sic] for proportional growth assessment. Acta Paediatr. Belg. 28: Suppl. 169-180, 1974.
27. Sprague, H.A.: The relationship of certain physical measurements to swimming speed. Paper presented at the Annual Meeting of A.A.H.P.E.R., Milwaukee, April 2, 1976.

28. Stepnicka, J.: Typologie sportovcu. Acta Univ. Carol. Gymnica 1:67-90, 1974.
29. Stepnicka, J.: Typological and motor characteristics of athletes and university students. (In Czech) Prague: Charles University, 1972.
30. Tanner, J.M.: The Physique of the Olympic Athlete. London:George Allen and Unwin Ltd., 1964.
31. Tittel, K.: Zur Biotypologie und funktionellen Anatomic des Leistungs-sportlers. Nova Acta Leopoldina, 30: No. 172. Leipzig:J. A. Barth, 1965.
32. Tittel, K. and Wutscherk, H.: Sportanthropometrie. Leipzig:J. A. Barth, 1972.

Prédiction de dispositions athlétiques remarquables: perspective structurale

Examen des trois genres de prédictions et de leurs limites, suivi d'une révision de la connaissance actuelle concernant l'anthropométrie et la prédiction des aptitudes athlétiques remarquables. On y conclut qu'en termes de somatotype absolu, de dimensions absolues et relatives des corps, et de la composition corporelle, il existe des types définis capables d'accomplir des exploits exigeant soit de la force, soit de la vitesse, soit de l'endurance. Au départ, un physique avantageux permet de se concentrer sur d'autres qualités nécessaires à un rendement supérieur. La prédiction du physique et du rendement d'un athlète adulte, à partir du physique d'un jeune athlète, ne peut être faite que par grandes catégories.

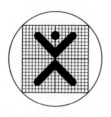

Aquatics and Human Performance

Activités aquatiques et performance humaine

Cardiorespiratory Adjustments to Swimming

Ingvar Holmér

Studies on the effects of swimming on man performed in a swimming flume is reviewed. Improved cardiorespiratory function and high maximal aerobic power adjustments occur. Thermoregulatory demands and hydrostatic and gravity effects may explain the small differences compared to land exercise. Hyperthermia, which is developed in lean swimmers more rapidly, may impair physical work capacity.

Introduction

In 1918 Liljestrand and Lindhard made the first attempt to measure cardiac output during swimming in man [24]. Their investigation was performed offshore at the Swedish westcoast. Conditions were difficult to control, methodological problems existed and the data then obtained were not very accurate. More than 50 years would pass before Dixon and Faulkner, using a CO_2 rebreathing method, determined cardiac output during swimming [9]. The inherent difficulties in making measurements on man while swimming have limited the possible physiological variables to be studied and probably acted as a deterrent to many scientists. During the last decade an increasing number of studies have produced a more detailed picture of the effects of swimming on man [15]. This review is intended to present some of those studies and mainly those performed in a swimming flume in our laboratory.

Experimental Procedures

In many studies tethered swimming has been used, which limits the prediction of free swimming conditions, since it is presently unknown in which respects tethered and free swimming are interchangeable. From a physiological point of view the differences

Ingvar Holmér, Department of Physiology, Gymnastik- och iddrottshögskolan, Stockholm, and Work Physiology Division, National Board of Occupational Safety and Health, Stockholm, Sweden.

between free and tethered swimming might be small or even negligible. After all, the swimming movements are quite similar and the muscles at work are probably the same. However, the transfer of energy produced in the working muscles to hydromechanical energy, especially propulsive energy, quite possibly differs between the two types of swimming. In terms of mechanical efficiency tethered and free swimming are extremely difficult to compare, as Goff et al [12] concluded from comparable data. Whenever data are used to evaluate or predict swimming performance, it is desirable that measurements be made during free swimming.

This is possible in a swimming flume [2] and in pools where the swimmer can be paced by a moving platform [8]. The swimming flume is a pool in which water can be circulated in a 2.5-meter wide, 1.2-meter deep and 4-meter long loop. Both water temperature (10 to 40 C) and water speed (0 to 2.0 m $\times$ s^{-1}) can be controlled. Experienced subjects are able to swim in essentially the same position in the flume for extended periods. Since 1968, metabolic, cardiorespiratory and biomechanical studies have been performed in the flume in our laboratory on swimmers of different standards.

Effects of Submergence

Before discussing cardiorespiratory adjustments to swimming a brief review of physiological responses to head-out immersion is relevant. During head-out immersion buoyant force almost cancels the effect of gravity on the body. The weight of the body in water amounts to a few kilograms. Body composition, amount of air in the lungs and depth of immersion are the most important factors determining the buoyant force [10]. The pressure of surrounding water and the buoyant force combine to produce certain respiratory and circulatory adjustments. Static dimensions of the lungs during head-out immersion compared with sitting in air are given for three subjects in Figure 1. Vital capacity (VC) was lowered by approximately 10%. Functional residual capacity was only 0.5-1.1 larger than residual volume (RV). In water tidal volume increases to a greater percent of TLC due to the utilization of the inspiratory reserve volume (IRV). In other words expiratory reserve volume (ERV) is reduced and breathing position is displaced toward RV.

Respiratory pressures and mechanics are affected during submersion [20]. However, during surface swimming the effects are probably too small to cause significant respiratory and circulatory disturbances. Buoyant force and hydrostatic pressure clearly offset

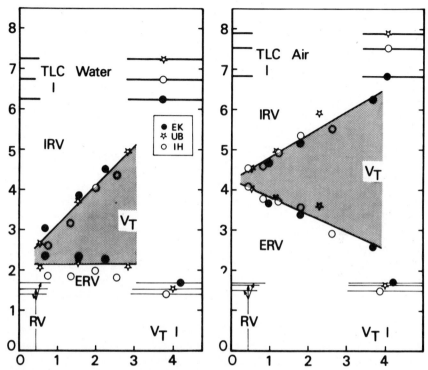

FIG. 1. Records of the volume of the lungs in air and during head-out immersion. Individual values stated for three subjects. (From von Döbeln and Holmér [10].)

the tendency of blood to pool in the lower portions of the body when in a vertical position on land. Central blood volume and venous return would be increased, presumably resulting in an increased stroke volume [1, 11, 23]. Head-out immersion in a vertical position in thermoneutral water produces a significant increase in cardiac output with little change in heart rate [1]. These adjustments are similar to those observed in air for the supine when compared to the standing position. Rennie et al [34] reported that resting heart rate and cardiac output were reduced when immersed head out in water below 34 C.

Respiration

If swimming caused restrictions on respiration it could affect the gas exchange in the lung. Respiration is normally synchronized with stroke rate. Furthermore, swimming involves a forced inspiratory phase against increased pressure on the thoracic cage and underwater expiration must overcome a high pressure (50 to 100 mm H_2O). Introducing a respiratory valve to the swimming subject may affect the normal breathing pattern. In our studies, however, the typical breathing pattern was usually preserved; e.g. blood gas determinations with and without valve during swimming did not reveal any significant differences [19].

Biomechanical Properties

To our knowledge only one investigation has examined the biomechanical properties of the lungs during swimming. Deroanne and colleagues [7] recorded esophageal pressure, air flow and tidal volume on three subjects during breaststroke and backstroke swimming and compared them with those recorded in a seated position out of water and in different positions in water. All measurements were carried out at about the same level of ventilation (50 l $\times$ min^{-1}). Values for lung conductance during swimming as well as during immersion, irrespective of body position, were 20% to 30% lower than on land. Lung compliance was decreased by approximately 30% during backstroke, but almost unchanged during breaststroke swimming when compared with land data. In other words airway resistances are increased during swimming, and elastic resistances are increased in backstroke swimming. It is obvious that many of these findings are readily explained by the factors mentioned above.

Ventilation

Although severe strain is imposed upon respiration, the swimmer displays normal ventilation rather than hypoventilation. In this respect the respiratory valve should facilitate breathing, indicating a relative hypoventilation during free swimming, which also has been claimed by some investigators [9, 25, 28]. However, this is not supported, based on blood gas data, as mentioned before, at least not for the breaststroke [19]. During maximal work in air most subjects react by a hyperventilation and consequently an increased ventilation coefficient. This is not seen during maximal swimming. Figure 2 depicts pulmonary ventilation and ventilation coefficient during maximal swimming and maximal running in elite swimmers. Although the biomechanical conditions are quite unfavorable for breathing in the supine position, backstrokers are reported to hyperventilate during maximal swimming [25]. Backstroke swimmers do not immerse their face and consequently may have

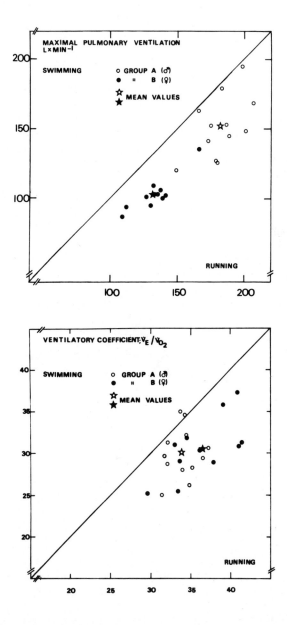

FIG. 2. Individual maximal values for pulmonary ventilation (*top*) and ventilatory coefficient (*bottom*) during swimming as compared to running. (From Holmér et al [18].)

undisturbed breathing pattern. Alveolar ventilation per breath was calculated to be higher during maximal swimming than maximal running [19].

Respiratory Gas Exchange

In a study of five subjects during swimming with indwelling catheters we were able to demonstrate that gas exchange was sufficient to maintain an oxygenation of the arterial blood similar to that observed in running [19]. Although the alveolar-arterial O_2-pressure gradient was lower during maximal swimming, O_2 saturation of arterial blood was about 91% or almost the same as in running (Fig. 3). Figure 3 also depicts the partial pressure of O_2 in arterial blood. Data obtained during maximal breaststroke swimming and maximal running were almost identical. Not only O_2 pressure, but also CO_2 pressure showed a remarkable similarity during submaximal as well as maximal swimming compared with running.

In summary, the strain imposed upon the respiratory system during swimming does not interfere with gas exchange, at least not during breaststroke swimming. Apparently a given alveolar ventilation is obtained at a lower total ventilation than in running. An adequate saturation of arterial blood is maintained during swimming. Consequently, it is unlikely that respiration is a limiting factor in the oxygen transport system to working muscles.

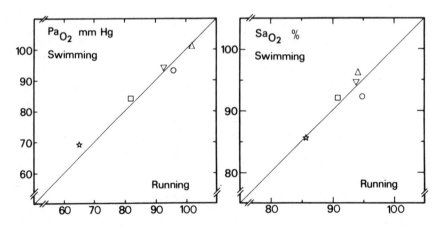

FIG. 3. Comparison of arterial O_2 tension (P_{aO_2}) and arterial O_2 saturation (S_{aO_2}) in five subjects during maximal work swimming and running. (From Holmér et al [19].)

Circulation

In a series of experiments cardiac output was determined with the dye-dilution technique in five subjects during breaststroke swimming [19]. A comparison was made with similar data obtained during running in the same subjects. Cardiac output, heart rate and stroke volume are related to $\dot{V}O_2$ in Figure 4 for the two subjects representing the lowest and the highest $\dot{V}O_2$ max from the group. Similar relationships were obtained in the other three subjects. These observations suggest that the cardiovascular system responds to increased workloads in a similar way during swimming and running despite dissimilar posture, respiratory mechanics, external pressure and thermal load between the two activities. An increased stroke volume due to better diastolic filling in the supine position has been advocated to explain the lowered heart rate at a given submaximal $\dot{V}O_2$ observed in swimming in some investigations [13, 28, 29]. However, subjects in our study did not attain lowered submaximal heart rates at similar $\dot{V}O_2$'s.

All five subjects in our study had lower maximal cardiac output swimming when compared to running, stroke volume being about the same. Mean arterial blood pressure (MBP) was increased by 10 to 20 mm Hg during both submaximal and maximal swimming when compared to running [19]. Heart rate during maximal swimming has been reported in several investigations to be lowered by 10 to 15 beats $\times$ min^{-1} when compared to running [9, 16, 25, 27] (Fig. 5), walking [28] and bicycling [3, 13, 16].

Differences in degree of training in swimming, in the size of muscle mass at work, in thermoregulatory demands for a skin circulation and in hydrostatic and gravitational effects upon the body can modify the circulatory response to swimming. Central cardiovascular reactions during submaximal swimming, as mentioned, are evidently not affected significantly by these factors, except for the increased mean arterial blood pressure. However, the lowered cardiac output during maximal swimming in our study should be explained by one or more of these factors. It should be emphasized that cardiac work (MPB $\times$ cardiac output) was essentially the same during maximal work swimming and running. In their study of tethered swimming, Dixon and Faulkner [9] demonstrated that trained swimmers attained the same maximal cardiac output swimming as running, heart rate being 13 beats $\times$ min^{-1} lower and stroke volume 5% higher. Recreational swimmers, however, attained 25% lower cardiac output, lower heart rate as well as lowered stroke

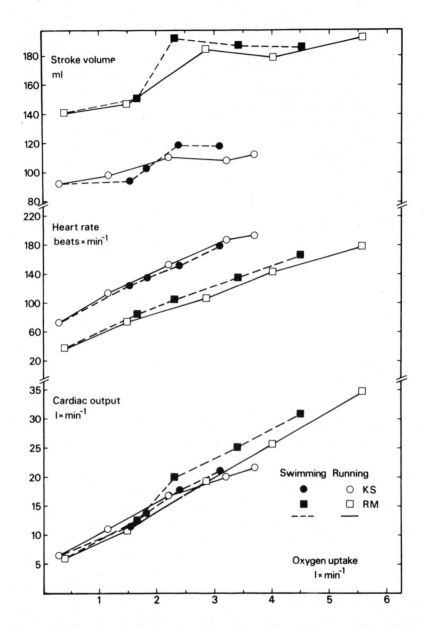

FIG. 4. Cardiac output, heart rate and stroke volume in two subjects during swimming and running. (From Holmér et al [19].)

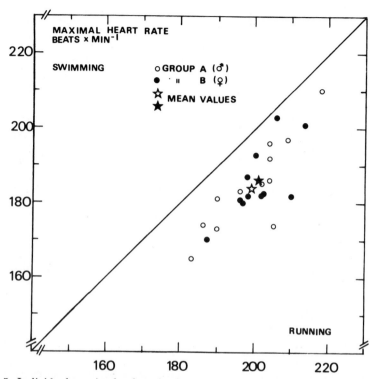

FIG. 5. Individual maximal values for heart rate during swimming as compared to running. (From Holmér et al [18].)

volume during swimming when compared to running. Our data do not fit any of their categories.

Thermoregulatory demands are known to provoke circulatory adjustments [33, 35]. In this respect the temperature of the water during swimming constitutes a crucial factor. This topic will be discussed later. The increased MBP indicates an increased peripheral resistance during swimming when compared to running at a given cardiac output. Thermoregulatory skin vasoconstriction may be one explanation for this phenomenon.

Arterial O_2 saturation (Fig. 3), blood gas tensions and pH (Table I) were remarkably similar during swimming and running, as mentioned previously. Values for O_2 content in arterial blood were almost identical during maximal swimming and running. O_2 extraction was equally high in both types of exercise, as indicated by very low O_2 content in femoral venous blood (about 2 vol%). In contrast, calculated O_2 difference between arterial and mixed venous

Table I. Blood Gas Tensions and pH in Four Subjects

	Submax Work		Max Work	
	Swimming	Running	Swimming	Running
PO$_2$ mm Hg				
Arterial	90 ± 5	86 ± 3	89 ± 11	86 ± 11
Venous	24 ± 1	24 ± 1	19 ± 4	18 ± 2
PCO$_2$ mm Hg				
Arterial	41 ± 3	39 ± 2	33 ± 5	34 ± 3
Venous	66 ± 5	62 ± 9	81 ± 8	81 ± 12
pH				
Arterial	7.36 ± 0.01	7.38 ± 0.03	7.20 ± 0.03	7.29 ± 0.07
Venous	7.27 ± 0.02	7.30 ± 0.02	7.08 ± 0.03	7.14 ± 0.05

Values are means ± SD. There was no significant difference between values for swimming and running during either submaximal or maximal work [19].

blood was significantly higher in maximal running (16.0 vol%) than in swimming (14.8 vol%) [19]. Regional blood flow data are lacking for a more sophisticated analysis of the hemodynamics of the two types of exercise.

Oxygen Transporting Capacity in Swimmers

Swimming makes great demands on the oxygen transporting system and elite swimmers display all the functional adaptations normally seen in persons partaking in endurance-type sports. Lung volumes and heart volume are increased and respiratory and cardiovascular functions are on high levels [3, 18, 25]. Very high values for $\dot{V}O_2$ max in swimming have been reported, mean value for 12 male swimmers 5.05 l × min^{-1} and for 11 girl swimmers 3.42 l × min^{-1} (Fig. 6). Although exceptionally well-trained swimmers, these boys and girls on the average produced 7% higher $\dot{V}O_2$ max for running. Similar findings have been reported in other studies [3, 16]. However, Magel and Faulkner [25] and Dixon and Faulkner [9] demonstrated that trained swimmers attained the same $\dot{V}O_2$ max during tethered swimming as running. As mentioned, there are several dissimilarities between the two types of exercise. Especially the fact that in part different muscle groups are activated in swimming than in running and that swimming is to a greater extent arm work complicates a more detailed comparison. High correlation between arm work capacity and swimming performance (free style) has been reported [4]. The different results obtained for $\dot{V}O_2$ max swimming when compared to running can be readily explained by

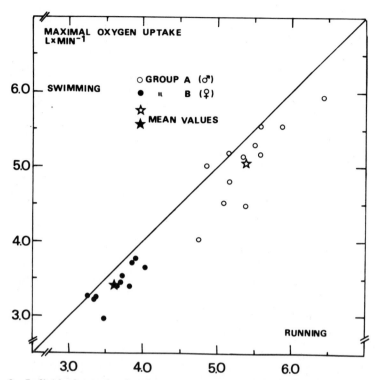

FIG. 6. Individual maximal values for oxygen uptake during swimming as compared to running. (From Holmér et al [18].)

different degrees of training in the two types of exercise. Magel and Faulkner's college swimmers may have been less trained in running than our swimmers, although training in running is a rare feature in the training program of our swimmers. The predictive value of the $\dot{V}O_2$ max while running for swimming performance is strongly questioned. In one of our elite swimmers, an Olympic gold medal winner, the $\dot{V}O_2$ max of swimming and running has been determined repeatedly during his career. As illustrated in Figure 7, apart from the first years, the $\dot{V}O_2$ max of running was constant. The high intensity swim training, however, produced significant variations in the $\dot{V}O_2$ max of swimming, variations which were demonstrated to be even larger in free-style arm swimming. The peaks in $\dot{V}O_2$ max while swimming coincide with the periods of his most successful performances. In a recent study by Magel and colleagues [26] the specificity of swim training in 15 recreational swimmers on $\dot{V}O_2$ max was further emphasized. They could demonstrate an 11% increase in

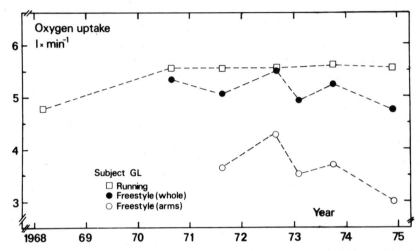

FIG. 7. Oxygen uptake during swimming and running at maximal intensities by one world-class swimmer over the past eight years (Holmér, unpublished results).

$\dot{V}O_2$ max swimming tethered, whereas no increase was seen in $\dot{V}O_2$ max running following a ten-week interval swim training period.

In summary, the $\dot{V}O_2$ max of swimming apparently entails adaptations unique to this training form, which suggests that a swimmer's training of $\dot{V}O_2$ max should take place in the water to the greatest possible extent.

Water Temperature and Thermoregulatory Demands

Thermoregulatory studies in swimming are few [31]. Immersion in water at a temperature of 30 C or lower involves a risk of eliciting a progressive hypothermia, especially pronounced in lean subjects [14, 17, 21, 30, 36]. During hypothermia a concomitant increase in $\dot{V}O_2$ at rest and during swimming at a given submaximal velocity due to shivering is observed [5, 14, 17, 21, 30-32, 34]. Man responds to cold with peripheral vasoconstriction and shivering. However, increased extremity blood flow in conjunction with shivering or muscular work accelerates the cooling rate of lean subjects in water at 18 to 20 C or colder [17, 22].

Compared to normal swimming in water at 26 C, swimmers attained about 10 beats $\times$ min^{-1} lower heart rate at a given submax $\dot{V}O_2$ in water at 18 C. Similarly, approximately 10 beats $\times$ min^{-1} higher heart rate was obtained in water at 34 C [17]. This increase in submaximal heart rate at a given $\dot{V}O_2$ with water temperature may provide for a greater cardiac output, which itself is a consequence of reduced peripheral resistance. However, Rennie et al [34] observed similar cardiac output during exercise in water at 22 to 36 C, heart rate being reduced. Further evidence was put forward in a recent paper by McArdle and colleagues [29] that stroke volume compensated entirely for the heart rate variations under similar conditions, thus keeping cardiac output constant. Dissimilarities in type of exercise and body posture somewhat limit the value of comparing these studies with free-swimming data.

In Figure 8 heart rate response to maximal swimming in water at three different temperatures is given. Heart rate seems to be related to internal body temperatures. In some of the subjects this relation could be partly explained by the concomitant variation in $\dot{V}O_2$. However, subjects with unchanged $\dot{V}O_2$ max while swimming also demonstrated lowered heart rates in cold water and increased heart rates in warm water (34 C).

In our studies in the swimming flume at different water temperatures reduced $\dot{V}O_2$ was obtained during maximal swimming

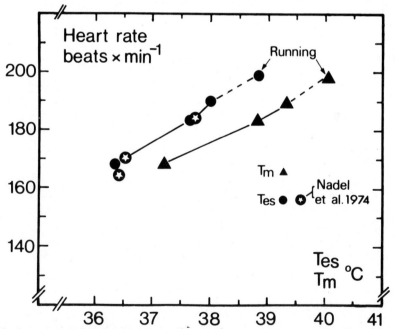

FIG. 8. Mean values for heart rate in five subjects during maximal swimming and maximal running in relation to esophageal (T_{es}) and muscle temperature (T_m) [17]. Also plotted are mean heart rates obtained in three subjects in a similar study by Nadel et al [30].

in subjects with lowered internal temperature (esophageal temperature below approximately 37 C) [17, 21].

During exercise with severe cold or heat stress thermoregulatory and metabolic demands will be in conflict. Our data suggest that during maximal swimming in cold or warm water thermoregulatory demands might supersede oxygen demands. The severity of the thermal load then determines the extent to which the cardiovascular system and physical work capacity are affected. Although a great part of the hemodynamic responses induced by temperature may be the effect of changes in the peripheral vasomotor tone, cold per se might have a direct effect upon cardiac function and its regulation. Davies and colleagues [6] demonstrated recently in hypothermic subjects performing maximal cycling that the decreased heart rate was unaffected by atropine.

Summary

Competitive swimmers are characterized by an excellent cardiorespiratory function and a high maximal aerobic power. Cardiorespiratory adjustments to swimming are determined by the rate of the work and degree of conditioning in swimming. Modifications, more or less pronounced, are brought about by thermoregulatory demands and hydrostatic and gravity effects. Dissimilarities in these respects can readily explain differences in cardiorespiratory adjustments in swimming when compared to exercise on land, differences that are remarkably small if studied under optimal conditions. Unfavorable breathing conditions do not prevent a normal oxygenation of arterial blood even at maximal swimming. $\dot{V}O_2$ max for swimming is superior to $\dot{V}O_2$ max for running as a reliable predictor of swimming performance. This fact also strongly suggests that the swimmer's training of the oxygen transporting system should be made by swimming. Hypothermia is rapidly developed in lean subjects during swimming in cold water. Thermoregulatory demands under severe cold stress and, presumably, hypothermia per se affect cardiorespiratory functioning in such a way that physical work capacity is impaired.

Acknowledgments

Sincere appreciation is extended to Per-Olof Åstrand and Ulf Bergh for their helpful comments in reviewing the manuscript, and to Stenberg-Flygt AB, Solna, for providing the swimming flume.

References

1. Arborelius, M. Jr., Balldin, U.I., Lilja, B. and Lundgren, C.E.G.: Hemodynamic changes in man during immersion with the head above water. Aerospace Med. 43:592-598, 1972.
2. Astrand, P.-O. and Englesson, S.: A swimming flume. J. Appl. Physiol. 33:514, 1972.
3. Astrand, P.-O., Engström, L., Eriksson, B.O. et al: Girl swimmers. Acta Paediatr. Suppl. 147, 1963.
4. Charbonnier, J.P., Lacour, J.R., Riffat, J. and Flandrois, R.: Experimental study of the performance of competition swimmers. Europ. J. Appl. Physiol. 34:157-167, 1975.
5. Craig, A.B., Jr. and Dvorak, M.: Thermal regulation of man exercising during water immersion. J. Appl. Physiol. 25:28-35, 1968.
6. Davies, M., Ekblom, B., Bergh, U. and Kanstrup-Jensen, I.-L.: The effects of hypothermia on submaximal and maximal work performance. Acta Physiol. Scand. 95:201-202, 1975.
7. Deroanne, R., Pirnay, F., Dujardin, J. and Petit, J.M.: Mechanical properties of the lungs during swimming. In Lewillie, L. and Clarys, J.P. (eds.): 1st Int. Symposium on Biomechanics in Swimming. Brussels. Université libre de Bruxelles, Laboratoire de l'Effort, 1971, pp. 207-215.
8. Di Prampero, P.E., Pendergast, D.R., Wilson, D.W. and Rennie, D.W.: Energetics of swimming in man. J. Appl. Physiol. 37:1-5, 1974.
9. Dixon, R.W. Jr. and Faulkner, J.A.: Cardiac outputs during maximum effort running and swimming. J. Appl. Physiol. 30:653-656, 1971.
10. Döbeln, W. von and Holmer, I.: Body composition, sinking force, and oxygen uptake of man during water treading. J. Appl. Physiol. 37:55-59, 1974.
11. Echt, M., Lange, L. and Gauer, O.H.: Changes in peripheral venous tone and central transmural pressure during immersion in a thermoneutral bath. Pfluegers Arch. 352:211-217, 1974.
12. Goff, L.G., Brubach, H.F. and Specht, H.: Measurements of respiratory responses and work efficiency of underwater swimmers utilizing improved instrumentation. J. Appl. Physiol. 10:197-202, 1957.
13. Goodwin, A.B. and Cumming, G.R.: Radio telemetry of the electrocardiogram, fitness tests, and oxygen uptake of water-polo players. Can. Med. Assoc. J. 95:402-406, 1966.
14. Hayward, J.S., Eckerson, J.D. and Collis, M.L.: Thermal balance and survival time prediction of man in cold water. Can. J. Physiol. Pharmacol. 53:21-32, 1975.
15. Holmer, I.: Physiology of swimming man. Acta Physiol. Scand. Suppl. 407, 1974.
16. Holmer, I.: Oxygen uptake during swimming in man. J. Appl. Physiol. 33 (4):502-509, 1972.
17. Holmer, I. and Bergh, U.: Metabolic and thermal response to swimming in water at varying temperatures. J. Appl. Physiol. 37:702-705, 1974.
18. Holmer, I., Lundin, A. and Eriksson, B.O.: Maximum oxygen uptake during swimming and running by elite swimmers. J. Appl. Physiol. 36:711-714, 1974.

19. Holmer, I., Stein, E.M., Saltin, B. et al: Hemodynamic and respiratory responses compared in swimming and running. J. Appl. Physiol. 37:49-54, 1974.
20. Hong, S.K., Cerretelli, P., Cruz, J.C. and Rahn, H.: Mechanics of respiration during submersion in water. J. Appl. Physiol. 27:535-538, 1969.
21. Keatinge, W.R.: Survival in cold water. Oxford & Edinburgh:Blackwell, 1969.
22. Keatinge, W.R.: The effect of work and clothing on the maintenance of the body temperature in water. Q. J. Exp. Physiol, 46:69-82, 1961.
23. Lange, L., Lange, S., Echt, M. and Gauer, O.H.: Heart volume in relation to body posture and immersion in a thermo-neutral bath. Pfluegers Arch. 352:219-226, 1974.
24. Liljestrand, G. and Lindhard, J.: Uber das Minutenvolumen des Herzens beim Schwimmen. Skand. Arch. Physiol. 39:64-77, 1919.
25. Magel, J.R. and Faulkner, J.A.: Maximum oxygen uptakes of college swimmers. J. Appl. Physiol. 22:929-938, 1967.
26. Magel, J.R., Foglia, G.F., McArdle, W.D. et al: The specificity of swim training on maximum oxygen uptake. J. Appl. Physiol. 38:151-155, 1975.
27. Magel, J., McArdle, W.D. and Glaser, R.: Telemetered heart rate response to selected competitive swimming events. J. Appl. Physiol. 26:764-770, 1969.
28. McArdle, V.D., Glaser, R.M. and Magel, J.R.: Metabolic and cardiorespiratory response during free swimming and treadmill walking. J. Appl. Physiol. 30:733-738, 1971.
29. McArdle, W.D., Magel, J.R., Lesmes, G.R. and Pechar, G.S.: Metabolic and cardiovascular adjustment to work in air and water at 18, 25 and 33° C. J. Appl. Physiol. 40:85-90, 1976.
30. Nadel, E.R., Holmer, I., Bergh, V. et al: Energy exchange of swimming man. J. Appl. Physiol. 36:465-571, 1974.
31. Neilsen, B.: Metabolic reactions to changes in core and skin temperature in man. Acta Physiol. Scand. 1976. (In press.)
32. Nielsen, B.: Metabolic reactions to cold during swimming at different speeds. Arch. Sci. Physiol. 27:207-211, 1973.
33. Nielsen, B.: Thermoregulation in rest and exercise. Acta Physiol. Scand. Suppl. 323, 1969.
34. Rennie, D.W., Di Prampero, P. and Cerretelli, P.: Effects of water immersion on cardiac output, heart rate, and stroke volume of man at rest and during exercise. Med. Sport 24:223-228, 1971.
35. Rowell, L.B.: Human cardiovascular adjustments to exercise and thermal stress. Physiol. Rev. 54:75-159, 1974.
36. Sloan, R.E.G. and Keatinge, W.R.: Cooling rates of young people swimming in cold water. J. Appl. Physiol. 35:371-375, 1973.

Les ajustements cardio-respiratoires survenant au cours de la nage sportive

L'auteur fait état de résultats de recherches effectuées en laboratoire aquatique et met un accent particulier sur les ajustements remarquables qui se font du côté de l'efficacité du système de transport de l'oxygène comme résultat de l'entraînement en natation de compétition. Les aspects pertinents de la thermorégulation et ceux des exigences particulières de déplacement en milieu aqueux sont discutés sur la base d'expériences avec des nageurs dont les niveaux de tolérance à l'hypothermie diffèrent et affectent la performance.

Energetics of Locomotion in Man

D. R. Pendergast, P. di Prampero, A. B.
Craig, Jr., and D. W. Rennie

Resistive forces that must be overcome while swimming at various velocities are presented and discussed. At given swimming speeds, frictional forces, form drag and wave formation constitute body drag which affects energy expenditure and mechanical efficiency. Oxygen uptake and blood lactic acid data on freestyle swimmers up to velocities of 2 m/sec are presented for the purpose of establishing total energy requirements under aerobic and anaerobic components. The differences between (as well as the interdependence of) drag and efficiency and the importance of their ratio are shown in subjects with different technical abilities and in both female and male skilled swimmers.

Introduction

The quantitative examination of the energetics of swimming has been hampered in the past by lack of data on the overall resistive forces that a swimmer must overcome while actually swimming and the total energy necessary to overcome water resistance while swimming at high velocities.

Under conditions of swimming at a constant velocity, [v], a propulsive force must be supplied by the swimmer that is equal and opposite to the resistance to progression called body drag, $[D_b]$, which we define as the sum of frictional forces, form drag and wave formation. The rate of external work, $[\dot{w}]$, or power of a swimmer is the product of D_b and v as shown in equation 1. Useful power is expressed in equation 2 in the familiar terms of overall energy

D. R. Pendergast, P. di Prampero, A. B. Craig, Jr. and D. W. Rennie, Department of Physiology, School of Medicine, State University of New York at Buffalo, Buffalo, N.Y., U.S.A.

At the time of our investigations, P. E. di Prampero was on leave from the Centro Studi di Fisiologia del lavoro Muscolare del CNR, Milan, Italy; A. B. Craig, Jr. was on leave from the Department of Physiology, School of Medicine at the University of Rochester, Rochester, New York.

The investigations reported in this presentation were supported in part by National Institutes of Health Grant 5-POI HL 14414.

expenditure and overall net mechanical efficiency, [e]. Since the units for external power can be expressed as $l\,O_2 \cdot min^{-1}$ equations 1 and 2 can be equated and rearranged as in equation 3. It is obvious from equation 3 that the energy cost of swimming, $\dot{V}O_2$, at a given velocity, v, (3a) or at a given distance (3b), is determined by the ratio of body drag to efficiency. These equations are further rearranged in equation 4 showing that the energy cost of swimming a given distance is equivalent to the ratio of D_b/e. Body drag and efficiency are influenced independently by many factors including body size and shape, body density, stroke selection, stroke mechanics and devices that aid the swimmer. Thus it is critical to measure body drag and efficiency independently while swimming in order to evaluate the energy cost of swimming.

$$\dot{W} = D_b \cdot V \tag{1}$$

$$\dot{W} = \dot{V}O_2 \cdot e \tag{2}$$

$$\dot{V}O_2 = v \cdot \frac{(D_b)}{e} \tag{3a}$$

$$\dot{V}O_2 = d \cdot \frac{(D_b)}{e} \tag{3b}$$

$$\frac{\dot{V}O_2}{d} = \frac{D_b}{e} \tag{4}$$

With the use of a doughnut-shaped swimming pool 60 meters in circumference and a revolving observation platform, swimmers were monitored continuously to determine the total energy cost, body drag and efficiency while swimming the freestyle up to velocities of 2 meters per second. Steady-state submaximal oxygen consumption was measured while subjects swam at constant velocities. The propulsive force that the swimmer had to provide was varied by either adding to the body drag or subtracting from the body drag known external forces that acted in the direction of swimming. Net oxygen consumption during the fifth minute of swimming was plotted as a function of the imposed external forces. As the external propulsive force was reduced, the swimmer's propulsive force had to increase, causing a linear increase of oxygen consumption. The energy required from the subject was always below maximum oxygen consumption; thus the total energy cost of the swim could be estimated by the measurement of oxygen consumption at the mouth. The energy cost of free swimming was determined by extrapolating the linear relationship of net oxygen consumption on the external force to zero external force. The body drag of swimming at a given speed was calculated by extrapolating this same relationship to the point where the net oxygen consumption was zero. Hence, the external propulsive force exactly offset body drag. Efficiency was calculated from the slope of the relationship between external force and net oxygen consumption at each velocity, $\dfrac{\Delta F \cdot v}{\Delta \dot{V}O_2}$ [4, 17]. This method for determining the total energy cost of free swimming has been validated by comparing the total energy cost of swimming predicted by extrapolation of the external force vs. net oxygen consumption relationship to zero external force with that observed directly where the total energy cost of swimming could be determined aerobically [17].

The total energy cost of swimming was studied in 12 university swimmers. Data for one representative swimmer up to his maximum swimming velocity are presented in Figure 1. The oxygen transport system is capable of supplying the total energy requirement up to 1.10 meters per second, about 60% of maximum velocity, in this subject. At faster velocities the oxygen transport system was not capable of generating enough metabolic power. The difference between the dashed and solid lines, oxygen deficit, at any velocity represents the metabolic power that must be supplied anaerobically, $\dot{V}O_2$an. Expensive and uncommon facilities are required to apply this method for determining total energy cost of swimming. To develop a method available to others, we compared our estimates of anaerobic power with the rate of lactic acid accumulation in venous blood using the method described by Margaria and others for running [3, 5, 11, 13].

Venous blood lactic acid concentration ($mM \cdot l^{-1}$) was determined as a function of swimming time for velocities ranging from 50% to 100% of maximum swimming speed for each subject. Lactic acid concentration was determined eight to ten minutes after the completion of the swim to insure equilibration and that the "peak" lactic acid value was determined. As for running [3, 5, 11, 13], at any given speed lactic acid concentration rose linearly with exercise time. For purposes of estimating anaerobic power, it is the rate of increase of lactic acid concentration at each velocity that is

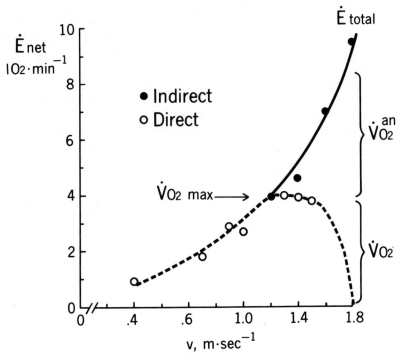

FIG. 1. Energy cost of actual swimming, in $1 O_2$ equivalents per minute, as a function of swimming velocity. The dashed line represents directly measured oxygen consumption and the solid line, total energy cost estimated by extrapolation [4, 17].

important, i.e., the slope of the regression of lactic acid concentration and swimming time for each velocity.

In Figure 2 data for the rate of rise of lactic acid as a function of swimming speed is added to the total energy cost and aerobic power data from Figure 1. It can be seen that when the demand (total energy requirement) exceeds the aerobic power, an increase in speed results in an increase in the rate of rise of lactic acid concentration. The velocity where there is a significant rate of rise of lactic acid represents about 90% of the swimmer's $\dot{V}O_2$ max. By determining the discrepancy between energy requirement and aerobic supply at any speed and relating this value to the rate of rise of lactic acid accumulation in venous blood, the oxygen equivalent for lactic acid accumulation was calculated. This value determined for the 12 subjects in this study was 2.6 ml O_2/kg mM, a value slightly lower than the value reported for running [5, 10, 13]. Utilizing this

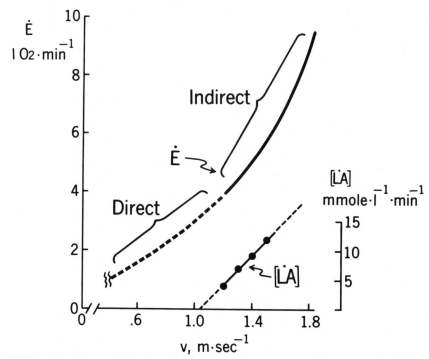

FIG. 2. Total energy cost, determined by extrapolation [4, 17] as a function of swimming speed and the rate of rise of venous blood lactic acid, determined eight minutes into the recovery from exercise, as a function of swimming speed for one skilled swimmer.

empirical relationship, the anaerobic component of swimming can be added to the aerobic component to determine the total energy cost of swimming at any given velocity.

As can be seen from Figure 1, the energy cost of swimming increases curvilinearly with velocity which (based on equation 4) suggests that the ratio of D_b/e is not constant as is the case for running [1, 9, 14].

The average energy cost to swim 1 km is presented for various velocity ranges for 32 male swimmers in Figure 3. For velocities up to 1.2 meters per second the energy cost of swimming 1 km was constant. This can be explained by the fact that the increased body drag resulting from increasing velocity was offset proportionally by increased swimming efficiency. However, when velocity was increased up to 1.7 meters per second, body drag increased disproportionally compared to the increase of efficiency. At still

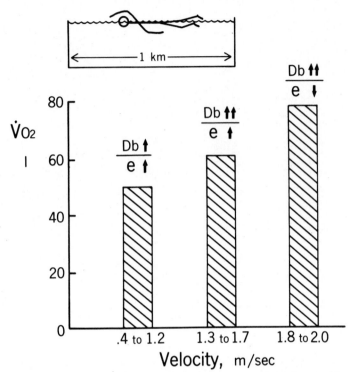

FIG. 3. The amount of energy, expressed as 1 O_2, to swim 1 km at velocities of .4 to 1.2, 1.3 to 1.7 and 1.8 to 2.0 meters per second. Above each level of energy requirement changes in drag and efficiency are indicated by arrows.

higher velocities there was an even greater increase in the energy cost of swimming due to an actual decrease in efficiency while body drag continued to increase curvilinearly.

Subjects of poorer technical ability were characterized by a higher energy cost per unit distance at any speed and the velocity where the energy cost per unit distance began to increase with increases in speed was lower. In general, the subjects with a lower energy cost per unit distance had a higher efficiency and lower drag than subjects with a higher energy cost per unit distance. However, in some individuals a low energy cost was a result of a high body drag being compensated for by a high efficiency while in others a low efficiency was counteracted by a low body drag, further emphasizing the importance of the ratio of body drag and efficiency, and not either alone in affecting the energy cost of swimming [17].

The independence of drag and efficiency and the importance of their ratio can be emphasized further by examining the effect of devices used to aid the swimmer. In Figure 4 the energy cost of freestyle swimming is compared with freestyle swimming with the legs floated but inactive and swimming with an aqueon. It can be seen that the energy cost was reduced in half despite the fact that the floats increased the swimmer's drag. A similar response was observed when the swimmer utilized an aqueon to assist propulsion with a disproportionally high efficiency being responsible for the reduced energy cost to swim 1 km.

The effect of decreasing or holding constant body drag was determined while fin swimming at the surface and swimming with SCUBA. The energy cost of swimming with fins at the surface or with SCUBA is 40% less than when freestyle swimming. In the case of fin swimming, body drag is reduced and efficiency is increased whereas during SCUBA, drag is not significantly different from

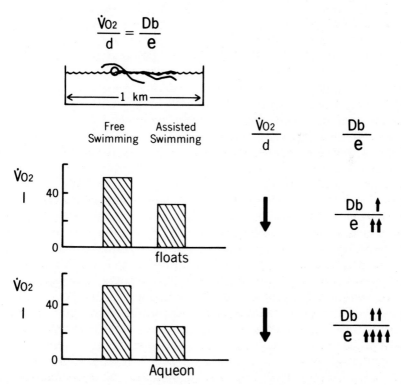

FIG. 4. The amount of energy, expressed as $1\ O_2$, to swim 1 km for free swimming and with feet floated and immobile in the upper plate and utilizing an aqueon in the lower plate. At the right, changes in $\dot{V}O_2/d$, D_b and e are indicated by arrows when compared with assisted freestyle swimming.

freestyle swimming, but it is a considerably more efficient form of propulsion. These comparisons establish both the independence of drag and efficiency and the importance of their ratio in determining the energy cost of swimming.

In another study the energy cost of swimming a given distance for 16 skilled female swimmers was found to be significantly lower than for their male counterparts, 34 and 50 l O_2 per kilometer, respectively. This difference was also shown for unskilled swimmers as well as for the breast stroke and back crawl. The body drag of the women was significantly lower at all speeds than men of similar competitive experience, 3.8 and 5.2 kg at 0.9 meters per second. The lower drag of women was only in part due to a smaller surface area. In addition to a lower drag the women had a significantly higher efficiency than the men, 4 and 3.5 at 0.9 meters per second. Thus, the reduced energy cost for women is due both to lower body drag and to increased e at all velocities up to 1.2 meters per second.

The difference in the body drag when women are compared to men can be accounted for by differences in body sizes and overall body density [18]. It has been shown [18] that the density of the lower extremities of women is less than that of men which allows the former to waste less energy on leg kicking, a factor in their higher efficiency. The differences between the energy cost to swim a given distance for men and women can be completely explained on the basis of body composition and its distribution.

It is well documented that body density increases with age up to maturity and that the density of boys and girls is not significantly different up to puberty. Basing ourselves on these data, we had 54 individuals from age 5 to 18 from a local swim club swim at 0.7 meters per second while determinations were made for the energy cost per unit distance. The energy cost of swimming when corrected for body size was not influenced by sex up to the 15-year-old group at which time there was a significant drop in the energy cost per unit distance of the women and an increase in the cost of the men, typical of the adult pattern observed. These changes could be a result of increased subcutaneous fat development in the women and increased musculature in men consistent with the hypothesis that body density and its distribution are critical factors in determining the energy cost of swimming.

Given the fact that women and younger swimmers expend less energy to swim a given distance than men or older swimmers, then why do men swim faster than women, and why do older swimmers swim faster than younger swimmers? By rearranging equation 3a, it is evident that the velocity of swimming is a product of two factors: (1) total energy input and (2) ratio of drag to efficiency. Evidently, men and adult swimmers can supply enough energy to more than compensate for the less effective relationship of drag and efficiency than is the case for women and younger swimmers. The results are faster swimming velocities at greater energy expense.

In conclusion, methods of determining the body drag, efficiency and total energy requirement during swimming have developed an empirical relationship between anaerobic power and the ratio of rise of venous blood lactic acid. It is clear that it is the ratio of body drag to efficiency that is important in determining the energy cost of swimming using the energy cost of swimming 1 km to express the proficiency or technical ability of the swimmer. Women expend less energy to swim than men, due to lower drag and higher efficiency, probably due to a more horizontal attitude in the water and smaller surface area. The sex difference appears at a time concurrent with subcutaneous fat development in women and increased musculature in men.

References

1. Astrand, P.O. and Rodahl, K.: Textbook of Work Physiology. New York:McGraw, 1970, pp. 545-546.
2. Cerretelli, P., di Prampero, P.E. and Piiper, J.: Energy balance of anaerobic work in the dog gastrocnemius muscle. Am. J. Physiol. 217:581-585, 1969.
3. Cerretelli, P., Piiper, J., Mangili, F. and Ricci, B.: Aerobic and anaerobic metabolism in exercising dogs. J. Appl. Physiol. 19:29-32, 1964.
4. di Prampero, P.E., Pendergast, D.R., Wilson, D.R. and Rennie, D.W.: Energetics of swimming in man. J. Appl. Physiol. 37:1-5, 1974.
5. di Prampero, P.E., Peeters, L. and Margaria, R.: Alactic O_2 debt and lactic acid production after exhausting exercise in man. J. Appl. Physiol. 34:628-633, 1973.
6. Holmér, I.: Physiology of swimming man. Acta Physiol. Scand. Suppl. 407:1-53, 1974.
7. Karpovich, P.V.: Mechanical work and efficiency in swimming crawl and back stroke. Arbeitsphysiologie 10:504-514, 1939.
8. Margaria, R., Aghemo, P. and Sassi, G.: Lactic acid production in supra-maximal exercise. Pflügers Arch.326:152-161, 1971.
9. Margaria, R., Cerretelli, P., Aghemo, P. and Sassi, G.: Energy cost of running. J. Appl. Physiol. 18:367-370, 1963.
10. Margaria, R., Cerretelli, P., di Prampero, P.E. et al: Kinetics and mechanism of oxygen debt contraction in man. J. Appl. Physiol. 18:371-377, 1963.
11. Margaria, R., Cerretelli, P. and Mangili, F.: Balance and kinetics of anaerobic energy release during strenuous exercise in man. J. Appl. Physiol. 19:623-628, 1964.
12. Margaria, R. and Edwards, H.T.: The removal of lactic acid from the body during recovery from muscular exercise. Am. J. Physiol. 107:681-686, 1934.

13. Margaria, R., Edwards, H.T. and Dill, D.B.: The possible mechanism of contracting and paying the oxygen debt and the role of lactic acid in muscular contraction. Am. J. Physiol. 106:689-714, 1933.
14. Margaria, R., Mangili, F., Cuttica, E. and Cerretelli, P.: The kinetics of the oxygen consumption at the onset of muscular exercise in man. Ergonomics 8:49-54, 1965.
15. McArdle, W.D., Glaser, R.M. and Magel, J.R.: Metabolic and cardiorespiratory response during free swimming and treadmill walking. J. Appl. Physiol. 30:733-738, 1971.
16. Pendergast, D.R. and Craig, A.B. Jr.: Biomechanics of flotation in water (Abstract). Physiologist 17:305, 1974.
17. Pendergast, D.R., di Prampero, P.E., Craig, A.B. Jr., et al: A quantitative analysis of the front crawl in men and women. J. Appl. Physiol. 43:475-479, 1977.
18. Saltin, B. and Astrand, P.O.: Maximal oxygen uptake in athletes. J. Appl. Physiol. 23:353-358, 1967.

Le coût énergétique de la locomotion en milieu aqueux

Présentation et commentaires sur les forces de résistance à surmonter en nageant à différentes vitesses. Lorsqu'on nage à une vitesse donnée, les forces de frottement, la friction sur le corps et la formation de vagues créent une résistance qui influe sur la dépense énergétique et l'efficacité mécanique. Présentation de données sur la consommation d'oxygène et la production d'acide lactique dans le sang de nageurs qui atteignent la vitesse de 2 m/s en style libre, dans le but d'établir le besoin total d'énergie en composantes aérobies et anaérobies. On y montre les différences entre la résistance et l'efficacité (de même que leur interdépendance) et l'importance de leur proportion chez des sujets ayant des aptitudes techniques différentes et chez des nageurs expérimentés des deux sexes.

The Expanding Spectrum of Aquatic Sciences

John A. Faulkner

Studies related to swimming tests and equipment; body composition of swimmers; physiological response during swimming; efficiency and biomechanics of swimming; conditioning for swimming; and thermal exchange are reviewed. It is concluded that despite the development of complex and sophisticated methods the studies in the last ten years do not appear to have made an impact on improved swimming performance.

Introduction

In a review article [13], I noted that swimming had not been subjected to the same intensity of scientific investigation as other physical activities. Scientific investigations of swimming have been restricted by the inaccessibility of the aquatic environment and the difficulty of monitoring variables in the water. Despite these difficulties, during the 1930s and 1940s Peter Karpovich and his co-workers [19-21] initiated a series of studies on body resistance during towing and the caloric cost of swimming. Meanwhile, Cureton and his associates [9, 35] used somatotyping to describe the body build of swimmers and fitness tests to assess their condition. Improved instrumentation and renewed interest resulted in a number of significant publications during the 1960s. Astrand and his associates [1] published a monograph on the physiology of girl swimmers and Pugh and his co-workers [31, 32] contributed several papers on the physiology of channel swimmers. More recently, Lewillie and Clarys [22] and Clarys and Lewillie [8] have edited the papers presented at two international symposia on the biomechanics of swimming.

John A. Faulkner, Department of Physiology, University of Michigan Medical School, Ann Arbor, Mich., U.S.A.

71

Swimming Tests and Equipment

The use of tethered swimming tests [23, 35], free swimming tests [1, 23, 32], the construction of swimming flumes [18] and swimming treadmills [10] and the development of telemetry equipment [15] have resulted in extensive data on the metabolism, circulation and respiration of recreational and competitive swimmers swimming. We have recently extended these observations to patients who have had a myocardial infarction (unpublished data, 1976). It is interesting that physiological data collected during tethered swimming is in good agreement with that collected in swimming treadmills and swimming flumes (unpublished data, 1976).

Although sophisticated physiological and biomechanical analyses have been made of swimmers swimming, the ultimate criterion of maximum performance is the athletic record book. Improvements in swimming velocity have occurred at all distances for both men and women. The result is a lower intercept for the distance time relationship but no change in the slope of the relationship. The improvements have resulted from improved physical endowment of swimmers, improved stroke mechanics, more rigorous and more highly specialized conditioning, increased competition, greater motivation and reduced swimsuit drag. Unfortunately, the data necessary for a precise evaluation of the relative impact of these contributing factors are not available.

Body Composition of Swimmers

Swimmers are taller and heavier and have less body fat than control subjects (10% body weight fat compared to 14%) of the same sex and age [12]. Channel swimmers are extremely high on endomorphy, although the winners and runner-ups in channel swims are less fat than the slower swimmers [32]. Compared to sprint swimmers, middle-distance swimmers tend to be fatter [12] and have a lower specific gravity [5]. It is unfortunate that somatotyping continues to be the most popular method of assessing the body builds of swimmers [17] and that more objective and sophisticated assessments have not been made.

Physiological Responses During Swimming

Oxygen uptake has been measured during tethered swimming [23, 35], during free swimming in open water [1, 23, 32], and during free swimming in flowthrough swimming flumes or treadmills in which the rate of water velocity could be controlled [10, 18]. The energy expenditure measured during swimming [12, 27, 32] appears to be a linear function of swimming velocity. The relationships of oxygen uptake, heart rate, stroke volume, cardiac output, arterio-venous oxygen difference and ventilation to increasing velocities of swimming or increased work rates during tethered swimming are similar to those observed during running or cycling.

When swimming velocity is increased up to power outputs close to maximum, a leveling off of the oxygen uptake and cardiac output is observed. As with running and cycling, the leveling off of oxygen uptake and cardiac output occurs simultaneously. The simultaneous leveling off of cardiac output and oxygen uptake in a variety of different physical activities (often at very different maximum values for cardiac output and for oxygen uptake) further substantiates the very basic relation between these two variables. The relationship appears to result from the rapid attainment of a maximum arteriovenous oxygen difference at low power outputs and the subsequent dependence of the oxygen uptake of contracting skeletal muscle upon blood flow.

Efficiency of Swimming

Efficiency is defined as the ratio of work performed divided by energy expended, with both expressed in the same units and then converted to a percentage. The difficulty in measuring the efficiency of swimming has been the problem of estimating the drag of the swimmer [12]. Karpovich and his co-workers reported efficiencies from 0.5% to 2.2% [21] and in a later study 1.7% to 4.0% [20]. For eight channel swimmers, Pugh et al [32] found an average efficiency of 2.8%.

In an ingenious study of the energetics of swimming, DiPrampero and his associates [10] measured net oxygen uptake of swimmers swimming at different velocities as they were alternatively pulled forward through the water by the addition of weights (negative drag) or pulled backward by the addition of weights (positive drag). At a given velocity, they found a linear relationship between net oxygen uptake and drag. The extrapolation of the net oxygen uptake-drag relationship back to a zero net oxygen uptake provided an estimate of the force which if applied would enable the swimmer to achieve that velocity with no increase in the expenditure of energy above the resting level. This force is equivalent to the thrust exerted by the swimmer at that swimming velocity, and at constant velocity the force would be equal to the water resistance or body drag. The mean for ten subjects was 3.4 kg at 33 m·min^{-1} and 6.54 kg or 54 m·min^{-1}. Each is significantly larger than the value for passive drag or for drag estimated from the Karpovich formula [19]. Since body drag during swimming was about twice the value for passive drag, the resistive forces appear to be increased by the swimming movements. The average efficiencies calculated from these data were 2.61% at 33 m·min^{-1} and 5.24% at 54 m·min^{-1}. The range was from 1.0% to 7.5%. The higher efficiencies are due to the increased estimates of the resistive forces.

Man's efficiency running is 25% to 30% [33] and the variability even between trained and untrained runners is only about 5% to 7% [25]. Efficiency varies widely during swimming, with as much as an eightfold difference between trained and untrained swimmers. Even among competitive swimmers major differences are observed and efficient stroke mechanics, as well as a high maximum oxygen uptake, is a major factor in competitive swimming performance.

Conditioning for Swimming

During training for swimming compared to training for running or cycling there are unique differences of an aquatic vs. terrestrial environment, a horizontal vs. erect posture, and predominantly arm and shoulder vs. leg muscle contractions for propulsion. These differences require that the evaluation of the maximum oxygen uptake and physical work capacity of swimmers be measured during swimming rather than during traditional laboratory tests [13].

The maximum oxygen uptakes of recreational swimmers swimming are 16% to 26% less than during walking, running or cycling (Table I). For competitive swimmers, some investigators have reported lower maximum oxygen uptakes swimming than in other activities, whereas we have seen no difference in the maximum oxygen uptakes of highly conditioned competitive college swimmers (Table I). The 26% decrement in maximum oxygen uptake of the recreational swimmer swimming compared to running was due to a 25% lower cardiac output swimming [11]. The arteriovenous oxygen differences were maximal in each exercise (160 and 156 ml/l, respectively).

In their classic study of the enzyme activity and fiber composition of the skeletal muscles of untrained and trained men, Gollnick et al [16] included five swimmers. Skeletal muscle fibers may be classified as slow twitch oxidative, fast twitch oxidative and fast twitch glycolytic [30]. During low tension-high repetition activities, the slow-twitch oxidative fibers are very resistant to fatigue, the fast

Table I. Maximum Oxygen Uptakes Measured During Swimming
and During Walking, Running, or Cycling

| Group | Maximum Oxygen Uptake (l/min) | | | Reference |
	Other Activity	Swimming	% Difference	
Recreational	4.36	3.79	13	Astrand and Saltin, 1961
Competitive female	2.74	2.59	5	Astrand et al [1]
Competitive male	3.83	3.36	12	McArdle et al [27]
Recreational	4.54	3.79	16	Holmer et al, 1974
Competitive	5.38	5.05	6	Holmer et al, 1974
Competitive	4.20	4.14	1	Magel et al [23]
Competitive	4.26	4.05	5	Dixon and Faulkner [11]
Recreational	3.58	2.66	26	Dixon and Faulkner [11]
Recreational	2.40	2.34	2	unpublished data, 1976
Post-MI Patients	1.72	1.36	20	unpublished data, 1976

twitch oxidative are moderately resistant to fatigue, and the fast twitch glycolytic fatigue very quickly [6]. Endurance runners with a mean maximum oxygen uptake of 72 $ml \cdot kg^{-1} \cdot min^{-1}$ have 59% slow-twitch oxidative fibers in the vastus lateralis muscle of the leg, and competitive swimmers have 74% slow-twitch oxidative fibers in the deltoid muscle of the arm. Normal percentages for untrained men are 36% and 46% for the legs and arms, respectively. The controversy as to whether the percentage of slow-twitch and fast-twitch fibers is genetically determined or adaptable to exercise regimens has not been resolved.

Unlike the twitch characteristics the oxidative capacity of skeletal muscle fibers is readily adaptable to training [3, 14, 26] or detraining [14]. Swimmers have an oxidative capacity for the arm muscles 2½ times higher than untrained men although their maximum oxygen uptake is slightly less than 2 times higher [16].

It is clear from these data that there is a high degree of specificity to the training for swimming. Recent studies on twins trained for running or for swimming [18] and on the training of a group of swimmers who had maximum oxygen uptakes during swimming 15% less than during running [24] support the concept of the specificity of training for swimming. The swimmers increased their maximum oxygen uptake during swimming by 11%, but showed no change in their maximum oxygen uptake running.

Swimmers have been included with other sportsmen in group comparisons of maximum oxygen uptake [2]. When swimmers are included as a group and maximum oxygen uptakes are normalized per kilogram of body mass, the swimmers appear to be poorly trained with a maximum oxygen uptake of 54 $ml \cdot kg^{-1} \cdot min^{-1}$ compared to the distance runners' maximum oxygen uptake of 80 $ml \cdot kg^{-1} \cdot min^{-1}$ (Fig. 1). However, on most swimming teams the majority of the swimmers are sprinters who swim events up to 100 meters or middle-distance swimmers who swim 200 to 400 meter races. On a given team, very few swimmers compete at the 1500 meter distance.

From our data on over 25 highly trained college swimmers we divided the swimmers into sprint, middle distance and distance categories. The absolute maximum oxygen uptakes in $liters \cdot min^{-1}$ of sprinters and distance swimmers are presented in Figure 1. The middle distance swimmers were not significantly different from the sprinters. The exception was 400 meter swimmers who also swam the 1500 meters. These swimmers were classified as distance swimmers. We did not normalize per kilogram of body mass because swimmers do not have to carry their body mass as runners do, and consequently the selection for swimmers is on the basis of absolute maximum oxygen uptake. On this basis, world class swimmers compare favorably with world class distance runners. Furthermore, sprint swimmers appear much better trained than sprint runners likely due to their conditioning by interval training.

Thermal Exchange

In air, man maintains thermal balance throughout a moderate range of environmental temperatures through minimal physiological adjustments [4]. Immersed in water, a water temperature of 33 C is necessary to maintain normal core temperature without an increase in heat production, body insulation or both [34]. The lowest temperature at which thermal balance can be maintained without an increase in heat production is 22 C for fat men and 32 C for thin men [7].

Molnar [28] has studied the interaction between seawater temperature and the duration of immersion on the number of

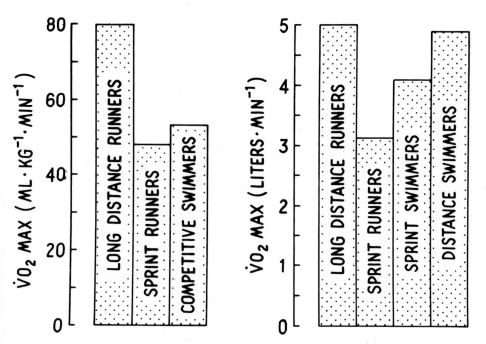

FIG. 1. The maximum oxygen uptakes of trained runners and trained swimmers expressed in ml·kg^{-1}·min^{-1} (A) and in liters·min^{-1} (B).

survivals following shipwrecks. The number of survivors decreased rapidly below a seawater temperature of 15 to 20 C. Channel swimmers swim from 12 to 22 hours in 15 to 16 C water, a seawater temperature at which shipwrecked persons survive only four to five hours. During 20 minutes of swimming, internal body temperature changes are related to water temperature, swimming intensity and body composition [29]. Between water temperatures of 18 and 33 C, the $\dot{V}O_2$ was inversely related to water temperature. The increased energy cost of swimming in cold water was due to shivering.

Biomechanics of Swimming

Equipment has been developed for a variety of cinematographical and biomechanical analyses of swimmers swimming [8, 22]. These have made possible sophisticated analyses of different techniques for the start of swimming races, the forces developed during the stroke cycles by highly trained and nontrained swimmers, patterns of hand movement during the arm stroke, analysis of propulsion by the arms and by the legs and the interaction of velocity and body drag.

Summary

The spectrum of aquatic sciences during the past ten years has expanded phenomenally into sophisticated physiological and biochemical studies of swimmers at rest and during swimming. Development of complex instrumentation has also facilitated biomechanical assessments of swimmers. Unfortunately, these advances do not appear to have made a serious impact on the teaching or coaching of swimming. The significant improvements in swimming records appear to have resulted more from improved recruitment of skilled performers into swimming and improvements in the art of coaching rather than a significant contribution of scientific knowledge.

References

1. Astrand, P.O., Eriksson, B.O., Nylander, I. et al: Acta Paediat. Suppl. 147, 75, 1963.
2. Astrand, P.O. and Rodahl, K.: Textbook of Work Physiology. New York:McGraw-Hill Book Co., 1970.
3. Barnard, R.J., Edgerton, V.R. and Peter, J.B.: J. Appl. Physiol. 28:762, 1970.
4. Belding, H.S.: In Newburgh, L.H. (ed.): Physiology of Heat Regulation and the Science of Clothing. Philadelphia:Saunders, 1949, p. 351.
5. Bloomfield, J. and Sigerseth, P.: J. Sports Med. Phys. Fitness 5:76, 1965.
6. Burke, R.E., Levine, D.N., Zajac, F.E. III et al: Science 174:709, 1971.
7. Cannon, P.: J. R. Naval Med. Serv. 49:88, 1963.
8. Clarys, J.P. and Lewillie, L. (eds.): Swimming II. Baltimore:University Park Press, 1975.
9. Cureton, R.K., Jr.: Physical Fitness of Champion Athletes. Urbana, Ill.:University of Illinois Press, 1951.
10. DiPrampero, P.E., Pendergast, D.R., Wilson, D.W. and Rennie, D.W.: J. Appl. Physiol. 37:1, 1974.
11. Dixon, R.W., Jr. and Faulkner, J.A.: J. Appl. Physiol. 30:653, 1971.
12. Faulkner, J.A.: In Falls, H.G. (ed.): Exercise Physiology. Springfield, Mo., 1968, p. 415.
13. Faulkner, J.A.: Res. Q. 37:41, 1966.
14. Faulkner, J.A., Maxwell, L.C. and Lieberman, D.A.: Am. J. Physiol. 222:836, 1972.
15. Glasser, R.M., Magel, J.R. and McArdle, W.D.: Res. Q. 41:200, 1970.
16. Gollnick, P.D., Armstrong, R.B., Saubert, C.W. IV et al: J. Appl. Physiol. 33:312, 1972.
17. Hebbelink, M., Carter, L. and DeGaray, A.: In Clarys, J.P. and Lewillie, L. (eds.): Swimming II. Baltimore:University Park Press, 1975, p. 285.
18. Holmer, I. and Astrand, P.O.: J. Appl. Physiol. 33:510, 1972.
19. Karpovich, P.V.: Res. Q. 4:21, 1933.
20. Karpovich, P.V. and Millman, N.: Am. J. Physiol. 142:140, 1944.
21. Karpovich, P.V. and Pestrecov, K.: Int. Z. Angew. Physiol. 10:504, 1939.
22. Lewillie, L. and Clarys, J.P. (eds.): Swimming I. Baltimore:University Park Press, 1971.

23. Magel, J.R. and Faulkner, J.A.: J. Appl. Physiol. 22:929, 1967.
24. Magel, J.R., Foglis, G.F., McArdle, W.D. et al: J. Appl. Physiol. 38:151, 1974.
25. Margaria, R., Cerretelli, P., Aghemo, P. and Sassi, G.: J. Appl. Physiol. 13:367, 1963.
26. Maxwell, L.C., Faulkner, J.A. and Lieberman, D.A.: Am. J. Physiol. 224:356, 1973.
27. McArdle, W.D., Glaser, R.M. and Magel, J.R.: J. Appl. Physiol. 30:733, 1971.
28. Molnar, G.W.: JAMA 131:1046, 1946.
29. Nadel, E.R., Holmer, I., Bergh, U. et al: J. Appl. Physiol. 36:465, 1974.
30. Peter, J.B., Barnard, R.J., Edgerton, V.R. et al: Biochem. 2:2627, 1972.
31. Pugh, L.G.C. and Edholm, O.G.: Lancet 2:761, 1955.
32. Pugh, L.G.C., Edholm, O.G., Fox, R.H. et al: Clin. Sci. 19:257, 1960.
33. Robinson, S.: In Bard, P. (ed.): Medical Physiology. St. Louis, Mo.:Mosby, 1961, p. 494.
34. Spealman, C.R.: In Newburgh, L.H. (ed.): Physiology of Heat Regulation and the Science of Clothing. Philadelphia:Saunders, 1949, p. 323.
35. Van Huss, W. and Cureton, T.K.: Res. Q. 26:205, 1955.

L'éventail des connaissances et des moyens scientifiques dans le secteur des activités aquatiques

L'auteur fait une revue analytique des études qui au cours des dernières décades ont porté sur les différentes spécialités de la nage sportive. Les travaux ont porté, entre autres, sur les caractéristiques physiques des nageurs, les adaptations physiologiques, les aspects biomécaniques, l'entraînement sous toutes ses formes et les ajustements thermiques. Il se dit d'avis que malgré une amélioration constante de l'équipement et des conditions de recherche, cette dernière ne semble pas avoir eu l'impact attendu sur l'amélioration des performances.

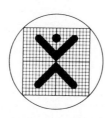

Acute and Chronic Effects of Exercise and Training

Effets aigus et chroniques de l'exercice et de l'entraînement physiques

Changes of Brain Wave During Physical Training

G. Ogihara and T. Negi

Jasper and Penfield [5] made it clear that a pure 25 c/sec beta rhythm which occurs in the rolandic region is blocked by voluntary movement similar to the blocking of occipital alpha rhythm with visual stimulation and attention. This blocking occurs only at the beginning and cessation of the act. Sustained blocking occurs only with continuous consecutive movements requiring sustained attention.

Gastaut [2, 3] and other researchers such as Magnus [9], Klass and Bickford [6] presented the concept "rythmes en arceau," "wicket rhythms," which are bursts of an average frequency of 9 c/sec waves in the rolandic region. Chatrian and his co-workers [1] made a precise research into this rhythm. This rolandic alphoid rhythm is blocked by passive, reflex and voluntary movement, and such mental activity as attention, but this effect is the longest and strongest in the case of voluntary movement and is produced in the contralateral hemisphere before muscular contraction.

For these phenomena, researchers considered that these blockings are caused by the preparation of the cerebral cortex for muscular contraction.

Since 1964, we have been studying the effect of hypnotic suggestion in physical education [10]. In the early stage, we studied physical changes, such as those in the cardiovascular system and oxygen intake of subjects and the effect of muscular strength, using an arm ergometer and a bicycle ergometer, in the hypnotic state caused by hypnotic suggestion. These studies gradually developed to electroencephalophysiology. The following experiments were made.

We investigated the relation between the intensity of stimulus and the amplitude of evoked potential and how the amplitude is affected by the verbal suggestion of stimulus intensity when the subject is in the hypnotic state. Results obtained were as follows:

G. Ogihara, Department of Physical Education, and T. Negi, College of General Education, Osaka University, Toyonaka, Osaka, Japan.

1. There is an approximately parallel relation among the intensity level (db) of auditory stimulus, the light area of optical stimulus and the amplitude of evoked potential.

2. When the subject is in the hypnotic state, the amplitude of vertex potential is greater if he is told that the stimulus is loud, and the amplitude is less if he is told that the stimulus is small.

3. When the subject is hypnotized, the amplitude of evoked potential in the occipital area increases and decreases according to the verbal suggestion that the light looks larger and smaller, respectively.

Our studies developed into research of brain waves of subjects in the hypnotic state.

Subjects, with eyes closed, were given bicycle ergometer load in the hypnotic state. The brain waves of the subjects were clearer when it was suggested that they can pedal easily than when it was suggested that their pedaling is difficult.

From these experimental results, we observed how brain waves change, especially in frequency, during the period of physical exercise training as subjects become more skilled.

In the first experiment, a 14-year-old schoolgirl was used as a subject. She had been unable to ride a bicycle and her brain wave showed no alpha blocking when her eyes were open. Using a radio-telemeter, her electroencephalograms were recorded every day for about ten days while she was learning to ride a bicycle.

We used four channel radio-telemeters made by Sanei-Sokki Co. in Japan. For the disposition of electrodes, we took the ten-twenty system, and small cup electrodes were connected with bentnite paste on the scalp, covered with cotton tampon and fixed with surgical tape for protection against shaking.

We always took bipolar recordings and recorded the brain waves in the frontal, central and occipital areas of subjects who were taking exercise. In most cases, we used the following bipolar recordings: $FP_2 - F_4$, $F_3 - C_3$, $P_3 - O_1$ and $P_4 - O_2$, or $F_Z - F_4$, $C_Z - C_4$, $P_4 - O_2$ and ECG. These recordings are considered to be the most effective to avoid the mixing of electromyograms of the scalp. Recording paper speed was 1.5 cm/sec, and sensibility was controlled to 50 μv/5 mm and time constant (low out) was 0.3.

Figure 1 shows the brain waves when subject is at rest with eyes closed and Figure 2 shows the brain waves when she is at rest with eyes open. Her brain waves show no alpha blocking when she keeps her eyes open.

As shown in the brain waves of the first day (Fig. 3) and the second day, she could not ride a bicycle at first. Her brain waves in

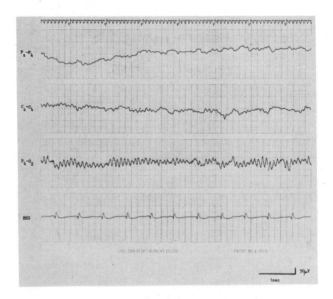

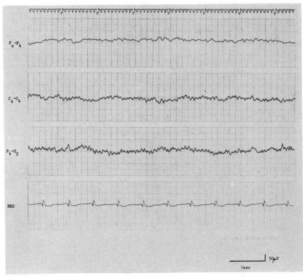

FIGURE 2.

the occipital region were complicated, because her riding was done
with voluntary effort and with the help of others. Brain waves on the
third day are seen in Figure 4.

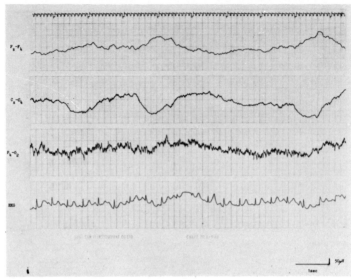

FIGURE 3.

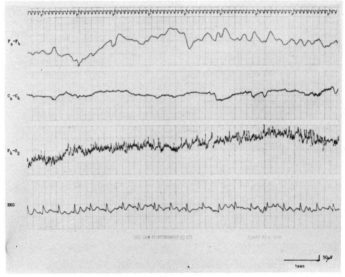

FIGURE 4.

On the fifth day, she could ride almost without help, but her electroencephalogram came to contain an electromyogram owing to her voluntary muscular movement of bicycle riding just like an electrocardiogram (Fig. 5).

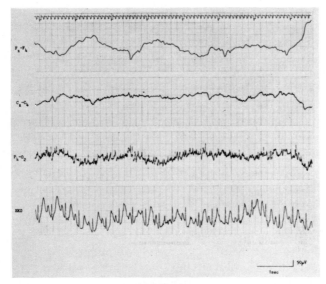

FIGURE 5.

Brain waves became simpler as she got used to riding, until alpha waves began to appear with an increase in her skill and smoothness of riding. Brain waves recorded on the tenth and last day of training (Fig. 6) show again alpha waves clearly similar to that at rest.

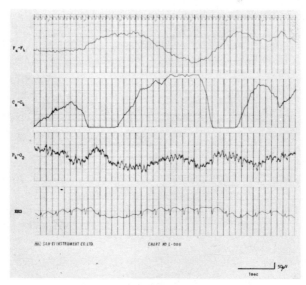

FIGURE 6.

Our second experiment, with a number of novice skiers as our subjects, was undertaken. We made electroencephalographical observations of them practicing on natural snow. For our subjects, we selected three medical students of Osaka University. They have brain waves of typical type, that is, alpha waves appear when their eyes are closed and alpha blocking occurs when their eyes are open. Figure 7 shows skier with an eye bandage. They were all cooperative for our difficult experiment. Brain waves were taken by using a radio-telemeter. The receiver was set in a house and the antenna in the middle of an approximate 70-meter slow descent course.

We recorded their brain waves during the descent skiing as they learned skiing every day. But it was difficult in the beginning to observe brain waves in the occipital area. Because of their closed eyes, they seemed to have some fear so that their brain waves were too complicated to analyze and were mixed with electromyographical fluctuations due to neck tenseness. This phenomenon is shown in Figure 8. On the third day, the electromyographical effect almost disappeared (Fig. 9). As the subjects became more skilled, their brain waves became more normal and simpler, until even alpha waves sometimes appeared during the smooth descent skiing. Indeed, brain waves recorded on the fourth day still showed the aspect of fast wave (Fig. 10), but alpha wave occasionally is found clearly in the brain wave recorded on the last day (Fig. 11).

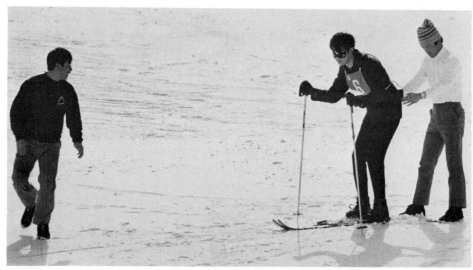

FIGURE 7.

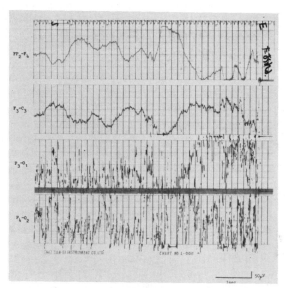

FIGURE 8.

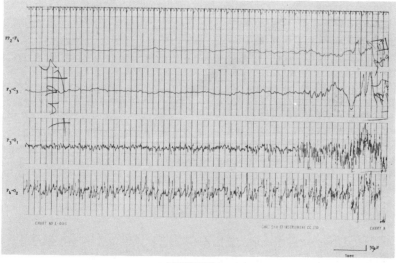

FIGURE 9.

As for the radio-telemetric recording of brain waves of subjects taking exercise, Hughes et al [4] made an observation in terms of football players playing games, and Walter et al [12] took a measurement of Contingent Negative Variation when subjects were

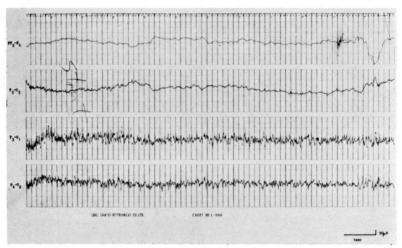

FIGURE 10.

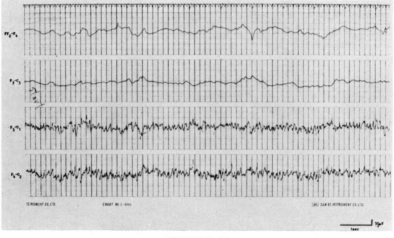

FIGURE 11.

walking. However, no research has been published as yet in regard to subjects who are beginning exercise and becoming skilled.

It is not quite clear yet how related our research is to Jasper and Penfield's beta wave in the rolandic region and Gastaut et al's "rythme en arceau" blocking owing to voluntary movement. However, the rolandic area is closely related to voluntary movement, and they say that it has something to do with the brain's preparation for body movement. There have been many such kinds of research to the present time.

No positive conclusion may be drawn on this problem in our case, because we have not yet precisely studied the time relation between alpha blocking and muscular contraction. It can be said that alpha wave, which most often occurs in the occipital area, shows the mental activity. This is verified by the fact that brain waves begin to contain slow wave when sleep becomes deeper. But in our experiment, it might be possible to suppose that alpha wave is blocked, which necessarily always exists owing to the subjects' mental activity, that is, concentrating attention, when they, novices, begin to learn new exercise.

Furthermore, according to Hirai, alpha wave appears in the case of "Zen" meditation. Ulett et al [11] could successfully indicate the depth of hypnosis by the rate of alpha wave occurrence. There is also an opinion that the alpha wave due to the closed eyes is caused by the phenomenon that the physical balance, which has been controlled by the sense of sight, turns into a proprioceptive reflex system.

When we learn new exercise, we need higher mental activity using the cerebral cortex in the beginning, but as we grow more skilled and more used to the exercise, our mental activity becomes a lower and reflexive one that does not require much cerebral cortex participation. Our experiment may be most useful if it is applied to the feedback training for those who begin to learn new exercise.

In our laboratory, successful results are being gained with the introduction of a frequency analyzer.

References

1. Chatrian, G.E., Petersen, M.C. and Lazarte, J.A.: The blocking of the rolandic rhythm and some central changes related to movement. Electroencephalogr. Clin. Neurophysiol. 11:497-510, 1959.
2. Gastaut, H.: Etude électrocorticographique de la réactivité des rythmes rolandiques. Rev. Neurol. 87(2):176-182, 1952.
3. Gastaut, H., Doniger, M. and Courtois, G.: On the significance of "wicket rhythms," "rythmes en arceau" in psychosomatic medicine. Electroencephalogr. Clin. Neurophysiol. 6:687, 1954.
4. Hughes, J.R. and Hendrix, D.E.: Telemetered EEG from a football player in action. Electroencephalogr. Clin. Neurophysiol. 24:183-186, 1968.
5. Jasper, H. and Penfield, W.: Zur Deutung des normalen Elektroencephlograms und seiner Veränderungen. Electrocorticograms in man; Effect of voluntary movement upon the electrical activity of the precentral gyrus. Arch. Psychiatr. Z. Neurol. 183:163-174, 1949.
6. Klass, D.W. and Bickford, R.G.: Observation on the rolandic arceau rhythm. Electroencephalogr. Clin. Neurophysiol. 9:570, 1957.
7. Lelord, G.: Different modalities of reaction of the central and anterior rhythms at 10 c/sec. Electroencephalogr. Clin. Neurophysiol. 9:561, 1957.

8. Maddocks, J.A., Sessions, R. and Rex, J.: Observation on the occurrence of precentral activity at alphafrequency. Electroencephalogr. Clin. Neurophysiol. 3:370, 1951.
9. Magnus, O.: The central alpha-rhythm ("rythme en arceau"). Electroencephalogr. Clin. Neurophysiol. 6:349-350, 1954.
10. Negi, T. and Ogihara, G.: Application of hypnotic suggestion to physical education. IV. (A study on the guidance of physical education using brain wave and hypnotic suggestion.) (In Japanese.) Jpn. J. Phys. Fit. Sports Med. 22(3):94-100, 1973.
11. Ulett, G.A., Akpinar, S.A. and Itil, T.M.: Quantitative EEG analysis during hypnosis. Electroencephalogr. Clin. Neurophysiol. 23:361-368, 1972.
12. Walter, W.G., Cooper, R., Grow, H.J. et al: Contingent negative variation and evoked responses recorded by radio-telemetry in free-ranging subjects. Electroencephalogr. Clin. Neurophysiol. 23:197-206, 1967.

Structure interne de certains paramètres de l'appareil neuromusculaire en liaison avec la capacité de travail ergométrique et sportive spéciale chez les sportifs de classe supérieure

R. Kossev

Le médecin pratiquant le diagnostic fonctionnel de l'appareil neuromusculaire rencontre de sérieuses difficultés lorsqu'il essaie d'établir la corrélation entre la capacité de travail physique et la capacité fonctionnelle de l'appareil neuromusculaire. Ceci se rapporte particulièrement aux charges physiques d'une puissance variable de l'effort, comme c'est le plus souvent le cas dans les conditions d'entraînement naturelles et lors de tests ergométriques diagnostiques largement pratiqués. Les résultats pratiques sont variés et divergents, et dans le meilleur des cas, coincident seulement au point de vue statistique avec la présomption théorique de la nécessité d'un lien très étroit entre l'appareil neuromusculaire et la capacité de travail physique.

Il est logique de chercher la contradiction entre la réalité et le modèle théorique dans la connaissance insuffisante que l'on a de l'information fournie par les méthodes diagnostiques. Autrement, il nous resterait à éliminer l'appareil neuromusculaire comme un facteur de la capacité de travail physique et à admettre que les limites sont dues à d'autres systèmes fonctionnels. Une telle position est au point de vue physiologique absurde. L'appareil neuromusculaire est le réalisateur de l'activité motrice et un terrain fondamental des processus métaboliques, tandis que les autres systèmes fonctionnels, et principalement le système cardiorespiratoire, ont des fonctions de régulation, d'approvisionnement et de transport, soumises au rythme et aux particularités du métabolisme de la musculature effectuant les

R. Kossev, Institut supérieur de culture physique, Sofia, Bulgarie.

efforts. Afin d'étudier l'informativité de certains paramètres de l'état fonctionnel de l'appareil neuromusculaire largement connus, nous avons soumis à une analyse corrélative une partie des 10,000 examens effectués pendant les dernières années dans les Départements d'étude de l'appareil neuromusculaire et de spiroergométrie du Laboratoire de recherches fonctionnelles sur des sportifs, à Sofia, Bulgarie. Nous avons mis en corrélation 4 paramètres de l'appareil neuromusculaire (rhéobase, chronaxie, rythme optimum et maximum de la labilité neuro-musculaire) avec 46 paramètres spiro-ergométriques, caractérisant la capacité de travail ergométrique, l'échange de gaz et la tension du système cardiovasculaire, certains indices biochimiques de l'état acido-basique, le poids corporel et d'autres valeurs directement mesurables ou dérivées. Les paramètres de l'appareil neuromusculaire ont été étudiés avant et après un chargement ergométrique à degrés, jusqu'à renoncement. La rhéobase et la chronaxie ont été mesurées selon les principes de l'électro-diagnostic classique, et la labilité selon la méthode d'électro-stimulation de Titov (1964), qui caractérise la reproductivité de fréquence optimum et maximum lors de stimulation à impulsions rectangulaires à courant continu. Le chargement ergométrique a été réalisé selon un programme, élaboré par le directeur du département, Dr. Iliev, qui prévoit une durée des degrés de 90 sec et une augmentation de l'intensité du travail par degré de 30 Watts, le degré de départ étant 60 Watts.

La corrélation directe, le procédé de corrélation partielle et multiple ont démontré, que la rhéobase, la chronaxie, le rythme optimum et maximum apportent une information générale sur l'état de l'appareil neuro-musculaire, mais reflètent aussi les mécanismes indépendants de l'aptitude fonctionnelle neuromusculaire. En résultat du chargement peuvent se produire des changements dans les valeurs de certains ou de tous les paramètres. Ces changements ont aussi un caractère général, mais concernent avant tout les mécanismes indépendants représentés par les différents paramètres. Ceci explique le variété soulignée des grandeurs mesurées après le chargement, menant dans certains cas à une contradiction évidente.

Les paramètres de l'aptitude fonctionnelle neuromusculaire démontrent une dépendance corrélative avec toutes les données de l'examen spiroergométrique. La corrélation partielle et multiple a montré cependant que la dépendance corrélative directe ne correspond pas dans tous les cas au lien fonctionnel. Après une introduction graduelle de différents paramètres constants, la corrélation directe primaire indique une tendance à modifier sa valeur et même son caractère. Ce fait nous a porté à admettre que "la présence corrélative" de l'appareil neuromusculaire, dans le plus grand nombre de cas, est due à un transfert d'information entre des paramètres à haute corrélation se trouvant hors du champ d'action de l'appareil neuromusculaire, et à considérer de ce fait la corrélation directe comme provoquée et non-informative. Nous avons établi de pareilles hautes corrélations directes provoquées également entre les paramètres de l'examen spiroergométrique; en physiologie sportive ces corrélations sont considerées comme soulignant des liens fonctionnels.

Les premières conclusions de cette analyse ont confirmé grossièrement l'importance autonome de l'appareil neuromusculaire comme facteur de la capacité de travail physique, mais elles n'ont pas localisé cette importance. Pour cette raison nous avons entrepris des recherches orientées vers une corrélation des paramètres neuromusculaires avec des indices de la tension individuelle de l'organisme lors du chargement. Comme paramètres les plus appropriés nous avons choisi les paramètres mathématiques, caractérisant les courbes individuelles "consommation d'oxygène — intensité de l'effort" et les phases relatives de capacité de travail qui en découlent. Nous avons utilisé le modèle de Dr. Iliev, qui a proposé de diviser la capacité de travail en trois phases — stable, compensée et non-compensée, en rapport avec le régime individuel de consommation d'oxygène au cours du programme de chargement par degrés. La phase stable correspond à la partie linéaire du début de la courbe individuelle "consommation d'oxygène — intensité de l'effort," la phase compensée à la partie suivante qui croît exponentiellement, et la phase non-compensée à la dernière section dans laquelle la consommation d'oxygène ne suit pas le cours théorique de sa partie exponentielle.

Nous avons établi que le rythme optimum est en haute corrélation avec la durée de la capacité de travail stable et en corrélation modérée avec la durée de la capacité de travail compensée, c'est-à-dire avec la capacité des processus métaboliques aérobies du tissu musculaire. Le rythme maximum est en haute corrélation avec les limites de la capacité de travail compensée et la durée de la capacité de travail non-compensée, et il reflète la capacité des composantes anaérobies. Nous avons en effet trouvé une corrélation partielle et multiple du rythme optimum avec les paramètres de l'examen spiroergométrique représentant la capacité des mécanismes métaboliques aérobies — capacité aérobie, consommation d'oxygène et fréquence cardiaque au début du chargement. Inversement, le rythme maximum s'est avéré en dépendance des paramètres en rapport avec la puissance anaérobie et la dynamique de la participation active des processus anaérobies dans l'accroissement de la consommation d'oxygène au cours des derniers degrés de chargement, avec l'intensité des processus de récupération et les paramètres biochimiques de l'équilibre acido-basique.

Les changements des valeurs des paramètres neuromusculaires, provoqués par le travail réalisé étaient en rapport avec la durée et la proportion entre les phases de la capacité de travail.

Nos résultats et nos conclusions présentés de manière schématique indiquent que les paramètres de l'appareil neuromusculaire sont en état de refléter réellement les aspects de son aptitude fonctionnelle qui concernent directement l'envergure de la capacité de travail physique. La dépendance entre eux est tellement importante qu'on pourrait pronostiquer avec une sûreté considérable la durée individuelle et les limites des phases de capacité de travail, le caractère et les paramètres de la courbe individuelle "consommation d'oxygène — intensité du chargement," les moments de participation active des processus métaboliques anaérobies et les possibilités de maintenir leur intensité.

Nous considérons que cette recherche confirme la place du diagnostic fonctionnel neuromusculaire dans un programme général des recherches fonctionnelles dans le sport. Considérées comme une expression de mécanismes physiologiques et métaboliques différents, la variété et la divergence des valeurs obtenues concernant les paramètres neuromusculaires et les données obtenues après les tests ou les charges d'entraînement naturelles perdent leur caractère contradictoire et reçoivent une explication logique. Les paramètres neuromusculaires ont ce caractère contradictoire et chaotique seulement en apparence, puisque leur vrai contenu est difficilement accessible à l'appréciation directe, à cause des relations d'information complexes avec d'autres paramètres déjà établis et ouvertement manifestes.

Effects of Work Bouts of Various Durations on Reaction Time

Ken Watanabe

The purpose of this study is to investigate what effects muscular activity has on the central nervous system when the work is done on the bicycle ergometer for various durations.

Figure 1 shows the experimental conditions. As a principal measurement of the central nervous function, we employed both single and choice reaction times. For stimuli of the single reaction we used a yellow lamp, while for the choice reaction we used a red or blue lamp. We made use of the Monark's bicycle ergometer as a physical work loading apparatus. Subjects carried out the whole experiment in a supine position.

The subjects were five healthy adult men aged 20 to 22, including a football player and a short-distance runner.

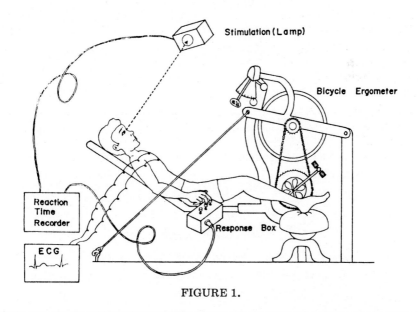

FIGURE 1.

Ken Watanabe, The Faculty of Liberal Arts, Yamaguchi University, Japan.

In addition to reaction time, we measured such psychophysio-
logical indices as flicker frequencies, heart rates, respiration rates,
blood pressure, finger blood flow by means of the occlusion method,
amplitude of pulse waves of the finger photocell plethysmograph,
change of the finger volume and the electroencephalogram.

Figure 2 shows the procedure for this experiment. The reaction
time measurement was repeated for five sessions before the physical
exercise, and it was measured for six sessions from 5 to 30 minutes
after completion of the exercise. Each session consisted of 12 trials
of single and choice reaction times, respectively, from which the
middle ten were taken into account omitting each one of the longest
and the shortest trials.

In this study, the work consisted of four series of different
durations: 0, 5, 12 and 54 (exhaustion) minutes. Each series of
experiments was done every three or four days in a random order.

The load for each subject was determined in such a manner that
the heart rate should reach 170 at 12 minutes from the start. As a
result, the average load adopted for all subjects was 660 kpm/min
with the maximum of 750 and the minimum of 600.

Procedure

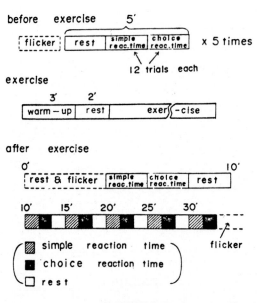

FIGURE 2.

The maximum heart rate achieved in the 5 minute exercise was 151.8; in the 12 minute exercise, 166.2; and in the all-out exercise, 189.6.

The average work intensity expressed by the levels of oxygen intake corresponded to 60% of the maximum value.

We obtained the following results: marked shortening of both simple and choice reaction times was seen after the 12 minute exercise and the all-out exercise. The shortening effect was most noticeable in the 10 to 15 minutes after the completion of the exercise, and yet it continued beyond 30 minutes.

Figure 3 shows the mean percentage of all reaction times after the exercise compared with the pre-exercise values. In one subject, reaction time was delayed after the 12 minute and the all-out exercise, but in the other four subjects, both of the simple and choice reaction times were apparently shortened about 10%.

Figure 4 shows the percentage of change in flicker frequencies compared with the pre-exercise value. The fact that immediately after the 12 minute exercise flicker frequencies increased about 0.9 and after the all-out exercise it increased 2.0 coincided with the shortening of reaction time.

Figure 5 shows the change of mean blood pressure in comparison with the resting value before commencement of the exercise. We can

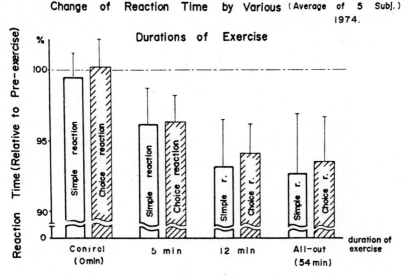

FIGURE 3.

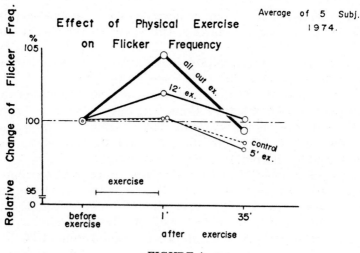

FIGURE 4.

observe essentially no effect from the reaction time trials themselves, but can observe a slight increase in mean blood pressure after the 12 minutes of exercise and obvious decrease after the all-out exercise owing to the depression of the diastolic blood pressure.

In Figure 6, change of the finger blood flow was compared with the resting value before commencement of the exercise. Here we find

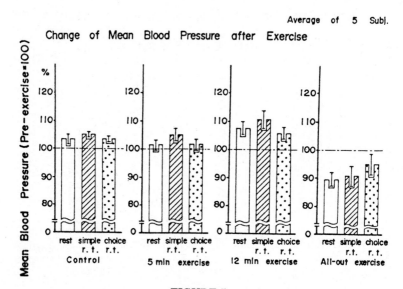

FIGURE 5.

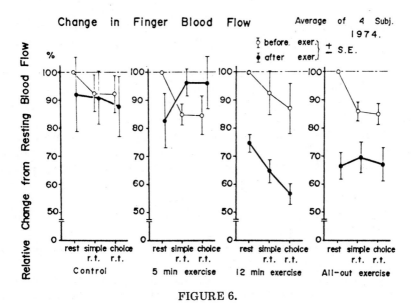

FIGURE 6.

a remarkable decrease of 5 to 8 ml/100 ml tissue/min after the 12 minute and the all-out exercise.

Figure 7 shows the decrement of the finger volume recorded in free blood flow condition by means of the water plethysmograph

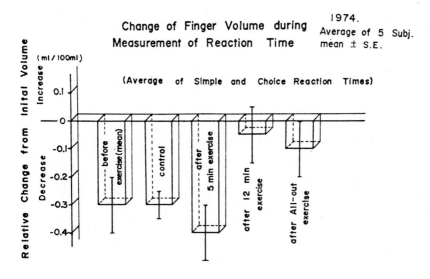

FIGURE 7.

during measurement of reaction times. Here we can observe that the degree of decrement of the finger volume became less after the 12 minute and the all-out exercise.

Figure 8 shows the change of the amplitudes of the finger photocell plethysmograph; in contrast with the blood flow, the longer the exercise continued the higher the amplitudes became after it.

Figure 9 shows the change of average alpha frequencies of EEG recorded on the P-O lead. Here we can also notice no essential change after the 0 and 5 minute exercise, but after the 12 minute and the all-out exercise we find marked increase of the alpha frequencies at rest and during measurement of reaction times.

Figure 10 shows the alpha indices of EEG, i.e., appearance ratio of alpha rhythms for a certain time.

It is especially noticeable that the alpha indices at rest after the all-out exercise clearly increased.

As mentioned above, both of the simple and choice reaction times were obviously shortened by the effect of the 12 minute and the all-out exercise on a bicycle ergometer. This effect was supported by the increase of flicker frequencies after these durations of exercise.

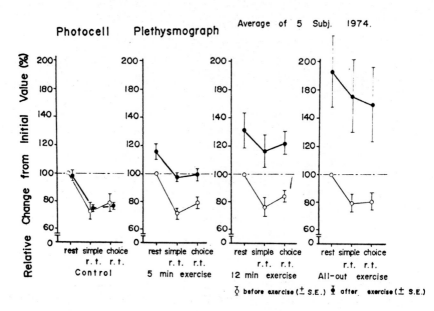

FIGURE 8.

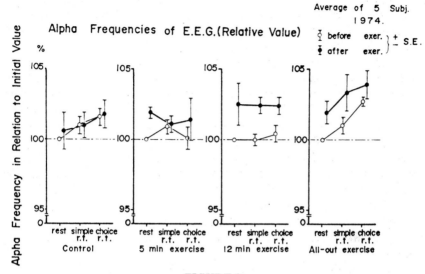

FIGURE 9.

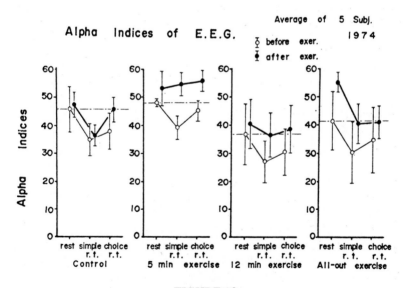

FIGURE 10.

The increase of the average alpha frequencies of EEG after these longer durations of exercise may also suggest the occurrence of the intracerebral activation.

Finally, we must consider the cause of discrepancy between the decrease of both finger blood flow and finger volume and the increase of the amplitudes of photocell plethysmograph. It can be explained that the blood vessels of the finger constricted even under the condition of large pulse pressure. It suggests that according to the activation of the central nervous system the function of the vasoconstrictor was also activated by the effect of physical exercise.

The Influence of Physical Loads on Muscle Mechanical Characteristics

F. M. Talishev and T. I. Fedina

The muscle being a movement effector possesses, like any other organism tissue, biological characteristics inherent to any living structure and mechanical properties inherent to a physical body. While biological properties of the muscle have been the subject of an extensive study, the significance of mechanical characteristics is still lacking scientific attention. During the last few years the increasing number of scientists working in the sphere of movement physiology and biomechanics have realized the important role of visco-elastic properties of the muscle in movement mechanisms [2-4, 6-8, 10, 11].

The present study attempts to find the dependence of visco-elastic indices upon the magnitude of the effort, the muscle length and physical load under actual training conditions.

Visco-elastic indices were measured with the help of the seismomyotonographic technique [5].

The influence of muscle efforts differing in value on visco-elastic indices was studied in the following ways. A subject in a prone position extended the talocrural (ankle) joint lifting a weight equal to 10%, 20%, 30%, 50%, 60% and 80% of the maximum effort with a 10- to 15-minute interval. The measurements were taken on musculus gastrocnemius. The results showed that the dependence between visco-elastic indices and the magnitude of the effort is asymptotic: $y = A - D \cdot 10^{-kx}$. However, while the elasticity index, beginning with low intensity efforts, exceeds the initial values and grows with the increase of effort magnitude, the viscosity index for low intensity efforts is 40% to 50% lower than initial values and then with the increase of loads it tends to the initial values (Fig. 1A). Starting with loads equal to 60% to 70% of maximum efforts, the rate of growth for both indices falls sharply and the increment remains small up to maximum efforts. But while the elasticity index for the maximum loads exceeds initial values by 90%, the viscosity index exceeds them by 10%.

F. M. Talishev and T. I. Fedina, All-Union Research Institute of Physical Culture, Moscow, U.S.S.R.

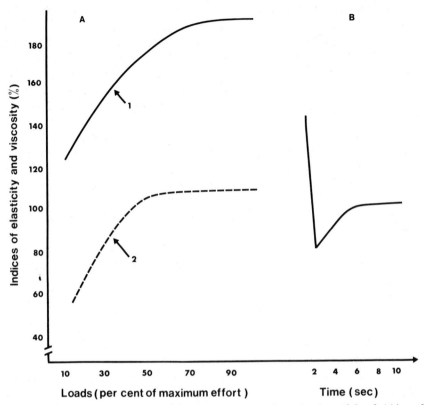

FIG. 1. Alteration of visco-elastic indices with the increase of load (A) and dynamics of the elasticity index after a maximum effort (B). 1 = index of elasticity and 2 = index of viscosity.

After a single maximum effort (Fig. 1B) the elasticity index, which immediately following the effort exceeded the initial values by 40%, sharply drops down to the value 30% to 40% lower than the initial figures. Then it slowly rises to the value 10% higher than the initial one. This dynamics of the elasticity index is very similar to the change of the muscle strain under conditions of unexpected unloading as described by Huxley and Simmons (1971).

The repeated reproduction of maximum effort with a 5-second interval gave a cumulative effect. During the effort the elasticity index increased to 260% and the viscosity index decreased to 80% as compared to initial values measured before the effort and taken for 100%.

A question arose: What changes in mechanical properties of a human muscle take place after different quantities of muscle work in sport? The measurements were taken from seven skiers before the start and after 10-km and 30-km races, as well as after work to a capacity, i.e., after the skiers had covered a maximum possible distance with a present movement speed. Mechanical indices of the muscles were measured of the gastrocnemius muscle for three positions of the ankle joint: (1) passive maximum plantar flexion; (2) intermediate or neutral position; (3) passive maximum dorsal flexion.

Measurements prior to the start showed that when the muscle length increases due to the changed angle in the ankle joint, elasticity index grows. Attenuation coefficient somewhat rises in the second position as compared to the first one and then goes down (third position), i.e., in case of muscle stretching attenuation coefficient reached its maximum when the muscle length corresponded to the neutral position of the ankle joint. These results are similar to those obtained by Truong (1974) who, when stretching a muscle of a frog, observed a maximum or a flex point at the attenuation coefficient curve.

The measurement of the same indices after the 10-km race yielded the following results: the elasticity index exceeded on the average the initial values for the three positions of the joint by 20%, 7% and 23%, respectively. After the 30-km race and the maximum distance races the elasticity indices differed little from those measured before the start, though the former had a tendency to drop lower than the initial values by approximately 3% to 5%. This stability of the elasticity index would have been a surprise had we not observed earlier that this index drops sharply after a single maximum effort of a certain duration (three seconds). We can assume that a similar phenomenon takes place after continuous effort but in different temporal intervals (our measurements were taken 10 to 15 minutes after the finish). It is also possible that the rate of this process depends upon the quantity of specific load, because after the 10-km race the elasticity index was higher than the initial values. It may be of interest to study the dynamics of these values after the finish.

The measurements of viscosity index after the finish revealed its average increase after the 10-km race by 51%, 40% and 38% for the three respective positions of the ankle joint. After the 30-km race the viscosity index for the first position does not practically differ from initial values, but for second and third positions it still exceeds the latter by 25% and 80%, respectively. After the maximum distance race the viscosity index decreases in comparison with the initial values by 36%, 9% and 164% for the three respective positions of the ankle joint. It seems likely that the direction of change in viscosity index values depends upon the duration of physical activity. It is worth noting that though nearly all the curves of viscosity index due to the muscle stretch reached their maximum at neutral position of the ankle joint, this maximum is better observed in measurements carried out after the load (Fig. 2).

It was already mentioned that the elasticity index grew with the increase of the muscle length. Its increment in stretching was individual for every subject.

When comparing the elasticity index increment in stretching to the length of maximum distance covered, the latter varying from 55 to 105 km for some athletes, we found the correlation between the values compared (r = +0.73), that is, the greater distance covered by the skier corresponded to the higher increase of the elasticity index in muscle stretching measured before the start.

As the elasticity index rises with stretching it is possible to assume that the more it grows the greater is the muscle stretchability. The hypothesis put forward by a number of authors [1, 2, 9] that, when stretched, the muscle can accumulate potential elastic energy which is then transformed into kinetic energy, utilized by contraction, allows us to assume that a muscle with greater stretchability has more functional potentialities. As far as our reasoning is correct, the

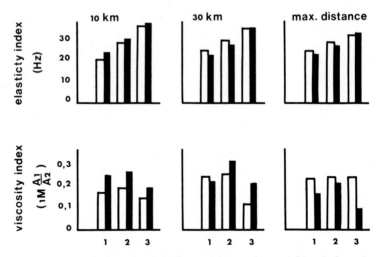

FIG. 2. Alteration of visco-elastic indices with muscle stretching before the start and after 10- and 30-km races and after a maximum possible distance. White = before the start; black = after the finish; 1 = passive maximum plantar flexion; 2 = intermediate or neutral position; and 3 = passive maximum dorsal flexion.

last statement accounts for the observed dependence between the elasticity index increment and a greatest possible distance covered by an athlete. In any case this fact is interesting and worthy of further study to allow its practical application in sports.

References

1. Asmussen, E. and Bonde-Petersen, F.: Storage of elastic energy in skeletal muscles in man. Acta Physiol. Scand. 91(3):385-392, 1974.
2. Cavagna, G.A.: Elasticity in sprint running. Abstracts of papers. XXth World Congress in Sport Medicine. Handbook, 14-17, 1974.
3. Cavagna, G.A., Dusman, B. and Margaria, R.: Positive work done by a previously stretched muscle. J. Appl. Physiol. 24:21-32, 1968.
4. Cavagna, G.A., Komarek, L., Gitterio, G. and Margaria, R.: Power output of the previously stretched muscle. In Medicine and Sport, 6. Biomechanics II, 189-167, Basel, 1971.
5. Fyodorov, V.L. and Talishev, F.M.: The apparatus for definition of visco-elastic muscle properties. Theory and Practice of Physical Culture, vol. 5, 1963.
6. Grillner, S.: The role of muscle stiffness in meeting the changing postural and locomotor requirements for force development by the ankle extensors. Acta Physiol. Scand. 86:92-108, 1972.
7. Lloyd, B.B. and Zacks, R.M.: The mechanical efficiency of treadmill running against a horizontal impeding force. J. Physiol. (Lond) 223:355-363, 1972.
8. Long, C., Thomas, D. and Crochetiere, W.J.: Objective measurement of muscle tone in the hand. Clin. Pharmacol. Ther. 5:909-917, 1964.
9. Marey, M. and Demeny, M.G.: Locomotion humaine, mécanisme du saut. G.R. Acad. Sci. (Paris) 101:489-494, 1885.
10. Wachholder, K. and Altenburger, H.: Beiträge zur Physiologie der willkür lichen Bewegung. VIII. Mitteilung. Uber die Beziehungen verschiedener synergisch arbeitender Muskelteile und Muskeln bei willkülichen Bewegungen. Pflügers Arch. Ges. Physiol. 212:666-675, 1926.
11. Wagner, R.: Uber die Zusammenarbeit der Antagonisten bei der Willkür-bewagung. II. Mitteilung: Gelenkfixierung und Versteifte Bewegung. Z. Biol. 83:120-144, 1925.

Recovery Pattern From Fatigue of Isometric Tension and $\dot{V}O_2$ for Dog Skeletal Muscle in Situ

B. A. Wilson and W. N. Stainsby

Introduction

When muscle is stimulated to contract either for prolonged time periods at low twitch rates or for short time periods at high twitch frequencies, a decrease in contraction force occurs [2, 4, 11]. This negative staircase or fatigue has been attributed to many factors. One of the major determinants of a muscle's ability to develop force is its phosphorylcreatine (PC) concentration which is highly correlated with developed tension in muscles under many experimental conditions [4, 5, 7]. It has also been demonstrated that both developed tension and oxygen consumption vary directly with changes in blood flow at a fixed isometric twitch rate [1]. This paper indicates that maximal metabolic rate during twitch contractions is normally limited by blood flow. The flow-related responses, however, were absent in fatigued muscle.

The purpose of the paper is to examine the oxygen consumption ($\dot{V}O_2$), tension, blood flow, relationships during recovery from fatigue in the dog gastrocnemius-plantaris muscle and to analyze the tension recovery pattern over time.

Methods

Mongrel dogs of either sex weighing between 9.5 and 17 kg were used in this study. They were each anesthetized with sodium pentobarbital, 30 mg/kg with additional 30- to 60-mg doses given when needed. Each animal's trachea was intubated with a cuffed

B. A. Wilson, Department of Human Kinetics, College of Biological Science, University of Guelph, Guelph, Ontario, Canada, and W. N. Stainsby, Department of Physiology, College of Medicine, University of Florida, Gainesville, Fla., U.S.A.

Paper prepared with the technical assistance of Donna T. Dolbier.
Supported by NIH Grant HL 14806-16.

endotracheal tube to insure a patent airway and a ready connection to a respirator if desired. Each animal's rectal and muscle surface temperatures were kept between 36 and 37 C by a heat lamp and a heating pad. The muscles were always covered with saline-soaked gauze and a piece of plastic film to prevent evaporative cooling and drying.

For the fatigue studies the left gastrocnemius-plantaris muscle was partially isolated. The insertion tendon and lower half of the muscle were uncovered and freed from surrounding tissue to provide free movement of that end of the muscle. The tendon was cut so as to be as long as possible and fitted into a small aluminum clamp. The clamp, in turn, was connected to a very stiff isometric lever which had a displacement of about 0.2 mm/50 kg. The lever was strutted via a turnbuckle to two bone nails in the head of the femur by the origin of the muscle to prevent movement of the lever and femur relative to each other. After each experiment the lever was calibrated with preweighted weights. The sciatic nerve was isolated in the mid thigh area, tied and cut as close to the spinal cord as possible and fitted into a tubular electrode holder made of dental acrylic containing silver electrodes. Stimulation was of 0.2 msec duration and 8 v intensity. In each experiment the voltage was decreased to 2 v temporarily. In every case there was no decrease in contraction force indicating supramaximal stimuli were being used.

Following an extensive pilot series the protocol for the fatigue series was established. First Lo was determined by changing initial length, Li, and observing the Li at which greatest developed tension (total tension-rest tension), Lo, for single twitches, was obtained, then Li was decreased below Lo just enough that we would be sure we were below Lo. Then the preparation was allowed to rest for 10 to 15 minutes. Next, the muscles were stimulated to contract at a basal frequency, $0.2 \, t \, sec^{-1}$, and contraction force followed for 3 to 4 minutes to be sure steady conditions were present. Then the muscle was stimulated at $8\text{-}14 \, t \, sec^{-1}$. These stimulations produced a partially fused tetanus contraction which was quite unstable with mean force increasing and then decreasing with time as the relative rates of contraction versus relaxation changed while fatigue developed. At intervals the stimulation frequency was returned to the basal rate to assess the degree of fatigue. Sometimes flow was reduced by partial arterial occlusion to speed up fatigue development. When the contraction force at basal rate of stimulation was 20% to 40% of the initial contraction force at that rate, it was accepted that sufficient fatigue was present and no further rapid stimulation was applied. From then on one series of muscles were left at rest with basal stimulation only at intervals to assess contraction force under basal conditions during recovery. Another series of the muscles contracted continuously at basal rate throughout recovery. While in the final control series there was no fatigue induced and the muscles either rested with intervals of basal rate stimulation or contracted at basal rate for the same period of time that recovery and fatigue were followed in the preceding three series.

For the metabolic studies the more complete muscle preparation was utilized [8]. The entire muscle except its origin on the femur was separated from surrounding tissue. All blood vessels not connected directly to the popliteal vein were tied and all branches of the popliteal vein which did not come from the muscle were tied. As a result the flow through the popliteal vein was the venous outflow from the muscle. The popliteal vein was cannulated and the flow directed via a cannulating-type electromagnetic flow meter to the jugular vein where it was returned to the animal's circulation. The venous blood could be sampled via a small tube threaded through the cannula wall to the tip of the cannula near the muscle. Arterial blood could be sampled via a cannula in the contralateral femoral artery. This cannula was also connected to a pressure transducer to monitor blood pressure. Coagulation of the blood was prevented by intravenous heparin, 25 mg/kg, two thirds given initially and the remainder after one hour.

Oxygen uptake was calculated as the product of the arteriovenous oxygen content difference and the venous blood flow at the time the A-V samples were drawn. The arterial and venous samples were 0.6 ml and were sealed after being drawn into the tuberculine syringes with mercury containing caps and iced. The mercury was for mixing just prior to analysis of oxygen content using a Lex O_2 Con. The Lex O_2 Con was compared to the traditional manometric method in well over 100 duplicate analyses over a wide range of O_2 content and agreement was excellent [10]. This calculated oxygen uptake rate was divided by the weight of the muscle, obtained after the experiment, and the stimulus frequency at the time the samples were drawn and expressed as microliter per gram contraction. Nerve isolation and stimulation parameters as well as the general protocol of the metabolic studies were like those of the mechanical studies.

Results

There was little fatigue at low frequencies of stimulation. For example, in the control series at 0.2 t sec^{-1} there was only a 2%

decrease in contraction strength after 3.5 hours of continued contraction. After 8 to 14 t sec^{-1} stimulation, contraction force at basal frequency decreased rapidly and was 30% to 40% of control by 30 minutes. Decreased blood flow during rapid contractions facilitated the development of fatigue roughly in proportion to the decrease in flow. However, this was not studied systematically. When flow was decreased to one third to one fourth of spontaneous values, contraction strength was decreased to about 25% of initial conditions in 15 to 20 minutes. There were occasionally odd contracture responses during the development of fatigue at reduced flow which were not further investigated.

Whichever way fatigue was created recovery was about the same. Recovery was slow; the shape of the contraction force with time is plotted in Figure 1. It appears roughly exponential. A muscle fatigued to 50% of initial contraction force at basal stimulation frequency recovered to about 80% of initial contraction force after 2.5 hours of recovery. Extrapolation of the recovery suggested that full recovery should have occurred in about 4.5 hours. Recovery was the same whether the muscle remained at rest with basal condition contraction force monitored at 5 to 15 minute intervals or was

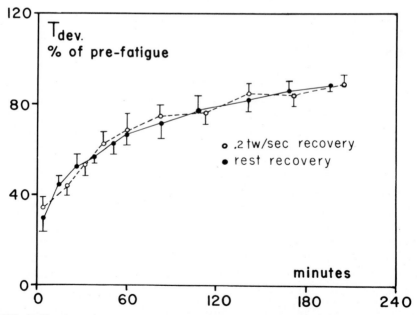

FIG. 1. Tension recovery pattern from fatigue. All points indicate mean tensions at .2 t sec^{-1} while bars indicate standard error of the mean.

allowed to contract at basal frequency continuously during recovery (Fig. 1).

In the metabolic studies initial resting oxygen uptake, blood flow, and arterial and venous blood oxygen concentrations were all within the range reported previously for this muscle preparation [3, 8]. Following the development of fatigue and 40 to 50 minutes of recovery resting oxygen uptake was slightly increased on the average. This was surely a result of recovery not being complete. Oxygen uptake was reduced in proportion to the developed isometric tension. When the oxygen uptake per contraction was expressed for each experiment as a percent of the oxygen uptake at 2 t sec^{-1} in that experiment and developed tension is expressed as a percent of the developed tension at 2 t sec^{-1}, the data from all the isometric experiments can be presented in a single figure (Fig. 2). All of the data fall along a single line. The data indicate a strong single relation between oxygen uptake and developed tension for changes in developed tension due to fatigue. The data also indicate that the relative coefficient of performance in muscles is constant with changes in contractile capacity due to fatigue.

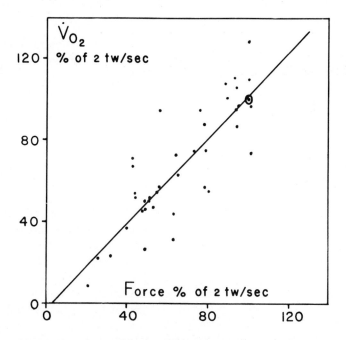

FIG. 2. Oxygen uptake, developed tension relationship for all .2 t sec^{-1} collections pre-fatigue and during recovery. (VO_2 = 1.07 × Tension–3.01).

Discussion

The data demonstrate a linear relationship between $\dot{V}O_2$ during recovery and developed isometric tension. It has been shown that phosphorylcreatine (PC) is correlated with the developed tension in muscle [4, 5] and suggested that repayment of PC is related to the aerobic capabilities of muscle [7]. The present data would support this suggestion as $\dot{V}O_2$, muscle blood flow and developed tension all increase in parallel during recovery.

The recovery pattern from fatigue for developed tension during continuous .2 t sec^{-1} contractions did not differ from the pattern of muscles recovering completely at rest. These data suggest that tension recovery, and therefore PC repayment, can occur equally well during rest or submaximal contractions. The exact twitch rate at which this relationship no longer exists requires further investigation.

The efficiency of the muscles in the present study was not affected by fatigue while in exercising man total body fatigue is accompanied by a decrease in work efficiency [6]. The present data indicate that this decrease in efficiency is not a result of individual muscle processes, but more probably due to total body substrate limits and/or lack of coordination in muscle groups as a result of total body fatigue.

The complexity of the recovery process is demonstrated by the prolonged time span, 4.5 hours for complete recovery in a single muscle. If a similar recovery pattern exists in human muscle, then this suggests that at least four hours must separate fatiguing work bouts if maximal muscular performance is expected.

Summary

Isometric force and muscle $\dot{V}O_2$ were studied during twitch (t) contractions using the in situ gastrocnemius-plantaris dog muscle preparation. Under isometric conditions basal contraction force was measured at a stimulation rate of 0.2 t sec^{-1}. A fatigued state was produced in two ways; either 30 minutes of isometric contractions at 10-14 t sec^{-1} or 10 minutes at a similar contraction frequency but with reduced blood flow. These treatments produced a 50% to 75% decrease in developed tension for the 0.2 t sec^{-1} level. The recovery from both types of fatigue was slow, requiring 2.5 hours for an 80% return in developed tension and an estimated 4.5 hours for complete recovery. The recovery pattern followed an exponential course over time. Oxygen uptake calculated from blood flow and arteriovenous oxygen content differences followed the relative contraction capability throughout recovery. The recovery patterns were not significantly different for the two types of induced fatigue. Nor was the recovery pattern significantly affected if the muscle was allowed to contract at the control rate of 0.2 t sec^{-1} during recovery. Application of these results to human muscular fatigue would suggest that approximately four hours must separate fatiguing physical work bouts if muscles are expected to perform at their maximal capability. The parallelism for the recovery of $\dot{V}O_2$ and developed isometric tension at a fixed twitch rate indicates that the coefficient of performance of this muscle was not altered by fatigue.

References

1. Barclay, J.K. and Stainsby, W.N.: The role of blood flow in limiting maximal metabolic rate in muscle. Med. Sci. Sports 7:116-119, 1975.
2. Del Pozo, E.C.: Transmission fatigue and contraction fatigue. Am. J. Physiol. 135:736-771, 1942.
3. Di Prampero, P.E., Cerretelli, P. and Piiper, J.: O_2 consumption and metabolic balance in the dog gastrocnemius at rest and during exercise. Pflugers Arch. 309:38-47, 1969.
4. Hudlicka, O.: In Keul, J. (ed.): Limiting Factors of Physical Performance. Stuttgart:Georg Thieme Publishers, 1973, p. 39.
5. Infante, A.A., Klaupiks, D. and Davies, R.E.: Phosphorylcreatine consumption during single working contractions of isolated muscles. Biochem. Biophys. Acta 94:504, 1965.
6. Robinson, S., Robinson, D.L., Mountjoy, R.S. and Bullard, R.W.: Influence of fatigue on the efficiency of men during exhausting runs. J. Appl. Physiol. 12:197-201, 1958.
7. Spronck, A.C.: In Ernst, E. and Straub, F.M. (eds.): Symposium on Muscle. Budapest:Akademiai Kiado, 1968, p. 181.
8. Stainsby, W.N.: Oxygen uptake for isotonic and isometric twitch contractions of dog skeletal muscle in situ. Am. J. Physiol. 219:435-439, 1970.
9. Stainsby, W.N. and Welch, H.G.: Lactate metabolism of contracting dog skeletal muscle in situ. Am. J. Physiol. 211:177-183, 1966.
10. Van Slyke, D.D. and Neill, J.M.: The determination of gases in blood and other solutions by vacuum extraction and manometric measurement. Int. J. Biol. Chem. 61:523-526, 1924.
11. Welch, H.G. and Stainsby, W.N.: Oxygen debt in contracting dog skeletal muscle in situ. Resp. Physiol. 3:229-242, 1967.

On the Fine Structural Changes of the Microvascular Beds in the Skeletal Muscle

Yoshio Ogawa

It is well known that endurance exercises produce moderate changes in the skeletal muscles, not only in the muscle itself but in its vascularizations. In the skeletal muscle, two or three types of muscle fibers are classified: red and white muscle fibers and intermediate muscle fibers.

There are many reports regarding these muscle fibers observed under light and electron microscopes. These reports respectively classified each muscle from the physiological and the morphological viewpoints. The classification of the muscle fibers is problematic because of the nonstandard methods employed. Despite the many investigations of the longitudinal and transverse sections in muscle specimens on the gastrocnemius muscle, for example, the above-mentioned types of muscle fibers are not yet precisely classified. However, the specimens in this experiment were perfused with Indian ink Ringer's solution through the blood vessels and, more or less, the microvasculatures in the muscles are easily observed.

In this report, the differences on the microvasculatures of the muscles after endurance exercises were mostly observed without reference to the musculatures.

Sixty male rats were used for the experiment and were divided into two groups: one group was a nonexercised group and the other an exercised group. The exercised group was given swimming exercises and treadmill running exercises starting two months after birth. The exercised group was given these exercises for about one hour every day during a 60-day period. After the 60-day period, Indian ink Ringer's solution was perfused into the bloodstream of the specimens. At the same time, specimens for electron microscopic observations were made.

Figure 1 shows a longitudinal section of the Indian ink perfused gastrocnemius muscle. It reveals a lesser degree of microvascularity.

Yoshio Ogawa, Yokohama City University, Yokohama, Japan.

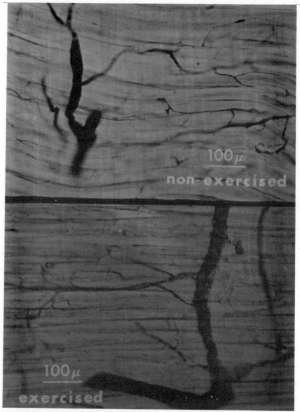

FIG. 1. The microvascularizations of white muscle in the gastrocnemius (longitudinal section) × 100.

Usually, these areas correspond to the white muscle fiber morphologically. The top area is of a nonexercised group, and the lower, of an exercised one.

Figure 2 of the same specimen shows a greater degree of microvascularity and is usually termed as red muscle fiber. The top of the figure is of a nonexercised group and the lower, an exercised one. The distributions of the minute blood vessels in these specimens are denser than in the Figure 1 specimens. In the lower area, tortuous capillaries are found surrounding the muscle fibers and the venules collect toward the small veins in broomlike arrangements.

Figure 3 is the transverse section of the gastrocnemius muscle. The relationship between the muscle fibers and the blood capillaries is clearly seen. In some places, a muscle fiber is very close to the

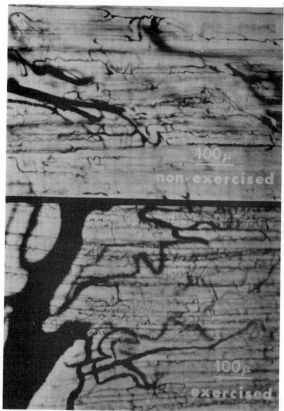

FIG. 2. The microvascularizations of red muscle in the gastrocnemius (longitudinal section) × 100.

capillaries, but in others, not so. The top of the figure is from a nonexercised group and the lower, from an exercised one.

Table I shows a comparison of the vascularity between the nonexercised group and the exercised one. In the red muscle fiber, the multiplication of the blood capillaries in the exercised group is statistically significant compared to the nonexercised.

It is important to discover how the blood capillaries multiply after long periods of endurance exercises, according to the observations of the electron microscopic specimens. A major change in the number of blood capillaries was noticed in the red muscles, according to the detailed investigations of the gastrocnemius, tibialis anterior and soleus muscles.

Figure 4 is the fine cross-sectional structure of a blood capillary in the gastrocnemius muscle from the exercised group. The endo-

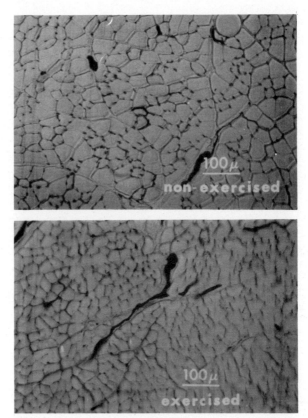

FIG. 3. The microvascularizations of red muscle in the gastrocnemius (cross-section) × 100.

Table I. Comparison of the Vascularity Between
Exercised Rats and Nonexercised Rats
(unit 1 mm^2)

	Capillary		Muscle Fiber	
	M	(S.D.)	M	(S.D.)
Red Muscle				
Exercised	379.5†	(30.5)	193.3†	(14.3)
Nonexercised	201.0†	(43.0)	102.5†	(14.3)
White Muscle				
Exercised	178.0	(18.5)	133.7*	(6.2)
Nonexercised	135.0	(46.4)	89.3*	(26.0)

*.05 level
†.01 level

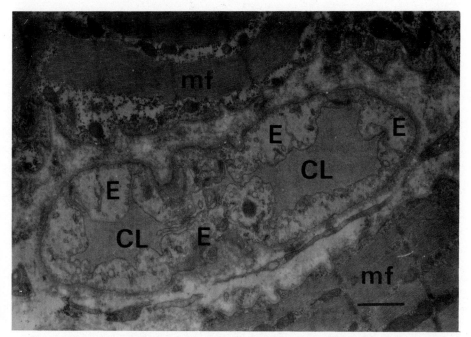

FIG. 4. The fine structure of the blood capillary in the gastrocnemius muscle (cross-section) × 7000. mf: miofibril, E: endothelium, CL: capillary lumen.

thelium is comparatively thick and many cell organelles are found. The many folds on the inner face of the capillary lumen, on opposite sides of the endothelial walls, approach and sometimes fuse to each other. After fusing, the capillary lumen is divided into two parts.

Figure 5 is a higher magnification of Figure 4. The central part of the capillary lumen is blocked by the swelling epithelial wall on both sides, and the capillary lumen is separated into two portions. On the left side of the center, a projection of the epithelium is fused; on the right, complete fusion has formed a tight junction.

Figure 6 shows a cross-sectional exercised specimen of the tibia anterior muscle. A blood capillary is constricted and fused tightly after extreme dilation, as seen on the left side. In this case, the endothelium is comparatively thin, but fine cell organelles and vacuoles can be observed. The capillary lumen is completely separated into two parts, one on the left side and the other in the middle of the figure.

Figure 7 is a transverse sectional specimen of the exercised soleus muscle. The capillary is extremely dilated, as seen in Figure 6. The constricted place is organically joined together in the center of the

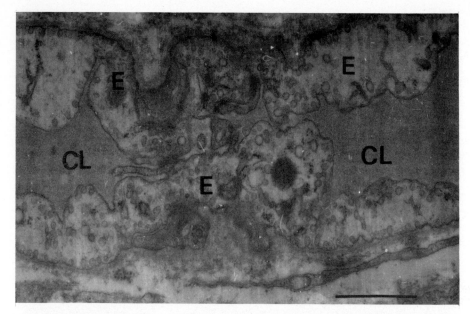

FIG. 5. The fine structure of the blood capillary in the exercised gastrocnemius muscle fusing in the central (cross-section) × 22,000. E: endothelium, CL: capillary lumen.

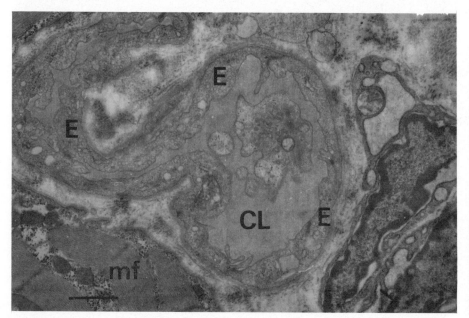

FIG. 6. The fine structure of the blood capillary in the exercised tibia anterior muscle constricted and tightly fused (cross-section) × 8,000. mf: miofibril, E: endothelium, CL: capillary lumen.

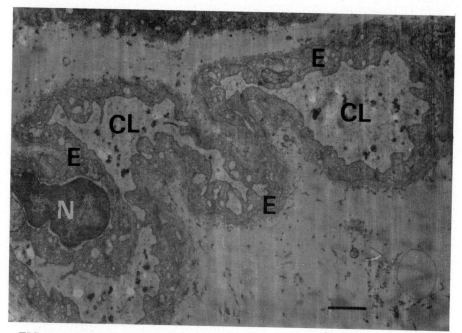

FIG. 7. The fine structure of the blood capillary in the exercised soleus muscle with the constriction organically divided (transverse section) × 6,000. CL: capillary lumen, E: endothelium, N: nucleus.

figure. In this case, Indian ink Ringer's solution was perfused into the bloodstream; therefore, the particles of Indian ink are found in both of the capillary lumens.

Figure 8 is a transverse sectional photograph of a capillary in the tibia anterior muscle belonging to the exercised group. The capillaries are completely divided, and each endothelium is observed to be thicker than in the case of Figures 6 and 7. This fact indicates that the function of each endothelium is returning to an original condition and the forms of the cell organelles reveal a normal condition. Then, this results in two capillary canals developing.

Based on the above explanations and figures, the multiplying patterns of the microvascularizations in the red muscle fibers are morphologically summarized in the schematic drawing of Figure 9.

This schema outlines the processes of the changing pattern in the formation of blood capillaries. The changes in the endothelium are shown by the active pattern on the left and the passive pattern on the right. At top of the schema is a normally formed blood capillary. The formation processes are classified in two stages.

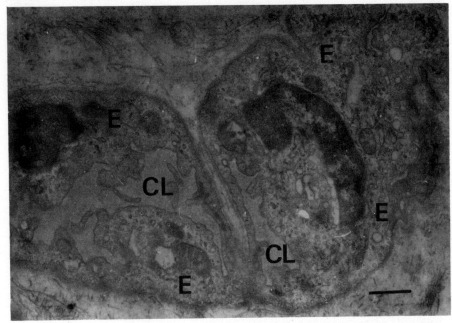

FIG. 8. The fine structure of the blood capillary in the exercised tibia anterior muscle with a completely divided capillary (transverse section) × 6,000. CL: capillary lumen, E: endothelium.

Stage one is the active pattern in which the endothelium grows thicker and the lumen becomes wider. Several projections begin to form on the inner face of the endothelium. Many kinds of cell organelles in the endothelium are found. In the center part of the capillary the projections on both sides of the inner face approach each other and fuse together. Stage two on the left side shows that the lumen is blocked and divides into two parts, eventually separating into two canals.

The passive pattern in stage one shows enlargement of the capillary lumen and the gradually thinning endothelium which is losing its cell organelles. Occasionally, fine cell organelles and vacuoles occur here and there.

In stage two of the passive pattern, the enlarged and thinner endothelium constricts in one part as the opposite sides approach each other. Finally, the constricting parts join and fuse together forming two separate canals.

In stage three both the active pattern and the passive pattern arrived at complete canalization, as seen in Figure 8.

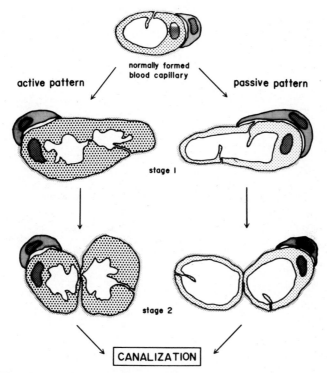

FIG. 9. The schema of the processes of the changing patterns in the formation of blood capillaries.

References

1. Ogawa, Y., Yusa, S., Takahashi, M. and Yamaguchi, H.: Distribution on the minute blood vessels of the skeletal muscle. J. Yokohama City Univ., Series C-44, No. 145, 1963.
2. Ogawa, Y.: A study of vascular pattern changes of muscular training. Kongressbericht: XVI Weltkongress fur sportmedizin, 1966, pp. 765-769.
3. Ogawa, Y.: Fine structural changes in albino rat's cardiac wall capillaries after endurance exercises. XXth World Congress in Sports Medicine, Congress Proceedings, 1974, pp. 275-277.
4. Ogawa, Y.: On the new formation of the blood capillaries in the skeletal and cardiac muscles due to endurance exercises. Proceedings of the Tenth International Congress of Anatomists, 1975, p. 350.
5. Satoyoshi, M. and Ogawa, Y.: On the changes of blood capillaries in the ventricular wall after endurance exercises. J. Yokohama City Univ., Series of Sport Sciences and Medicine, 4:1-34, 1975.

Adaptional, Pathological and Compensatory Processes in Skeletal Muscles Under Great Physical Stress

P. Z. Gudz

Muscles comprise 40% of the untrained human body, reaching 50% of that of the sportsman. For each 70 kg of body weight physical training gives a 7 kg increase of total muscular mass. What is the morphological nature of this muscle hypertrophy? Gepp was the first to pose the question in 1853.

Forty years later Morpurgo, investigating morphologically dog's musculus sartorius under intensive running exercises, suggested that the thickening of muscular fibers itself is responsible for the muscular mass increase. He strongly denied any increase in fiber number, proceeding from the generally accepted idea that the muscular tissue due to its great differentiation is incapable of deep rearrangements in the postnatal ontogenesis. Many scientists stick to the opinion even now.

However, numerous clinical examinations and experiments revealed great plasticity of the muscular tissue in various conditions. This sheds some light on the mechanism of muscular hypertrophy.

While experimenting with animals we found that the muscular mass increase results not only from the hypertrophy of existing fibers but also from their hyperplasia. The increase in fiber number is brought about in various ways. The longitudinal division of many hypertrophied fibers into two and three of smaller diameter occurs first. A thin fiber splitting from the hypertrophied fiber, followed by its thickening, is then observed. Finally, new muscular fibers develop from mioblasts formed from the fragments of dedifferentiating muscular fibers. Each of these processes can be explained as follows.

The muscle fiber hypertrophy can be attributed to the increase of miofibrils, sarcoplasma accumulation, hypertrophy and increase of mitochondria and muscular nuclei via amitosis. Motor nerve endings of such fibers expand and quantity of terminal branches and their

P. Z. Gudz, Kiev Institute of Physical Culture, Kiev, U.S.S.R.

nuclei increases. The capillary network expands, too, with new capillaries being formed. Their electron microscoping revealed broadening of frontier between endothelial cells, increasing of pinocytosis activity of the cytoplasm and growing of single and multiple cytoplasma in the space between capillaries, pointing out to the increase of the functional state.

Reaching the definite level of the rearrangement many of the hypertrophied muscular fibers start longitudinal division. The sarcolemma partitions grow inside the fibers dividing them into two or more thin ones. The splitting of a thin muscle fiber occurs similarly.

The possibility of the fiber increase under physical stress has long been under discussion, but as far as we know, we are the first to pose the question about innervation mechanism of newly formed muscular fibers.

We found additional dividing hypertrophied fibers. This ending develops from the collateral branch end, growing from the preterminal part of the motor axon. At first, such a nerve ending seems a primitive contact of a fiber and a nerve branch, later changing to a differentiated motor nerve ending. The slit of the fiber longitudinal division is between the two old and new motor endings, thus the new muscular fiber acquires its own motor nerve ending.

Under great physical stress both the adaption rearrangement and pathological changes of many fibers take place. Single or multiple contraction nodes appear on muscular fibers near and far off the motor nerve ending. Transverse striping disappears in the nodes due to actin and miosin miofilament ruining. The muscular fiber is being stretched between the nodes.

The result of this phenomenon may be varied. In some cases the structure of fibers changed sites is restored, in others the waxy degeneration of a fiber or its part takes place. Collagenal fibers of endomysia grow into the intact part of the fiber provided the motor nerve ending remains unaffected there. Such a fiber exists as ending in endomysia.

Under physical stress of a prolonged action leading to considerable pathological changes, the dedifferentiation in some muscular fibers may occur. The transverse striping disappears giving rise to the fiber splitting into transverse fragments. These fragments can form mioblasts changing into miosymblasts, muscular tubes and, finally, into muscular fibers. This results in the so-called microplastic operation of the intensively functioning muscle, thus compensating the fibers lost by degeneration.

In case of muscular overstraining various adaptational, pathological and compensatory reactions proceed in the nervous and vascular systems of the muscle. Arteriolovenous anastomoses of muscles in well-trained organism are closed thus providing transportation of all blood to muscular capillaries. In case of chronic fatigue they open and part of the blood goes out of a vena, leaving these capillaries aside.

Review of literature and our observations give every reason to say that the systematic training by intensive physical exercises leads to the profound restructuring of the muscles, giving rise to the qualitatively new structural elements, insuring high efficiency of muscle functioning. Furthermore, as our investigation on well-trained animals (later subjected to the hypokinesis regimen) showed, some stress on the muscles is necessary to maintain structural balance of the latter.

However, it would be wrong to believe that skeletal muscles' adaptional reaction and resources are inexhaustible. In case of chronic fatigue degenerative processes prevail over the processes of adaptation, regeneration and compensation. The sites of connective tissue develop on the degenerated fibers in the muscle. The muscle mass does not grow but decreases. Correspondingly, the operational efficiency of the muscle is reduced. With this in view an adequate selection of optimal physical stress, stimulating adaptional processes in the muscle without any pathological change, is of primary importance.

Histological Study on the Effect of Training Upon Skeletal Muscle Fibers

Kunio Kikuchi and Minoru Wada

Introduction

The skeletal muscle fibers of the mammal have from the past been generally classified into red muscle fibers and while muscle fibers according to the amount of myofibril and sarcoplasm, but recently the existence of medium (intermediate) muscle fibers having features intermediate between the foregoing from the standpoint of morphology, size and color has attracted much attention.

Ogata and Mori [6] have classified skeletal muscle fibers into red muscle fibers, white muscle fibers and medium muscle fibers according to the action intensity of oxidative enzymes. Henneman and Olson [2] have grouped skeletal muscle fibers into three types according to the activity level of mitochondrial ATPase, while Stein and Padykula [10] did similarly according to the response of succinic dehydrogenase (SDH).

A good deal of data are available at the cellular level on the effect of muscular training on skeletal muscle fibers, dating back to the work of Morpurgo [5] and Petow and Siebert [7]. This has been pursued more recently by Reitsma [8]. However, no data have been reported in the literature on the effect of muscular training on skeletal muscle fibers by type, that is, on red, white and medium muscle fibers.

In this study, a review was first made on the morphological characteristics of skeletal muscle fibers, that is, on the morphology, size and color, together with their distribution, which was followed by a histological study on the effect of dynamic muscular training, primarily isotonic muscular contraction, on skeletal muscle fibers classified into red, white and medium muscle fibers.

Kunio Kikuchi and Minoru Wada, Department of Health and Physical Education, Faculty of Integrated Arts and Sciences, Hiroshima University, Japan.

Method

Fourteen Wistar strain rats of the same venter approximately 30 days old were used in this study. They were divided into the training group and the control group on the basis of body weight. For the training the animals were placed in a treadmill each day for 90 days with a daily running distance of 250 meters at a speed of 40 meters/min. On completion of the training the rats were killed. Microscopic specimens were prepared of m. tibialis anterior, and then stained with Sudan black B stain.

For the measurement of the cross-section of the muscle fibers, microscopic photographs (Fig. 1) of the entire cross-section area of m. tibialis anterior were taken. Then the skeletal muscle fibers were cut out by type, weighed on a balance and then converted into cross-section area.

Results

Color, Shape and Size of the Skeletal Muscle Fibers

Figure 2 is a microphotograph of the entire cross-section of m. tibialis anterior. When the skeletal muscle fibers were stained with Sudan black B stain, red muscle fibers appeared deep blue, white skeletal muscles white and medium muscle fibers light blue. Red muscle fibers appeared round in shape, white polygonal in shape and medium intermediate between the foregoing in shape.

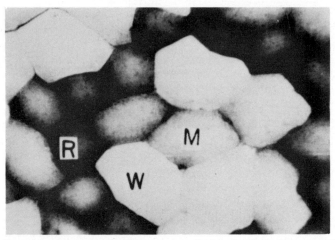

FIG. 1. Cross-section of M. tibialis anterior. Sudan black B stain × 400. R: red muscle fiber; M: medium muscle fiber; and W: white muscle fiber.

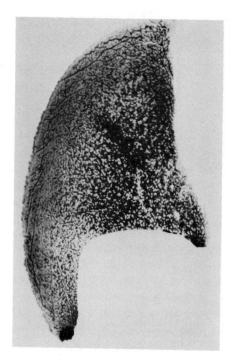

FIG. 2. Entire cross-section of M. tibialis anterior × 20.

Table I shows the average cross-section area and diameter per muscle fiber in the peripheral region and innermost region of m. tibialis anterior classified into red, white and medium muscle fibers. The cross-section area of red, white and medium muscle fibers in the peripheral region showed values higher than those in the innermost region. The average cross-section area of m. tibialis anterior as a whole showed the highest value in white muscle fibers, followed by medium and red.

Distribution of Muscle Fibers

The percent distribution of muscle fibers is shown in Figure 3. The distribution of red muscle fibers was low in the peripheral region and high in the innermost region, while the distribution of white muscle fibers was high in the peripheral region and low in the innermost region. The distribution of medium muscle fibers did not show a remarkable difference between the peripheral region and innermost region with the value ranging from 14.5% to 22.4%.

Table I. Average Cross-section Area and Diameter per Fiber in Various Regions of Tibialis Anterior Muscles of Rats

	N	Peripheral Region			Innermost Region			Whole Region		
		Red	Medium	White	Red	Medium	White	Red	Medium	White
Average area of cross-section per fiber (μ^2)	11	1280.6	1724.2	2803.5	962.6	1194.4	1716.1	1074.7	1428.4	2434.5
Average diameter of fiber (μ)	11	40.4	46.8	59.8	35.0	39.0	46.7	37.0	42.6	55.6

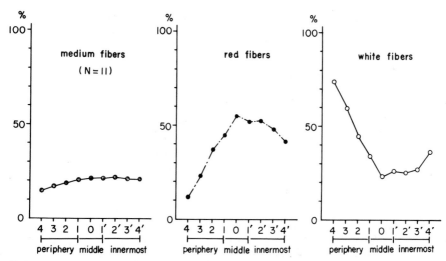

FIG. 3. Distribution of skeletal muscle fibers of tibialis anterior muscles of rats.

Effect of Training on the Skeletal Muscle Fibers

Effect on the entire cross-section area. Table II shows the effect of training on m. tibialis anterior classified into the peripheral region and innermost region and compares the rate of hypertrophy of red, white and medium muscle fibers. The rate of hypertrophy of the muscle fibers in the peripheral region was remarkably high in white muscle fibers, followed by medium and red. The rate of hypertrophy of muscle fibers in the innermost region did not show any apparent difference between red, medium and white muscle fibers. The average rate of hypertrophy of m. tibialis anterior as a whole was 33.0% in white, 19.1% in medium and 18.0% in red muscle fibers with the rate being remarkably high in white muscle fibers. The rate of hypertrophy of medium muscle fibers showed a value close to that of red.

Effect on the average cross-section area per fiber. The effect of training on the average cross-section area per muscle fiber showed almost the same trend as observed on the entire cross-section area.

Discussion

To study the effect of muscular training on the morphology of skeletal muscle fibers, Morpurgo [5] observed the enlargement of m. sartorius in dogs following two months of intensive treadmill exercise and noted the rate of hypertrophy per muscle fiber to be 53.2% to

Table II. Effect of Training on the Entire Cross-section Area in the Peripheral, Innermost and Whole Regions of Tibialis Anterior Muscles

	Group	N	Peripheral Region			Innermost Region			Whole Region		
			Red	Medium	White	Red	Medium	White	Red	Medium	White
Entire area of cross-section (mm²)	Training	7	2.34	2.23	15.31	3.29	1.87	4.14	5.63	4.11	19.45
	Control	7	1.99	1.86	11.30	2.71	1.53	3.38	4.77	3.45	14.62
Rate of hypertrophy (%)			16.2	19.9	35.5	21.3	22.2	22.5	18.0	19.1	33.0

55.0%. Reitsma [8] studied the hypertrophy of m. rectus femoris, m. plantaris and m. soleus in rats following treadmill exercise and reported that hypertrophy was observed in all the muscles examined.

The authors [3, 4] in studying hypertrophy of red muscle fibers (including medium muscle fibers) and white muscle fiber by changing the mode of training observed that by dynamic muscular training involving chiefly isotonic muscular contraction the rate of hypertrophy of white muscle fibers was greater than that of red and that by static muscular training involving chiefly isometric muscular contraction the rate of hypertrophy of red muscle fibers was greater than that of white. The trend of the rate of hypertrophy of red and white muscle fibers by dynamic muscular training employed in the current study was the same as that of the foregoing, but the rate of hypertrophy of medium muscle fibers showed a value close to that of red. These differences in rate of hypertrophy of muscle fibers by type are considered to be due to the difference in nerve supply by type of muscle fibers as advocated by Edstrom and Kugelberg [1], that is, to the difference in the level of adaptability to the burden attributable to dynamic muscular training due to the difference in nerve muscle unit of red, white and medium muscle fibers.

The following is one of the reasons why the rate of hypertrophy of white muscle fibers was greater than that of red. Sréter [9] has reported in his study of water volume and ion concentration of sodium and potassium within and without the cells of the mammals that dehydration and ionic change immediately following prolonged electrical stimulation were more remarkable in white muscle fibers than in red. Since the functional characteristics of medium muscle fibers have yet to be adequately elucidated, no discussion can be made on why the rate of hypertrophy of medium muscle fibers showed a value close to that of the red. We will pursue this as a future project.

Summary

Sudan black B staining was made on specimens obtained from m. tibialis anterior of Wistar strain rats and a histological study was conducted on the morphological characteristics of muscle fibers, their distribution and the effect of training on these muscle fibers. The following results were obtained.

1. Red muscle fibers appeared round in shape, white muscle fibers polygonal in shape, and medium muscle fibers a shape intermediate between the foregoing. White muscle fibers were the largest in size followed by medium and red.

2. The peripheral region of the muscles was abundant with white muscle fibers, while the innermost region was abundant with red. There was no remarkable difference in distribution of medium muscle fibers between the peripheral and innermost regions, being rather evenly distributed.

3. The rate of hypertrophy of the entire cross-section area of m. tibialis anterior was the highest in the white muscle fibers followed by medium and red.

4. The rate of hypertrophy of the average cross-section area per muscle fiber of m. tibialis anterior showed a trend similar to that of the entire cross-section area of the various muscle fibers.

References

1. Edström, L. and Kugelberg, E.: Properties of motor units in the rat anterior tibial muscle. Acta Physiol. Scand. 73:543-544, 1968.
2. Henneman, E. and Olson, C.B.: Relations between structure and function in the design of skeletal muscles. J. Neurophysiol. 28:581-598, 1965.
3. Kikuchi, K.: Histological study of muscular training — Comparison of effect of static and dynamic muscular training upon skeletal muscle fibers. Res. J. Phys. Educ. 16(2):67-74, 1971.
4. Man-i, M., Ito, K. and Kikuchi, K.: Histological studies of muscular training. Report I. Effect of training upon skeletal muscle fibers. Res. J. Phys. Educ. 11(3):153-165, 1967.
5. Morpurgo, B.: Uber Activitats-Hypertrophie der willkürlichen Muskeln. Virchows Arch. 150:522-554, 1897.
6. Ogata, T. and Mori, M.: Histochemical study of oxidative enzymes in vertebrate muscles. J. Histochem. Cytochem. 12(3):171-182, 1964.
7. Petow, H. and Siebert, W.: Studien über Arbeitshypertrophie des Muskels. Z. Klin. Med. 102:427-433, 1925.
8. Reitsma, W.: Skeletal muscle hypertrophy after heavy exercise in rats surgically reduced muscle function. Am. J. Phys. Med. 48(5):237-258, 1969.
9. Sréter, F.A.: Cell water, sodium, and potassium in stimulated red and white mammalian muscles. Am. J. Physiol. 205(6):1295-1298, 1963.
10. Stein, J.M. and Padykula, H.A.: Histochemical classification of individual skeletal muscle fibers of the rats. Am. J. Anat. 110:103-121, 1962.

The Effect of Acute Exercise on the Serum Cholesterol Esters at Different Metabolic Stages

David Montgomery and A. H. Ismail

Introduction

The association of hyperlipidemia with the atherosclerotic process is well documented in a wide range of experimental animals [3] and in man [7]. Of the different lipids, the cholesterol ester fraction is the most markedly discriminating variable between "normal" individuals and individuals with arteriosclerosis [15, 17].

Since a sedentary life style has been found to be associated with an increased incidence of heart disease, it has been suggested that physical activity may retard circulatory deterioration [6]. Most investigations into the effect of exercise on the serum lipids have been concerned with changes in the concentration of the different total lipid fractions. Few studies have examined the profile of the fatty acids in the cholesterol ester fraction. The purpose of the present study was to investigate the effect of a fitness program on the serum cholesterol ester fatty acid profile in adult men at different metabolic stress levels.

Methods

Twenty-four men ranging in age from 24 to 65 years were selected from 100 men who participated in the physical fitness program at Purdue University. All subjects had clinically normal serum glucose — 70 to 120 mg% [8] and triglycerides — 30 to 200 mg% [20] levels.

The physical fitness program was conducted three days each week for 1½ hours each session for a four-month period. The program consisted of calisthenics, jogging and recreational activities such as basketball, volleyball, swimming, squash and handball.

David Montgomery, McGill University, Montreal, Quebec, Canada, and A. H. Ismail, Purdue University, Lafayette, Indiana, U.S.A.

The subjects were tested at the beginning and at the end of the four-month physical fitness program. Age, height, weight and skinfold measurements were recorded by the same tester on two separate days preceding the treadmill test. The percent lean body weight was obtained utilizing the skinfold and anthropometric estimation of body density established by Wilmore and Behnke [21].

Each subject reported to the laboratory in the postabsorptive state. After a ten-minute bed rest, a venous blood sample was drawn from the antecubital vein. The treadmill elevation was lowered to 0% and the subject commenced running at a speed of 6 mph. Again, the percent grade was increased 2% every two minutes during the run up to a maximum of 10% elevation. The heart rate was continually monitored by an electrocardiogram. When the subject indicated that he could continue for only two minutes longer, the respiratory equipment was attached and a gas sample collected during the last 30 seconds of the run. The heart rate was also determined for this period and considered as the maximal heart rate. The CO_2 and O_2 percentages were determined directly from a 120-liter Tissot spirometer using Beckman analyzers. The analyzers were calibrated periodically using standard commercial gases. After the maximal run, the "Maximal I" blood sample was drawn from the antecubital vein. At the post test, this run was repeated in terms of time run and percentage elevation.

On the post test, all subjects were able to run a further distance during which a new maximum was obtained. This metabolic period was referred to as "Maximal II." The same procedures were followed as described in Maximal I performance. After the maximal run, the subject rested on a bed for a 15-minute recovery period after which the recovery blood sample was drawn from the antecubital vein. This terminated the treadmill test.

Seven individual cholesterol esters were identified and measured by gas-liquid chromatography. The total lipids were extracted by a modified Folch procedure [5], then the lipids were separated by thin-layer chromatography. The cholesterol esters were scraped from the thin-layer plate and methylated using boron trifluoride-methanol. The methyl esters were then analyzed on a gas-liquid chromatograph (Hewlett Packard, Model 5700A) using six-foot columns, 6.25 mm in diameter containing 3% HI-EFF on Gas Chrom Q, 100-200 mesh, with a column temperature of 180 C and a detector temperature of 250 C.

The identification of the methyl esters was made by comparing the retention times of the serum sample with those of two known reference standards. Quantitative results with NHI Fatty Acid

Standard GLOOOD agreed with the stated composition with a relative error less than 5% for major components (> 10% of the total mixture) and less than 10% for minor components (<10% of the total mixture).

Data were analyzed with an analysis of variance technique. The Newman-Keuls method [11] was used for mean comparison whenever the ANOVA results yielded significance at the .10 level. T-tests for related measures were used to see if the changes (in the descriptive data) from the pre to post tests were significant.

Results

The means and standard errors of selected descriptive data for the pre and post physical fitness tests are presented in Table I. The mean age of the 24 subjects was 44.9 years. There were no significant changes in weight or percent lean as a result of the four-month program. The physical fitness score increased significantly from 350.8 on the pre test to 379.1 on the post test. On the pre test, the subjects ran for a mean time of 10.5 minutes at a 6.3% grade, whereas on the post test, the subjects had improved significantly to a mean time of 14.0 minutes at 7.3% elevation.

The means and standard errors of the serum total cholesterol, total cholesterol esters and the seven individual cholesterol esters at different metabolic stages are presented for the pre test in Table II and for the post test in Table III. The ANOVA results are summarized in Table IV. It was necessary to present two analyses of

Table I. Anthropometric, Physiological and Biochemical Values (Means and S.E.) of the Pre and Post Physical Fitness Tests for the 24 Subjects

| Variable | Pre Test | | Post Test | | |
	$\overline{X}$	S.E.	$\overline{X}$	S.E.	t
Age (yr)	44.9	2.0	––	––	
Height (in)	69.9	0.5	––	––	
Weight (kg)	78.8	2.1	78.2	2.1	1.95
% Lean (%)	83.2	1.0	83.6	1.0	1.89
Physical fitness score	350.8	13.8	379.1	11.1	5.88†
Max heart rate (beats/min)	169.2	2.8	174.5	2.4	1.55
Max $\dot{V}_{O_2}$ (ml/kg/min)	42.7	2.2	45.2	1.7	1.82
Grade (%)	6.3	0.8	7.3	0.7	2.77*
Time run (min)	10.5	1.2	14.0	0.9	7.05†
Serum glucose (mg%)	90.6	1.4	90.2	1.6	0.22
Serum triglycerides (mg%)	124.7	14.0	117.3	10.2	0.79

*Significant at the .05 level (23 df)
†Significant at the .01 level (23 df)

Table II. Pre Test Values (Means and S.E.) of the Serum Cholesterol
Variables at Four Metabolic Stages

Variable	Rest	Submax. Ex.	Max. Ex.	Recovery
Total chol (mg%)	236.8 ± 9.4	246.9 ± 9.5	271.2 ± 9.9	239.5 ± 9.4
Total chol ester (mg%)	180.1 ± 7.4	186.0 ± 7.6	202.6 ± 8.1	179.9 ± 7.2
Chol myristate (%)	1.0 ± 0.1	0.8 ± 0.1	1.0 ± 0.1	1.0 ± 0.1
Chol palmitate (%)	14.4 ± 0.5	13.5 ± 0.6	13.8 ± 0.5	13.7 ± 0.5
Chol palmitoleate (%)	5.8 ± 0.5	6.0 ± 0.5	6.1 ± 0.4	5.8 ± 0.5
Chol stearate (%)	1.4 ± 0.2	1.1 ± 0.1	1.1 ± 0.1	1.2 ± 0.1
Chol oleate (%)	22.2 ± 1.0	22.5 ± 0.9	22.1 ± 0.8	21.5 ± 0.7
Chol linoleate (%)	48.7 ± 1.6	49.8 ± 1.9	49.9 ± 1.6	50.0 ± 1.7
Chol arachidonate (%)	5.2 ± 0.5	5.8 ± 0.6	5.5 ± 0.5	5.9 ± 0.5

variance tables for each variable so that the degrees of freedom for the F tests would not be fictitious as would be the case if five metabolic levels were used and Maximal I was repeated in the pre test to correspond with Maximal II in the post test.

There were significant differences ($P < .01$) between the metabolic stages for both total cholesterol and total cholesterol esters. There was a significant increase in the total cholesterol and total cholesterol esters from the resting state to the submaximal exercise, and a further significant increase during maximal exercise with a significant decrease during the recovery period.

For the individual cholesterol esters, the differences among the metabolic stages were significant for the serum cholesterol myristate percentage ($P < .05$), serum cholesterol stearate percentage ($P < .05$) and serum cholesterol palmitate percentage ($P < .10$). For the three saturated cholesterol esters, there was a decrease in percentage ester during the submaximal exercise in comparison with the resting level. The decrease was followed by an increase in ester percentage during the maximal exercise. There were no significant changes among the metabolic stages for any of the other cholesterol ester percentages.

Discussion

The serum total cholesterol response of the 24 subjects during exercise was similar to that reported in other studies [4, 10, 12, 14, 16, 19] as a result of acute exercise bouts. In an eight-month physical fitness program reported by Ismail et al [10], the mean serum total cholesterol level increased from 203.6 mg% at rest to 245.8 mg% during maximal exercise on the pre test in 54 subjects (mean age = 39.7 years) who worked on bicycle ergometers. On the

Table III. Post Test Values (Means and S.E.) of the Serum Cholesterol
Variables at Five Metabolic Stages

Variable	Rest	Submax. Ex.	Max I Ex.	Max II Ex.	Recovery
Total chol (mg%)	232.0 ± 10.7	250.1 ± 11.4	273.5 ± 12.1	276.3 ± 12.0	245.3 ± 10.5
Total chol ester (mg%)	178.0 ± 8.2	189.9 ± 8.5	206.2 ± 9.2	209.0 ± 9.1	186.6 ± 7.9
Chol myristate (%)	0.9 ± 0.1	0.9 ± 0.1	1.0 ± 0.1	1.0 ± 0.1	1.0 ± 0.1
Chol palmitate (%)	14.2 ± 0.5	13.6 ± 0.5	14.3 ± 0.5	13.8 ± 0.5	14.2 ± 0.5
Chol palmitoleate (%)	6.0 ± 0.5	6.3 ± 0.4	6.4 ± 0.5	6.6 ± 0.4	6.3 ± 0.4
Chol stearate (%)	1.2 ± 0.1	0.9 ± 0.1	1.1 ± 0.1	1.1 ± 0.1	1.1 ± 0.1
Chol oleate (%)	22.4 ± 0.7	22.2 ± 0.9	22.1 ± 0.8	22.4 ± 0.7	22.5 ± 0.7
Chol linoleate (%)	49.4 ± 1.7	49.9 ± 1.8	49.4 ± 1.6	49.2 ± 1.6	49.5 ± 1.6
Chol arachidonate (%)	5.1 ± 0.6	5.7 ± 0.7	5.6 ± 0.5	5.9 ± 0.6	5.6 ± 0.6

Table IV. F Values of the Serum Cholesterol Variables
at Four Stages of Metabolic Stress

Variable	F_1 Observed (Using Max I Data)	F_2 Observed (Using Max II Data)
Total chol (mg%)	99.37‡	101.25‡
Total chol ester (mg%)	53.85‡	55.47‡
Chol myristate (%)	3.43†	3.80†
Chol palmitate (%)	2.75*	2.67*
Chol palmitoleate (%)	0.30	0.57
Chol stearate (%)	3.84†	3.98†
Chol oleate (%)	0.32	0.83
Chol linoleate (%)	0.94	0.98
Chol arachidonate (%)	2.12	2.38*

F Value Necessary to be Significant

Level	F (3,60)
* .10	2.18
† .05	2.76
‡ .01	4.13

post test, the total cholesterol level increased from 191.8 mg% at rest to 239.6 mg% during maximal exercise.

In a study of 14 athletes (mean age = 34.1 years) who ran 42 km in a mean time of 2 hours 50 minutes, Hurter et al [9] reported plasma cholesterol levels of 205.1 mg% at rest and 217.6 mg% after the race. The blood samples were collected within ten minutes of the end of the race.

In the present study, the serum total cholesterol levels increased from 236.8 mg% at rest to 271.2 mg% during maximal exercise on the pre test and 232.0 mg% at rest to 276.3 mg% during maximal exercise on the post test. After the 15-minute recovery period the serum total cholesterol decreased to 239.5 mg% at the pre test and 245.3 mg% at the post test.

Cholesterol esters make up approximately two thirds of total cholesterol. Hence, it is no surprise that the serum total cholesterol esters followed a similar pattern in the different metabolic stages as the total cholesterol.

One other study by Hurter et al [9] has reported on the changes in the fatty acid profile of the cholesterol esters after exercise. After a 42 km race, 14 athletes had a significant (P <.05) increase in cholesterol palmitate (12.31% at rest to 13.36% after exercise) and a significant (P <.05) decrease in cholesterol linoleate (57.42% at rest to 55.41% after exercise). The authors explain the results by indicating that "there seemed to be preferential oxidation of unsaturated components in the complex lipids."

The results of the present study found a significant (P <.05) decrease in the saturated cholesterol esters during submaximal exercise and an increase during the maximal exercise. The 24 subjects ran for 10.5 minutes at a treadmill elevation of 6.3% during the pre test and 14.0 minutes at 7.3% during the post test. In the study by Hurter et al [9], the 14 athletes ran for a mean time of 2 hours and 50 minutes. Hence, the intensity as well as the duration may account for the differences in results. Also, the physical fitness condition of the subjects may partly explain differences in the response. In this study, the 24 subjects were of varying physical fitness levels, whereas the 14 subjects in the study by Hurter et al [9] were all of very high physical fitness level.

Since the plasma does not contain enzymes that hydrolyze cholesterol esters [18], and since only the side chain and not the ring carbon of cholesterol is degraded [1, 13], it is doubtful that there is preferential oxidation of unsaturated cholesterol esters in the plasma. The plasma cholesterol is part of an exchangeable pool of cholesterol consisting of many compartments with different rates of equilibration. It is estimated that normal man has about 1 gm of exchangeable cholesterol per kilogram body weight. During exercise, it is probable that the increase in cholesterol mobilization is due to an addition of cholesterol from other compartments. If so, then the serum cholesterol esters will resemble the cholesterol esters from the source of the additional cholesterol. The source of this cholesterol ester compartment cannot be conclusively stated without additional studies using labeled cholesterol.

References

1. Chaikoff, I.L., Siperstein, M.D., Dauben, W.G. et al: C^{14}-cholesterol. II. Oxidation of carbons 4 and 26 to carbon dioxide by the intact rat. J. Biol. Chem. 194:413-416, 1952.
2. Cholesterol Determinations. Houston, Texas:Hycel Incorporated.
3. Clarkson, T.B.: Atherosclerosis — Spontaneous and induced. Adv. Lipid Res. 1:211-252, 1963.
4. Fitzgerald, O., Heffernan, A. and McFarlane, R.: Serum lipids and physical activity in normal subjects. Clin. Sci. 28:83-89, 1965.
5. Folch, J., Lees, M. and Stanley, G.H.S.: A simple method for the isolation and purification of total lipids from animal tissues. J. Biol. Chem. 226:497-509, 1957.
6. Fox, S.M. and Skinner, J.S.: Physical activity and cardiovascular health. Am. J. Cardiol. 14:731-746, 1964.
7. Friedman, M.: Pathogenesis of Coronary Artery Disease. New York: McGraw-Hill Book Company, 1969, p. 269.
8. Glucose Determination. Philadelphia, Pa.:Harleco Incorporated.

9. Hurter, R., Swale, J., Peyman, M.A. and Barnett, C.W.H.: Some immediate and long-term effects of exercise on the plasma-lipids. Lancet 2:671-675, 1972.

10. Ismail, A.H., Corrigan, D.L., MacLeod, D.F. et al: Biophysiological and audiological variables in adults. Arch. Otolaryngol. 97:447-451, 1973.

11. Keuls, M.: The use of the "Studentized range" in connection with an analysis of variance. Euphytica 1:112-122, 1952.

12. Mock, G.W.: The effects of a four-month physical fitness program on selected free fatty acids. Unpublished Ph.D. Dissertation, Purdue University, 1972.

13. Myant, N.B. and Lewis, B.: Estimation of the rate of breakdown of cholesterol in man by measurement of $^{14}CO_2$ excretion after intravenous ($26\text{-}^{14}C$) cholesterol. Clin. Sci. 30:117-127, 1966.

14. Naughton, J. and Balke, B.: Physical working capacity in medical personnel and the response of serum cholesterol to acute exercise and to training. Am. J. Med. Sci. 247:286-292, 1964.

15. Portman, O.W.: Atherosclerosis in nonhuman primates: Sequences and possible mechanisms of change in phospholipid composition and metabolism. N.Y. Acad. Sci. 162:120-136, 1969.

16. Sannerstedt, R., Sanbar, S.S. and Conway, J.: Metabolic effects of exercise in patients with Type IV hyperlipoproteinemia. Am. J. Cardiol. 25:642-648, 1970.

17. Schade, W., Boehle, E. and Biegler, R.: Humoral changes in arteriosclerosis investigations on lipids, fatty acids, ketone bodies, pyruvic acid, lactic acid and glucose in the blood. Lancet 2:1409-1416, 1960.

18. Swell, L. and Treadwell, C.R.: Cholesterol esterases. III. Occurrence and characteristics of cholesterol esterase of serum. J. Biol. Chem. 185:349-355, 1950.

19. Teraslinna, P.: Effect of exercise on selected serum lipids and their relationships to certain variables of body structure and function. Unpublished Ph.D. Thesis, June 1966.

20. Tri-Chol Principle. Foster City, Calif.:Oxford Laboratory.

21. Wilmore, J.H. and Behnke, A.R.: An anthrometric estimation of body density and lean body weight in young men. J. Appl. Physiol. 27:25-31, 1969.

Relationships Between Physical Exercise and Concentration of Plasma Lipids

W. G. McTaggart and F. Ribas-Cardus

Introduction

High plasma lipid concentrations are considered to be associated with coronary atherosclerosis. Efforts by many investigators have been directed toward methods of reducing plasma lipids with the prospect of reducing the incidence and consequences of this disease. In this respect, data in the literature regarding the reduction of plasma lipids through physical exercise are inconclusive and contradictory.

The results reported in this paper represent one more attempt to study the relationships between plasma lipids and physical exercise. A better understanding of changes induced by physical exercise in plasma lipid concentrations would be valuable in designing reconditioning exercise programs in general and in particular for patients with a history of myocardial infarction going through a rehabilitation program.

Methods

Determinations of plasma total lipids (TL), total esterified fatty acids (TEFA), triglycerides (T), total cholesterol (TC), cholesterol esters (CE), free cholesterol (FC) and phospholipids (P) were made on 506 male subjects prior to the administration of a work-tolerance evaluation. The evaluation consisted of interviews, a physical examination and an exercise stress test. After analysis of the data, the subjects were classified as either healthy (363 subjects), patients with clinical or electrocardiographic signs of ischemic heart disease

W. G. McTaggart and F. Ribas-Cardus, Department of Rehabilitation, Baylor College of Medicine, Houston, Texas, U.S.A.

This investigation was supported by Project SRS 16-P-56813/6-12 of the Social and Rehabilitation Service, Department of Health, Education and Welfare, Washington, D.C.

(IHD) but without evidence or history of myocardial infarction (67 patients) and patients with evidence of IHD who also had a history of a previous myocardial infarction (76 patients).

The plasma biochemical parameters were determined by conventional colorimetric procedures and expressed in milligrams percent. Blood samples for the determination of biochemical parameters were obtained after an overnight fast of from 10 to 15 hours. In addition to the blood sample taken before the exercise stress test, a second sample was taken from each of 62 subjects within one minute after conclusion of exercise. Determinations of plasma lipids and glucose concentrations were made on each of these 62 blood samples.

The procedure for exercise stress testing employed a bicycle ergometer on which each subject exercised at increasing workloads up to a level corresponding to approximately 85% of the expected maximum age-adjusted heart rate for each individual subject. The extrapolation to this maximum level was made by linear regression [2]. Workloads are expressed in kilopond-meters/minute (kpm/min).

A select group of 13 subjects with ischemic heart disease has been participating in a reconditioning exercise program for lengths of time varying from one to three years. These subjects have been evaluated periodically for changes in physical work capacity and plasma lipid concentrations.

Results

The biochemical data obtained in the 506 initial studies and the age at which the subject was first studied are summarized in Table I. Comparison of the three subject groups (healthy, IHD patients without a previous MI and IHD patients with a previous MI) shows the mean ages of the two patient groups to be greater (p < 0.003) than that of the healthy subjects. Plasma lipid concentrations in the two groups of patients are higher than in the healthy subjects.

The mean plasma concentrations of cholesterol and triglycerides for each decade of age of these subjects are presented in Figure 1. Cholesterol values show a tendency to increase with age. No significant differences were found for the mean cholesterol values on comparing either group of patients to healthy males of the same age. Triglyceride values throughout the age range of our subjects appear to be the most variable of the lipid components. No trends in the mean values for plasma triglycerides relative to subjects' ages were observed on inspection of the data.

Table I. Summary of Blood Lipid Data

| Subject Class | Number | | Mean Age (yr) | TL | TEFA | Lipid Fraction,[a] Milligram Percent | | | | |
						T	TC	CE	FC	PL
Healthy	363	Mean	41.2	654	365	142	236	169	66	248
		S.D.[b]	±9.8	±184	±147	±140	±51	±40	±24	±56
Ischemic without MI[c]	67	Mean	48.2	673	372	144	251	181	69	251
		S.D.[b]	±9.1	±125	±104	±73	±48	±39	±22	±43
Ischemic with MI	76	Mean	51.8	732	437	190	257	180	74	262
		S.D.[b]	±6.9	±156	±128	±110	±55	±40	±24	±54

[a]TL = Total lipids; TEFA = total esterified fatty acids; T = triglycerides; T C = total cholesterol; CE = cholesterol esters; FC = free cholesterol; PL = phospholipids

[b]S.D. = standard deviation

[c]MI = myocardial infarction

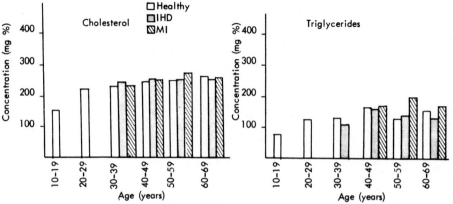

FIG. 1. Changes in concentration of plasma cholesterol and triglycerides with age.

The mean maximal physical work capacity (WLmax) of the two patient groups was significantly lower (p < 0.003) than that of the healthy subjects (Table II). The subjects who had a history of a previous MI had the lowest physical work capacity. A decrease in WLmax with increasing age of the subjects is evident in Table III, which shows a comparison of the mean WLmax for each decade of age. Patients having IHD without a MI had a work capacity similar to healthy subjects of the same age, while the patients of the same age group who had had a MI show a mean physical work capacity considerably reduced. The regression of WLmax on age is illustrated in Figure 2 where the mean WLmax for each age decade is plotted against the mean age of subjects within that decade. The age-adjusted limits equivalent to Åstrand's [1] performance classification of

Table II. Means and Standard Deviations for
Maximal Physical Work Capacity

Subject Class	Number	Maximal Physical Work Capacity, Kpm/min[a]
Healthy	348	1093 ± 227
Ischemic patients without MI[b]	67	946 ± 202
Ischemic patients with MI[b]	74	735 ± 355

[a]Significance of comparison between the mean of groups
corresponds to a p-value less than 0.003

[b]MI = myocardial infarction

Table III. Maximum Working Capacity According to Age Range

Age Range, Years	Healthy Subjects			Ischemic Subjects, no MI[a]			Ischemic Subjects with MI[a]		
	No.	Age, Yr. Value ± S.D.[b]	Max. Work Capacity, kpm/min Value ± S.D.[b]	No.	Age, Yr. Value ± S.D.[b]	Max. Work Capacity, kpm/min Value ± S.D.[b]	No.	Age, Yr. Value ± S.D.[b]	Max. Work Capacity, kpm/min Value ± S.D.[b]
10-19	3	18.3 ± 0.6	1453 ± 692						
20-29	33	26.9 ± 1.9	1296 ± 263				1	28.0 ± 0.0	984 ± 0
30-39	127	35.0 ± 2.8	1132 ± 314	12	34.2 ± 2.8	992 ± 143	2	39.0 ± 0.0	1043 ± 164
40-49	125	44.2 ± 2.8	1046 ± 291	21	44.7 ± 2.5	998 ± 226	24	45.9 ± 2.5	788 ± 258
50-59	51	53.6 ± 2.8	979 ± 263	26	53.4 ± 2.3	913 ± 203	36	54.0 ± 2.7	727 ± 325
60-69	7	62.0 ± 2.1	850 ± 264	8	63.1 ± 2.6	874 ± 258	11	62.2 ± 2.2	565 ± 244

[a]MI = myocardial infarction

[b]S.D. = standard deviation

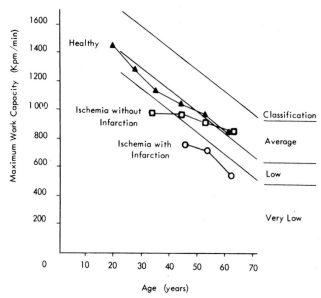

FIG. 2. Regression of maximum work capacity on age compared to performance classification of Åstrand.

average, low and very low are indicated on the graph. The decrease in WLmax of our healthy subjects closely parallels the limits of the low performance class of Åstrand. An inverse linear relationship between age and WLmax is apparent for each class of subjects.

The healthy subjects of our study were classified according to their maximal physical work capacity adjusted for age. Characteristics of maximum work capacity, age and concentration of plasma lipids (cholesterol and triglycerides) for each physical performance class are given in Table IV. No significant differences were found in the mean age of the subjects of the different performance classes. The differences in mean cholesterol and triglyceride concentrations were found to be also insignificant.

Biochemical data obtained before and within one minute after acute exercise are summarized in Table V. Mean values and standard deviations of total lipids, triglycerides, total cholesterol and plasma glucose are shown according to each subject class. Plasma lipids and glucose concentrations increased immediately after exercise. Mean value differences are statistically insignificant. The response of glucose concentrations to acute exercise varied. Some subjects showed increased glucose values while others exhibited either no change or a decrease.

Table IV. Age, Maximum Work Capacity and
Lipid Concentrations of Healthy Subjects
According to Performance Classification

		Astrand Performance Classification[a]				
		Very Low	*Low*	*Average*	*High*	*Very High*
Number of Subjects		144	64	103	19	16
Age, years	Mean	39.3	42.5	41.1	39.9	44.9
	S.D.[b]	±8.6	±8.7	±9.3	±10.7	±7.4
Maximum work	Mean	838	1048	1294	1548	1763
capacity, kpm/min	S.D.[b]	±161	±150	±181	±173	±222
Cholesterol	Mean	236	231	233	252	235
mg%	S.D.[b]	±53	±51	±45	±49	±63
Triglycerides	Mean	143	169	115	139	121
mg%	S.D.[b]	±115	±187	±62	±84	±62

[a]The work performance classifications were made according to work-level ranges
after an appropriate transformation from Astrand oxygen uptake values.
[b]S.D. = standard deviation

Changes in the plasma total lipids, triglycerides and cholesterol,
body weight and predicted WLmax for those persons on a reconditioning exercise program are summarized in Table VI. Changes in
the parameters were taken as the difference between initial values
and those most recently obtained. These differences are statistically
insignificant. No statistical trends were found which would support a
direct relationship between improved WLmax and plasma lipid
concentrations.

Table V. Average Values of Total Lipids, Triglycerides, Total Cholesterol
and Blood Glucose Taken Before and One Minute After Exercise

			Blood Fraction, Milligrams Percent							
Subject Classifi- cation	*No.*		*Total Lipids*		*Tri- glycerides*		*Total Cholesterol*		*Glucose*	
			Pre	*Post*	*Pre*	*Post*	*Pre*	*Post*	*Pre*	*Post*
Healthy subjects	24	Mean	634	714	109	112	208	231	93	94
		S.D.[a]	±142	±160	±61	±63	±50	±61	±13	±13
Ischemic with- out MI[b]	4	Mean	830	846	327	328	203	217	97	103
		S.D.[a]	±521	±442	±503	±476	±61	±84	±14	±12
Ischemic with MI[b]	34	Mean	665	710	148	157	215	226	107	110
		S.D.[b]	±126	±130	±81	±42	±42	±42	±51	±60

[a]S.D. = standard deviation
[b]MI = myocardial infarction

Table VI. Change in Body Weight, Plasma Lipids and Maximum Work Capacity (WLmax) for Persons in a Cardiac Recondition Exercise Program

Sub- ject	Diagnostic Class[a]	Initial Values					Observation Time	Latest Values				
		WT^b lbs	TL^b mg%	T^b mg%	TC^b mg%	$WLmax^b$ Kpm/min		WT^b lbs	TL^b mg%	T^b mg%	TC^b mg%	$WLmax^b$ Kpm/min
PW	Healthy	134	577	53	195	466	3 yrs 4 mo	137	562	80	228	811
EW	Healthy	160	870	174	223	740	2 yrs 7 mo	155	638	100	212	843
WA	Healthy	173	650	91	283	960	10 mo	173	698	115	290	756
FM	Healthy	175	643	65	237	954	1 yr 3 mo	162	768	68	300	868
DM	IHD w/o MI	162	799	287	222	520	3 yrs 0 mo	163	543	90	199	617
RP	IHD w/o MI	152	551	78	220	1498	3 yrs 3 mo	157	628	87	238	1300
VJ	IHD c̄ MI	168	899	405	217	812	1 yr 5 mo	163	519	207	183	930
CY	IHD c̄ MI	154	850	365	236	571	4 yrs 1 mo	154	594	155	202	627
DN	IHD c̄ MI	180	970	218	256	1265	3 yrs 0 mo	168	567	109	219	1065
JB	IHD c̄ MI	177	776	225	278	615	2 yrs 4 mo	180	420	192	226	645
JM	IHD c̄ MI	156	506	52	173	906	3 yrs 8 mo	155	667	103	169	1009
FH	IHD c̄ MI	155	671	116	243	555	2 yrs 9 mo	149	694	180	273	514
HS	IHD c̄ MI	168	768	295	187	717	2 yrs 10 mo	160	719	288	237	697
	Mean	162.6	733.1	186.5	228.5	813.8		159.7	616.7	136.5	228.9	821.7
	± S.D.[c]	12.7	144.8	122.7	32.6	304.0		10.8	95.2	64.2	39.4	216.6

[a]IHD w/o MI = ischemic without myocardial infarction; IHD c̄ MI = ischemic with myocardial infarction
[b]WT = weight; TL = total lipids; T = triglycerides; TC = total cholesterol; WLmax = maximum work capacity
[c]S.D. = standard deviation

Discussion

Patients with clinical or electrocardiographic signs of IHD but without MI had higher plasma lipids concentrations compared to those observed in healthy subjects. Patients with MI had also higher lipid concentrations. Epidemiological and clinical studies support the contention that patients with coronary heart disease have a high prevalence of hyperlipidemia as compared to healthy subjects without the disease. The difference in cholesterol concentrations between healthy persons and those with coronary heart disease has been reported to be greater in younger persons [6]. Concomitant with the increased lipid concentrations, patients with coronary heart disease exhibited a decreased physical work capacity. In our data, no significant correlations were found between the lipid values and WLmax when all subjects were treated jointly or as groups having comparable age.

When comparisons are established between patients and healthy males of comparable age, the differences in lipid concentration disappear. This lack of differences in lipid concentrations between our patients with MI and healthy subjects may have, at least in part, occurred as a result of dietary manipulation. The patients with MI were referred for evaluation two or more months after having their infarction. During this time they were subjected to diets low in fats and cholesterol. An increase in plasma lipids with age was found. This finding is in agreement with Fredrickson et al [3] who documented an increase in concentration of plasma lipids with increasing age. Patients having functional signs of IHD were older than the healthy subjects. The differences in lipid concentrations between patient groups and healthy subjects correspond with the differences in ages. This is especially true for values of total cholesterol. Plasma triglycerides being more variable did not show a definite trend with age.

Age differences with subjects composing the groups may in part account for the differences in physical work capacity between groups. The physical work capacity of individuals was shown by Åstrand to decrease with age. For the healthy males of the present study, the regression of work capacity on age closely parallels that predicted by Åstrand's data. Only small differences occurred in physical work capacity of our IHD patients without a previous MI and healthy subjects of the same age. The IHD patients without a MI were on the average older than the healthy subjects and should be expected to have a lower capacity for physical work. For those patients of this study having a previous MI, an age-related decrease in work capacity was observed, although the values were considerably lower than those observed in patients without MI and healthy subjects. The patients with MI were older than the other two groups, but the age difference would not account totally for the lower WLmax. An impairment of their capacity for physical work is probably the consequence of their clinical condition.

The healthy persons of this study were of varied physical condition with the majority exhibiting a very low WLmax. The mean ages and cholesterol values of the five physical performance classes do not show an apparent distinction with physical work performance. It seems logical to assume that the person of above average daily physical activity would fall within a higher physical performance class, while the less active would fall in a lower class. If this assumption is true, then it would follow that above average daily physical activity does not reduce plasma cholesterol concentrations. Triglycerides tend to be lower in the classes of highest work performance. The lower triglyceride values may be a response to the higher physical activity of this group, for it has been shown [4] that the free fatty acids of triglycerides are energy substrates during energy demands of working muscles.

Acute exercise in this study was found not to effect a significant change in the concentration of plasma lipids and glucose. The changes were found not to correlate with the attained heart rate, maximum work performed, nor the total amount of work performed. Keppler et al [5] reported that the form of exercise is important in eliciting changes in plasma free fatty acids and glucose. Short periods of exercise (six minutes or less) and interval exercise (exercise interrupted by rest) were found not to induce changes in either glucose or free fatty acids. Each period of the exercise stress test lasts for six minutes or less and is interspersed by a rest period of the same duration.

All persons participating in the reconditioning exercise program showed subjective improvement in their physical well-being. Although most of these have shown an improved capacity for physical work, others have remained stable, or even decreased. The prime factor for not improving or actually showing a decreased tolerance to physical work appears to be a lack of adherence to the prescribed program. No statistical trends were found to support a direct relationship between a change in WLmax and changes in plasma lipid concentrations. In general, plasma total lipids decreased while in the program. It would be speculative to assume that these changes are entirely the result of exercise, since other factors such as improved dietary habits and weight loss may have intervened in the lipid change process.

Summary and Conclusions

The subjects included in this study showed an increase in plasma lipids with increasing age. When comparisons were made between healthy subjects and those with ischemia of a comparable age, no difference in plasma lipid concentrations was found. The physical work capacity of all subjects decreased with increasing age. Small differences in physical work capacity were found when comparing the healthy subjects with those of the same approximate age but with clinical or electrocardiographic signs of ischemia and no history of myocardial infarction. Patients having had a previous myocardial infarction demonstrated a greatly reduced capacity for physical work.

No direct correlation between plasma lipid concentrations and WLmax was observed. The healthy subjects regardless of the level of the WLmax exhibited similar concentrations of plasma lipids. When the healthy subjects were classified into five groups according to their WLmax (very low, low, average, high and very high), the mean age of the groups was practically the same. This suggests that the absence of statistical difference in plasma lipid concentrations among groups which exhibited significant differences in work capacity was most probably due to the fact that the mean age of the groups was the same. Thus, age is a factor to be taken into consideration when comparing program results.

Active participation in a reconditioning exercise program resulted in an increased working capacity over time for some subjects. There was a decrease in plasma lipids, particularly triglycerides, in over half the subjects participating in the reconditioning program but this was not related to changes in work capacity.

The effect of acute exercise on plasma lipids or glucose, as it might be evidenced by measurements taken before and after the exercise stress test, was not statistically significant. In a few subjects who demonstrated marked change in one or more lipid values, the change was not related to either the intensity or duration of work performed. The fact that each level of exercise was of brief duration may have contributed to the lack of plasma lipid changes.

References

1. Astrand, P. and Rodahl, K.: Textbook of Work Physiology. New York: McGraw-Hill Book Company, 1970.

2. Cardus, D.: A computerized unit for a cardiac rehabilitation program. Arch.
   Phys. Med. Rehab. 52:416-421, 1971.
3. Fredrickson, D.S. et al: Fat transport in lipoproteins — an integrated
   approach to mechanisms and disorders. N. Engl. J. Med. 276:151, 1967.
4. Froberg, S.O.: Metabolism of lipids in blood and tissue during exercise. *In*
   Poortmans, J.R. (ed.): Biochemistry of Exercise, Vol. III. Baltimore:
   University Park Press, 1968, pp. 100-113.
5. Keppler, D., Keul, J. and Doll, E.: The influence of the form of exercise on
   the arterial concentrations of glucose, lactate, pyruvate, and free fatty acids.
   In Poortmans, J.R. (ed.): Biochemistry of Exercise, Vol. III. Baltimore:
   University Park Press, 1968, pp. 130-136.
6. Page, I.H. and Stamler, J.: Diet and coronary heart disease. Mod. Concepts
   Cardiovasc. Dis. 9:119, 1968.

The Effects of Variation in Diet and Intensity of Exercise on Blood Lactate Levels and Performance Time

B. C. Scully

Introduction

Several investigations have found that a high-carbohydrate diet will enhance performance by increasing muscle glycogen stores [2, 6, 19, 25]. Recent studies indicate that the white, intermediate and red muscle fiber loses its ability to produce tension as glycogen is depleted [5, 10, 11, 20, 25]. Other investigations suggest that the accumulation of lactic acid will inhibit performance [13, 14, 16, 17, 24, 30], and a few studies have reported that blood lactate is affected by diet [26, 29].

It is known that glycogen is the primary substrate for energy metabolism when energy requirements approach the limit of an individual's maximum aerobic capacity. Hultman and others [19] have shown that ingesting a high-carbohydrate diet two to three days prior to an endurance event will enhance performance. Little is known of the effect of diet on short exhaustive performances such as those which have great energy requirements for a few minutes. Such performances would necessitate anaerobic energy metabolism, glycogenolysis, and could be limited by substrate availability. Some investigators have stated that increasing glycogen stores would not enhance performance [14]. Others have reported an increase in anaerobic performance when subjects "carbohydrate loaded" [1].

The gap in the available information about diet, lactic acid accumulation and performance during acute exercise has generated the need for this investigation. The purpose of this investigation was to determine the effect of three dietary treatments (normal mixed, low carbohydrate, and high carbohydrate) and two intensities of exercise (85% of subjects' $\dot{V}O_2$ max and 110% of subjects' $\dot{V}O_2$ max) on blood lactate levels and performance times.

B. C. Scully, Department of Health and Physical Education, University of New Orleans, New Orleans, Louisiana, U.S.A.

Dietary Assignments and Procedures

Informed consent was obtained from 12 male University of Northern Colorado students enrolled in the graduate physical education program. The subjects' ages ranged from 23 to 36. The subjects' maximum aerobic capacity ($\dot{V}O_2$ max) was determined by administering a modified Balke running $\dot{V}O_2$ max test on a horizontal, motor-driven treadmill. The subjects' expired gas was collected in a 120-liter tissot gas collection tank. The analysis of subjects' expired gas was made by the Scholander micrometric technique [28]. The subjects' $\dot{V}O_2$ max was expressed in milliliters per minute per kilogram of body weight (ml/min/kg). The maximal capacities for the subjects ranged from 39.38 to 65.25 ml/min/kg with a mean of 52.93 ± 8.5 ml/min/kg. The weight of the subjects was between 65.23 and 97.73 with a mean of 76.05 ± 9.2 kg.

Relative workbout intensities of 85% $\dot{V}O_2$ max and 110% $\dot{V}O_2$ max were calculated using the Balke energy cost approximation method [3, 23]. The duration of each exercise bout was five minutes or until the subject became fatigued. Fatigue was defined as the point at which the subject was unable to keep pace on the treadmill.

All subjects were randomly assigned to three different dietary treatments: normal mixed (NM) which consisted of approximately 65% carbohydrates, 25% to 30% protein and 5% to 10% fat; high carbohydrate (HC) which contained 90% carbohydrate with the remainder protein and fat; low carbohydrate (LC) which was composed of 95% proteins and fats and 5% carbohydrates.

Food lists and their respective protein, fat and carbohydrate values were taken from a publication prepared by the Scripps Research Institute [8] and paralleled those of previous investigations [2, 6, 18, 26].

The subjects ingested each diet for one full week to insure adequate adaptation [25, 27]. The first exercise bout, either 85% of $\dot{V}O_2$ or 110% of $\dot{V}O_2$ max, whichever was randomly assigned, was performed on the fifth day of the assigned diet and the second exercise bout was performed on the seventh day of that diet. After both workbouts had been completed, the subject began the next dietary assignment.

Test Methods and Procedures

The experimental proceedings lasted approximately one month, or until each subject had completed the three different dietary treatments. Each subject performed his running exercise bouts in a postprandial state. The bed of the treadmill was horizontal and the speed of the bed corresponded to the treatment prescribed as stated above. At the command, "Go," the subject began running his five-minute exercise bout. The subject was timed throughout the exercise bout to insure exercise bout length or to determine performance time to fatigue. During the fourth minute of the workbout, or when the subject signaled oncoming fatigue, the subject's expired gas was collected and analyzed for CO_2 content and O_2 content to determine the energy cost for each workbout.

A blood sample was taken by the prewarmed fingertip puncture method using a lancet. The blood was collected in micropipettes three to four minutes after the exercise bout had terminated. This has been shown to be sufficient time for blood lactate to peak [24].

The blood sample was deproteinized in TCA, spun down in a centrifuge, and the supernate analyzed using the Barker-Summerson Technique [4]. The optical density of each sample was read on a Basch-Lomb 600 series spectrophotometer at wave length 560. The blood lactate data and time of workbouts were subjected to an analysis of variance as described by Lindquist [22]. Probability levels were recorded.

Results

A three-way analysis of variance, treatment by levels by subjects, was used to determine treatment differences on blood lactate levels. Table I shows measures of central tendency on blood lactate levels.

Blood lactates were significantly higher at 110% $\dot{V}O_2$ max than at 85% $\dot{V}O_2$ max, $P < 0.01$. Treatment differences produced an F which was significant at $P < 0.01$. The Duncan Multiple Range test

Table I. Effect of Diet and Intensity of Exercise
on Blood Lactate Levels

Treatments	$\overline{X}$ (Mean)	S.D. (Standard Deviation)	S.E. (Standard Error)
T_1 (85%; N.M.)	47.75	13.515	3.901
T_2 (110%; N.M.)	83.75	36.159	10.438
T_3 (85%; L.C.)	45.23	11.116	3.208
T_4 (110%; L.C.)	85.83	26.652	7.694
T_5 (85%; H.C.)	48.58	13.178	3.804
T_6 (110%; H.C.)	108.53*	23.570	6.804

* $p < 0.01$.

was used for multiple comparisons to determine which treatments accounted for the significant F. There were no significant differences between treatment blood lactate means at 85% of $\dot{V}O_2$ max. At 110% $\dot{V}O_2$ max, the HC blood lactate mean was significantly higher (P < 0.01) than the 110% $\dot{V}O_2$ NM or LC blood lactate means. There was no significant difference between blood lactate mean scores for the NM treatment and LC treatment at 110% of $\dot{V}O_2$ max. Figure 1 illustrates the mean blood lactate response to dietary treatment and intensity of exercise.

All subjects were able to perform the five minute exercise bout at 85% $\dot{V}O_2$ max regardless of their dietary treatment. A two-way analysis of variance for treatment performance times produced a between-treatment F which was significant, P < 0.04. The Scheffé multiple comparison was used to determine treatment differences of mean performance times. Table II shows measures of central tendency of treatment performance times.

There was no significant difference between performance times for the LC and NM diets at 110% $\dot{V}O_2$ max. There was no significant difference between performance for NM and HC diets at 110% $\dot{V}O_2$ max. There was significant difference between the HC and LC mean performance time, P < 0.04. Figure 2 illustrates the mean treatment performance time at 110% of $\dot{V}O_2$ max.

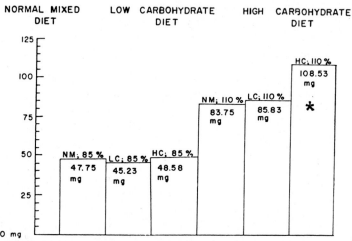

FIG. 1. Histogram of mean blood lactate levels relative to diet and intensity of performance. (mg/100ml Hb) *P < 0.01.

Table II. Mean Performance Treatment Time (in sec.) at 110% $\dot{V}O_2$ Max

Treatment	$\overline{X}$ (mean)	S.D. (Standard Deviation)	S.E. (Standard Error)
Normal Mixed; 110%	194.25	69.763	20.1389
Low Carbohydrate; 110%	186.85	71.1288	20.5331
High Carbohydrate; 110%	199.767*	65.0766	18.786

* p < 0.04

MEAN PERFORMANCE TIMES AT 110% MAX $\dot{V}O_2$
RELATIVE TO DIETARY TREATMENT

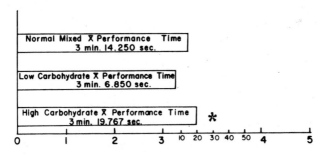

FIG. 2. Histogram of mean treatment performance times (in sec) at 110% $\dot{V}O_2$ max. *P < 0.04.

Discussion

The phenomenon of muscle fatigue has been an area of intense investigation by researchers for many years. In sports performances which are of an endurance nature, fatigue may be due to the following: lactic acid accumulation in the muscle, hypoglycemia, dehydration, excessive electrolyte losses in sweat, hyperthermia, depletion of muscle glycogen [9]. ⌐

In sports activities which require maximum exertion for approximately 30 seconds or less, the performer is dependent upon the intracellular stores of adenosine triphosphate (ATP) and creatine-phosphate (CP) and the rate of ATPase [12]. In performances which predominantly rely upon anaerobic glycolysis for energy transformation, fatigue may be related to the accumulation of metabolic end products, the lack of metabolic substrates or a combination of the above [14].

More recently Asmussen et al have hypothesized that the inhibition of the glycolytic pathway during supramaximal workloads is a result of the inhibition of the glycogen → glucose-1-phosphate reaction, caused by the accumulation of lactate [1]. Asmussen et al based their hypothesis on the Michaelis-Menton Theory which is applicable to enzyme kinetics and enzyme saturation with substrate [21]. Gollnick et al have hypothesized the possibility of reduced glycogen stores in the white muscle fibers as a limiting factor to supramaximal exercise [15].

The biochemical state of a performer undergoes a complex series of reactions during supramaximal exercise in order to maintain a level of homeostasis. The mechanisms of fatigue in a glycolytic performance may be caused by an accumulation of lactic acid causing an inhibition of pH sensitive enzymes, the concentration of enzymes which oxidize the glycolytic substrates, the concentration of substrate present in the individual muscle fibers, the intrinsic catalytic property of the enzyme-substrate set, i.e., Km and V max, or a combination of the above.

Due to the similarity in results between the present study and the work of Asmussen et al [1], the control of the glycolytic pathway could not be entirely governed by the accumulation of lactic acid. The variability in the dietary treatment mean scores of blood lactate indicates that the accumulation of lactate at the same relative workload is substrate dependent. Apparently intramuscular pH is not involved to a great extent, since the fatigue occurred at widely varying concentrations of lactate in the same individuals for the different dietary treatments.

According to the Michaelis-Menton Theory, the concentration of enzymes which oxidize the glycolytic substrates is dependent upon the concentration of substrate present. When there is a low concentration of substrate in the muscle fibers, as in such cases as depleted muscle glycogen stores from work or by diet, there may be a low concentration of catabolic enzymes in the glycogenolytic pathway [21]. The opposite may also be true, i.e., that an increase in endogenous glycogen stores might increase the catabolic enzymes involved in the oxidation of that substrate. The significance of this mechanism, should it occur, has yet to be established.

Based on the results of this study, the results of Asmussen et al and the work of Burke and Edgerton [7], it is suggested that the principal limiting factor to a single anaerobically glycogenolytic exercise bout to the fatigue point is the pre-exercise concentration of glycogen in the motor units involved.

Conclusions

It is apparent that the traditional practice of ingesting high protein-low carbohydrate diets for the purpose of enhancing athletic performance does indeed inhibit the performer by detracting from available substrate stores. When an athletic performance is anaerobic by virtue of the oxygen requirement for that task, increased glycogen stores will increase performance. The present investigation revealed no significant difference in anaerobic exercise bouts between NM and HC dietary treatment even though the HC mean performance time was 5.517 seconds longer than the NM dietary treatment. The poorest performance times were produced when subjects ingested LC diets and exercised at 110% $\dot{V}O_2$ max. This is suggestive that individuals who engage in such sport performances which are highly dependent upon anaerobic glycolysis should consume a diet which is high (80% plus) in carbohydrates for at least 48 to 60 hours prior to that performance. This will insure enough time to replenish or increase endogenous glycogen stores in those muscle fibers which have a lower oxidative capacity [25].

Acknowledgments

This paper was part of a doctoral dissertation completed at the University of Northern Colorado, Greeley, Colorado, April 1975. Special thanks are given to Richard A. Peterson, Ph.D., who acted as research adviser. Appreciation is expressed to Mrs. Becky Mayo and Mrs. Yvonne Cullen for their assistance in the preparation of this manuscript.

References

1. Asmussen, E., Klausen, K., Nielson, L.E. et al: Lactate production and anaerobic work capacity after prolonged exercise. Acta Physiol. Scand. 90:731-742, 1974.
2. Astrand, P.-O. and Rodahl, K.: Textbook of Work Physiology. New York:McGraw-Hill Book Company, 1970.
3. Balke, B.: Personal Communication.
4. Barker, S.B. and Summerson, W.H.: The colorimetric determination of lactic acid in biological material. J. Biolog. Chem. 35:535-537, 1941.
5. Bergstrom, J., Guarnieri, G. and Hultman, E.: Carbohydrate metabolism and electrolyte changes in human skeletal muscle. J. Appl. Physiol. 30:122-125, 1971.
6. Bergstrom, J., Hermansen, L., Hultman, E. and Saltin, B.: Diet, muscle glycogen and physical performance. Acta Physiol. Scand. 71:140-150, 1967.
7. Burke, R.E. and Edgerton, V.R.: Motor unit properties and selective involvement in movement. In Wilmore, J.H. (ed.): Exercise and Sport Sciences Reviews. New York:Academic Press, 1975.

8. Chemical Composition of Food Materials. Scripps Clinic and Research Foundation, La Jolla, Calif., 1970.
9. Costill, D.L.: Muscular exhaustion during distance running. Physician Sports Med. 36-41, October, 1974.
10. Costill, D.L., Gollnick, P.D., Jansson, E.D. et al: Glycogen depletion patterns in human muscle fibres during distance running. Acta Physiol. Scand. 89:374-383, 1973.
11. Edstrom, L. and Kugelberg, E.: Histochemical composition, distribution of fibres and fatigability of single motor units: Anterior tibial muscle of the rat. J. Neurol. Psychiat. 31:424-433, 1968.
12. Faulkner, J.A.: Muscle fatigue. In Briskey, E.J., Cassens, R.G. and Marsh, B.B. (eds.): The Physiology and Biochemistry of Muscle as a Food. Madison, Wisc.:University of Wisconsin Press, 1970.
13. Fitts, R.H. and Booth, F.W.: Relationship between muscle fatigue and muscle lactic acid, high energy phosphates and glycogen in electrically stimulated frog muscle. Med. Sci. Sports 6:76, 1974.
14. Gollnick, P.D. and Hermansen, L.: Biochemical adaptations to exercise: Anaerobic metabolism. In Wilmore, J.H. (ed.): Exercise and Sport Sciences Reviews. New York:Academic Press, 1973.
15. Gollnick, P.D., Piehl, K. and Saltin, B.: Selective glycogen depletion pattern in human muscle fibers after exercise of varying intensity and at varying pedaling rates. J. Physiol. 241:45-57, 1974.
16. Hermansen, L. and Olson, B.-J.: Blood and muscle pH after maximal exercise in man. J. Appl. Physiol. 32:304-308, 1972.
17. Hill, A.V. and Lupton, H.: Muscular exercise, lactic acid, and the supply utilization of oxygen. Q. J. Med. 16:135-171, 1923.
18. Hultman, E.: Physiological role of muscle glycogen in man with special reference to exercise. In Chapman, C.B. (ed.): Physiology of Muscular Exercise. New York:American Heart Association, Inc., Monograph 15, 1967, pp. 101-112.
19. Hultman, E.: Studies on muscle metabolism of glycogen and active phosphate in man with special reference to exercise and diet. Scand. J. Clin. Invest. 19, Supplement 94, 1967.
20. Kugelberg, E. and Edstrom, L.: Differential histochemical effects of muscle contractions on phosphorylase and glycogen in various types of fibres: Relation to fatigue. J. Neurol. Neurosurg. Psychiat. 31:415-423, 1968.
21. Lehninger, A.L.: Biochemistry, ed. 3. New York:Worth Publishers, Inc., 1971.
22. Lindquist, E.F.: Design and Analysis of Experiments in Psychology and Education. Boston, Mass.:Houghton Mifflin Co., 1953.
23. Nagle, F., Balke, B., Baptista, G. et al: Compatability of progressive treadmill, bicycle and step tests based on oxygen uptake responses. Med. Sci. Sports 3:149-154, 1971.
24. Osnes, J.-B. and Hermansen, L.: Acid-base balance after maximal exercise of short duration. J. Appl. Physiol. 32(1):59-63, 1972.
25. Piehl, K.: Glycogen storage and depletion in human skeletal muscle fibers. Acta Physiol. Scand. Suppl. 401, 5-32, 1974.
26. Pruett, E.D.R.: Glucose and insulin during prolonged work stress in men living on different diets. J. Appl. Physiol. 28:199-208, 1970.

27. Saltin, B. and Hermansen, L.: Glycogen stores and prolonged severe exercise. Symposium on Nutrition and Physical Activity. Uppsula:Almquist and Niksell, 1967, pp. 32-46.
28. Scholander, P.F.: Analyzer for accurate estimation of respiratory gases in one-half cubic centimeter samples. J. Biol. Chem. 167:No. 1, January 1947.
29. Wasserman, K.: Lactate and related acid base and blood gas changes during constant load and graded exercise. Can. Med. J. 96:775-779, 1967.
30. Weiser, P.C.: Alteration in enzyme activity in work and fatigue. *In* Simonson, E. (ed.): Physiology of Work Capacity and Fatigue. Springfield, Ill.: Charles C Thomas, 1971.

Effects on Fractionated Reaction Time of Sustained Movement to Deplete Metabolic Carbohydrate

John D. Brooke

Introduction

It has been noted over the years [6, 9] that when sustained hard exercise over hours results in depletion of body carbohydrate (CHO) stores, provision of dietary digestible CHO at exhaustion results subsequently in further exercise being possible, even though changes are not seen in the proportions of CHO to fats combusted at the active skeletal muscle. Also Brooke, Davies and Green [4] and Benade et al [2] note that with the provision of glucose syrup or sucrose drinks during such sustained exercise, the efficiency of work increases (decreased $\dot{V}O_2$ per W external) beyond that expected by application of the common calorimetry formula for kJ energy provision per l O_2 per RQ, e.g., Carpenter [8]. In such conditions it may be proposed that while local supply of muscle glycogen plays a major limiting role, part of the effect of metabolic availability of CHO may be upon neural function [1]. Glucose is the primary fuel for nerve cells and at blood glucose levels below approximately 75 mg 100 ml^{-1} hypoglycemic symptoms can occur [12]. Therefore, it was decided to investigate neural change in the intact normal human maintaining such sustained movement, specifically: Is there a deleterious effect upon the reaction time (RT) and upon its premotor and motor components of exercise depletion of body CHO stores and does dietary digestible CHO supplementation during and after such exercise limit this deterioration?

Method

Six male racing cyclist subjects in training, mean age 23 years, took part in four trials with ten days between each trial. Subjects worked in the evenings in groups of three, with onsets of exercise being approximately 15 minutes apart.

John D. Brooke, Department of Human Kinetics, College of Biological Science, University of Guelph, Ontario, Canada.

Pre and post (P-P) each exercise session measures were taken of blood glucose (G) by micro sampling of capillary blood, with duplicate sample replicability and also accuracy ± 2.0 mg 100 ml^{-1}, resting respiratory quotient (RQ) [4] by Douglas bag collection, within trial replicability 0.65 and FRT [6]. For the latter measure a Mingograf 81 ink-jet recorder was used at a paper speed of 250 mm sec^{-1}. Assessed against the 50 Hz mains cycle the time variation was less than 0.4% over 180 mm. Recordings were made at 700 Hz with a 500 μ V 10 mm^{-1} amplitude shift. Within trial replicability is shown in the standard errors reported in Table II.

A light source reaction time stimulus of duration ls was used with response via flexor digitorum 3 to a micro-switch, minimum depression force 53.3 gm. Prior to the stimulus a preparatory interval randomly varied in the range of 2.0 to 4.0 s was used via a warning light. The electromyogram of the active flexor was obtained using two 10-mm domed silver disc surface electrodes sighted 20 mm apart over the belly of the muscle. The skin site was prepared as described by Brooke et al [3] so that interference from skin resistance was low, as shown in Figure 1. It can be seen from Figure 1 that for data analysis the total reaction time (RT) was split into premotor (PMT) and motor (MT) components by reference to the onset of the neural activity. RT measures were made immediately before and 30 minutes after the exercise.

Before RT measures, subjects rested quietly for 20 minutes, were equipped with emg electrodes over five minutes and then were

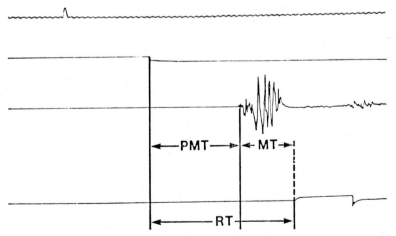

FIG. 1. Recording of reaction time (RT) premotor time (PMT) and motor time (MT), paper speed 250 mm s^{-1}.

tested. Ten habituation measures were made followed without break by 23 measures of which the first 20 were used as data. Where recording was unclear the measure(s) were discarded and the three reserve measures in serial seniority were used. The data from the measures were obtained by measurement to 0.5 mm from the paper trace.

The movement for each subject was standardized across treatments. Subjects rode their own racing cycles coupled to Ergowheel cycle ergometers [5] at a load to elicit a heart rate of approximately 160 beats min^{-1} (i.e., approximately 70% $\dot{V}O_2$ max evoked) until incapable of further movement at that load. The mean trial time was 186 minutes, standard deviation 41 minutes.

Before trials, subjects followed an approximate seven-hour fast alleviated by limited sugarless coffee or tea ingestion. Three dietary regimens were allocated randomly to subjects over trials to obtain a complete design. In one regimen (A), no food was taken during or after the exercise, i.e., prior to the postexercise measure of reaction time. In a second regimen (B), a drink of 66 ml of 30% wv^{-1} glucose syrup solution (energy value 240 kJ) was taken by subjects every 20 minutes during exercise. In a third regimen (C) 66 ml of such drink was taken at the cessation of exercise. Following the third trial and in the light of the stable individual differences appearing, a fourth regimen (D) was presented in a similar manner as before to subjects and constituted a further control of 66 ml of low energy drink (> 5 kJ) taken by subjects as in (B). Diets were under double-blind control. Water was available ad libitum during all rides. Over the experiment, the laboratory ambient temperature was maintained in the range 22 C to 25 C and air fans were used to keep subjects cool.

RT data were analyzed by two-way analyses of variance to assess the significance of differences between mean values for the four treatments (diets) and the two conditions (pre vs. postexercise) with 20 data points per treatment condition per subject. When significance relevant to the research problem resulted, orthogonal comparisons of treatment means were made [10]. Due to marked and stable differences between subjects in time of reaction, the statistical analyses were made for each subject separately.

Results

P-P changes over treatments, means and standard errors for subjects as a group are shown for G in Figure 2 and for RQ in Table 1.

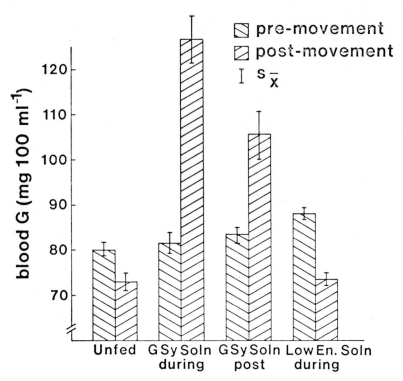

FIG. 2. Mean blood glucose pre vs. postsustained movement under four dietary regimens (n = 6).

Table I. Change in Respiratory Quotients P – P Movement
Under Four Dietary Regimens (n = 6)

	Unfed		Glucose During Work		Glucose Post Work		Low Energy During Work	
	$\bar{x}$	$s_{\bar{x}}$	$\bar{x}$	$s_{\bar{x}}$	$\bar{x}$	$s_{\bar{x}}$	$\bar{x}$	$s_{\bar{x}}$
Pre-post fall	0.05		0.08		0.10		0.06	
Pre value	0.82	0.07	0.90	0.05	0.91	0.05	0.89	0.10
Post value	0.77	0.03	0.82	0.03	0.81	0.01	0.83	0.15

P-P changes in RT, PMT and MT, means and standard errors, for subjects separately over treatments are shown in Table II. Resulting significant differences between means of treatments and of conditions are recorded in Table III.

Table II. Descriptive Statistics for Fractionated Reaction Time (ms) (n_t = 20) on Four Diets (A, B, C, D)

| Subject | Condition | Stat. | Reaction Time | | | | FRT Component | | | | | | | |
| | | | | | | | Premotor Time | | | | Motor Time | | | |
			A	B	C	D	A	B	C	D	A	B	C	D
1	Pre	$\bar{x}$	285	298	287	304	218	219	211	241	68	79	74	63
		$s_{\bar{x}}$	6.5	4.1	4.8	3.0	5.9	4.4	3.9	3.2	1.6	1.7	2.1	1.5
	Post	$\bar{x}$	256	323	299	355	200	245	230	274	57	78	69	81
		$s_{\bar{x}}$	3.5	7.2	10.1	8.9	3.4	7.1	9.6	9.4	1.3	3.6	1.7	2.2
2	Pre	$\bar{x}$	262	250	309	323	201	189	205	219	62	58	104	105
		$s_{\bar{x}}$	4.8	6.4	8.8	7.5	4.2	4.3	5.3	4.3	4.7	4.8	7.7	6.5
	Post	$\bar{x}$	417	291	356	376	277	193	222	252	141	99	137	123
		$s_{\bar{x}}$	21.1	12.6	15.4	8.5	21.4	4.5	4.8	5.4	10.5	12.1	13.9	5.8
3	Pre	$\bar{x}$	400	386	390	400	289	277	275	276	117	109	115	124
		$s_{\bar{x}}$	17.6	15.9	10.1	7.6	8.2	13.8	10.5	4.5	13.4	6.0	8.8	5.3
	Post	$\bar{x}$	472	383	390	438	290	269	257	300	180	114	133	131
		$s_{\bar{x}}$	14.1	11.4	14.7	22.2	9.6	8.8	10.7	17.2	9.4	4.3	12.0	7.7
4	Pre	$\bar{x}$	316	323	323	275	178	209	202	188	122	113	120	86
		$s_{\bar{x}}$	14.6	15.4	15.0	9.1	3.2	8.2	5.6	3.8	14.7	13.0	13.8	8.3

Table II. Descriptive Statistics for Fractionated Reaction Time (ms) (n_t = 20) on Four Diets (A, B, C, D) (Continued)

Subject	Condition	Stat.	Reaction Time				FRT Component Premotor Time				Motor Time			
			A	B	C	D	A	B	C	D	A	B	C	D
	Post	$\bar{x}$	312	339	328	311	203	191	189	182	109	148	139	129
		$s_{\bar{x}}$	12.2	17.8	11.3	20.9	5.5	5.9	3.6	4.0	9.1	17.4	11.6	18.9
5	Pre	$\bar{x}$	277	328	324	274	201	265	255	214	74	73	70	60
		$s_{\bar{x}}$	6.6	7.7	12.0	7.1	6.0	7.2	11.2	6.2	2.0	2.3	2.8	1.5
	Post	$\bar{x}$	317	312	326	290	218	241	259	216	99	73	68	74
		$s_{\bar{x}}$	9.7	9.5	9.3	10.9	9.3	8.0	9.2	8.6	6.9	2.3	1.6	4.9
6	Pre	$\bar{x}$	319	319	317	300	232	216	227	173	88	103	90	128
		$s_{\bar{x}}$	8.6	11.3	10.9	15.1	8.0	6.1	12.3	6.6	2.9	9.1	3.7	13.3
	Post	$\bar{x}$	355	347	335	305	238	243	225	205	125	107	116	100
		$s_{\bar{x}}$	18.6	15.3	17.3	12.3	8.0	13.6	7.6	12.5	13.6	8.2	12.8	5.3

Table III. All Significant Effects (p ≥ .01 or ≥ .05) From Orthogonal Comparisons of Hypothesized Differences Between Means

	Temporal Component of Responses											
	Reaction Time				Premotor Time				Motor Time			
	Pre-Post Diet				Pre-Post Diet				Pre-Post Diet			
Subject	A	B	C	D	A	B	C	D	A	B	C	D
s_1	.01 (+)	.01 (−)		.01 (−)	.05 (+)	.01 (−)	.01 (−)	.01 (−)	.01 (+)			.01 (−)
s_2	.01 (−)*	.01 (−)	.01 (−)	.01 (−)*	.01 (−)†			.01 (−)†	.01 (−)	.01 (−)	.01 (−)	
	Overall P-P .01 (−)				Overall P-P .05 (−)				Overall P-P .01 (−)			
s_3	.01 (−)			.05 (−)					.01 (−)			
s_4					.01 (−)	.05 (+)						
s_5	.01 (−)					.05 (+)			.01 (−)			.01 (−)
s_6								.05 (−)	.01 (−)			.05 (+)

* post values A vs. D sign. diff. p.05
† post values A vs. D sign. diff. p.01
p change hypothesized (see text)
(+) post faster than pre value
(−) post slower than pre value

Discussion

From the G and RQ measures, it is clear that the metabolic status of the subjects corresponded to their dietary intake, with much raised G levels and raised RQ after diets during work and somewhat raised G and RQ after one glucose syrup intake postwork. Without dietary supplementation or with low energy intake, levels of CHO available or combusted were characteristically low after exercise.

From Table III it can be seen that significant pre vs. postchanges in mean values for reaction time or its subcomponents occur for a number of subjects. In only one case, S_2, is an overall P-P deterioration seen and that in all 3 FRT components. Other P-P changes are linked to either CHO diet or ingestion vs. no ingestion. Subject 2 shows in premotor time the hypothesized deterioration under such metabolic CHO depletion, with alleviation of the effect by in- or postmovement feeding of digestible CHO, the latter being not simply an ingestion experimental effect. The same subject in reaction time shows similar deterioration, with a dietary alleviation of this effect occurring that appears to be partly an experimental effect of ingestion and partly attributable to the CHO ingestion.

Similarly S_5 in motor time and S_3 in reaction time show effects in the direction hypothesized and the responses of S_4 in premotor time may be interpreted in the same way. For the latter, movement-evoked CHO depletion deteriorates PMT, CHO ingestion during the sustained movement reverses the effect and mere ingestion has an experimental effect which is significantly less than that for CHO ingestion and which merely eliminates the P-P deterioration of the unfed condition. In these cases for subjects 2, 3, 4 and 5 deterioration of response time occurs with movement-evoked depletion of metabolic CHO, with the deterioration completely or partly alleviated by digestible CHO ingestion.

In contrast, S_1 shows a reverse effect. For RT and PMT metabolic CHO depletion speeds up response time, and ingestion, stomach filling or subsequent processes per se (CHO or low energy) result in deterioration of response. This effect for this subject is stable (note standard error) and significant.

Extending further the discussion of individual differences, S_6 shows little change that can be considered meaningful.

It is clear that in the present results stable individual differences exist in (a) overall susceptibility to the effect of metabolic CHO depletion under the present regimen, (b) in the appearance of this effect when it occurs and (c) in its alleviation by appropriate diet. This is not wholly unexpected, for McDonald [13] suggested in the context of CHO ingestion and disease that only a proportion of the population may be "sensitive" to CHO. The present results taken from "normal," i.e., clinically healthy, humans in "normal" performance support such a suggestion.

These individual differences are not related to differences in the postexercise levels of blood glucose or RQ, CHO fed or not, nor are they related to work times before exhaustion or to total power output.

As with other evidence of individual differences in carbohydrate metabolic pathways, e.g., those seen in glucose tolerance, it is clear that with the present marked differences between the subjects and between the temporal components of response attention must be given to characterizing such "normal" differences, for example, by hormone profile, by previous adaptation, by identification of threshold levels of other control mechanisms, etc., in order to interpret adequately the effects at present uncovered.

It should be noted that when effects of CHO depletion occur, they are not necessarily attributable to direct CHO effects on nerve cells. There is substance for considering in addition both changes in central nervous transmitter levels [14] and also attention-commanding effects from the feelings of distress and exhaustion produced by the CHO depletion. Such considerations would account for the continuing postexercise deterioration of S_2 under fed treatments when exhaustion resulted from depletion of active local muscle stores of glycogen with however ample metabolic CHO overall in body stores and in circulation. It would also be in keeping with Brooke, Hamley and Stone's report [7] of reduced sensitivity resulting from exercise exhaustion through partial anaerobiosis.

Acknowledgments

The research was supported by grants from the Science Research Council and from Beecham Products (UK) and was made possible by the cooperation of Mr. H. Nelson (British Cycling Federation Coach), his colleagues and his riders.

References

1. Astrand, P.O.: Interrelations between physical activity and metabolism of carbohydrate, fat and protein. *In* Bliss, G. (ed.): Nutrition and Physical Activity. Uppsala:Almquist and Wikells, 1967.
2. Benade, A.J.S., Wyndham, C.H., Strydom, N.B. and Rogers, C.G.: The physiological effect of mid-shift feed of sucrose. S. Afr. Med. J. 45:711-718, 1971.

3. Brooke, J.D., Cooper, D., Hamley, E.J. and Saville, B.F.: An electromyographical analysis of noxious ischaemic work. Bull. Br. Assoc. Sports Med. 3:26, 1967.
4. Brooke, J.D., Davies, G.J. and Green, L.F.: Nutrition during severe prolonged exercise in trained cyclists. Proc. Nutr. Soc. 31:93, 1972.
5. Brooke, J.D. and Firth, M.S.: Calibration of a simple eddy current ergometer. Br. J. Sports Med. 8, 2:120-125, 1974.
6. Brooke, J.D. and Green, L.F.: The effect of high carbohydrate diet on human recovery following prolonged work to exhaustion. Ergonomics 17:489-497, 1974.
7. Brooke, J.D., Hamley, E.J. and Stone, P.T.: Disturbances of attention and metabolic homeostasis during the performance of an exhausting physical activity. In Whiting, H.T.A. (ed.): Readings in Sports Psychology. London: Kimpton, 1972, pp. 198-211.
8. Carpenter, T.C.: Tables, Factors and Formulas for Computing Respiratory Exchange and Biological Transformations of Energy. Washington:Carnegie Institute, 1964.
9. Christensen, E.H. and Hansen, O.: IV Hypoglykamie, Arbeitsfahigkeit und Ermudung. Scand. Arch. Physiol. 81:137, 1939.
10. Edwards, A.L.: Experimental Design in Psychological Research, ed. 4. New York:Holt, Rinehart and Winston, 1972.
11. Green, L.F.: Blood glucose measurements in field trials. Br. J. Sports Med. 6:116, 1972.
12. Keele, C.A. and Neil, E.: Sampson Wright's Applied Physiology, ed. 12. London:Oxford, 1971.
13. McDonald, I.: Atheroma in various forms of essential hyperlipidaemia. In Stewart, S.S. (ed.): Sugar and Human Health. Maryland: I.S.R.F., 1972, pp. 44-49.
14. Wurtman, R.J. and Fernstrom, J.D.: Effects of the diet on brain neurotransmitters. Nutr. Rev. 32,7:193, 1974.

The Proportion of Proteins, Hemoglobin and Erythrocytes in Urine Subsequent to Overlong Endurance Performances

J. I. Karvonen and A. L. Karvonen

Introduction

The excretion of protein in urine in connection with severe physical strain is considered a normal phenomenon [1, 10]. According to some authors [6, 8] the presence of protein, hemoglobin and erythrocytes in urine may be due to the fact that during physical exertion there is an impairment of renal blood flow and of glomerular filtration, since the blood flow in functioning muscles increases. There is vasoconstriction of the renal arteries resulting in hypoxia of the kidneys as well as a decrease in the blood pH.

The training of an endurance athlete includes running tens of kilometers daily. Thus, according to normal criteria, heavy physical strain is part of the daily routine. In the present study, regularly training endurance athletes were investigated for proteinuria and hematuria during training, i.e., running over 25 km at a high, constant speed and during competition.

Material and Methods

The material comprised 25 competing athletes with long-distance running as their specialty. The urine samples were collected from them after a training run of 25 km or after discontinuing or completing the 100 km of the Suomi-juoksu* race. They were compared with urine samples collected at rest before the events. In addition to albumin, hemoglobin and erythrocytes, ketone bodies,

J. I. Karvonen and A. L. Karvonen, Sport Clinics of Deaconnes Institute, Oulu, Finland.

*Suomi-juoksu is an international running competition which takes place in Hartola, Finland, every year in July. The distance covered is 100 km.

glucose and the specific gravity of the urine were also determined from the samples. The time of disappearance of proteinuria was observed after the 25 km training run. The athletes covered the following distances: eight athletes 25 km, eight athletes 26 to 80 km (those who discontinued the Suomi-juoksu) and nine athletes 100 km.

The urine samples were collected immediately after the performance, stored at +4 C overnight and analyzed in a laboratory on the following morning. After the Suomi-juoksu of 100 km, only one urine sample from each athlete was taken. After the training run of 25 km, the changes in urinary values were followed up for 24 hours. All samples were taken from midstream urine, since the use of a catheter could not be considered in field conditions. The urinary protein was analyzed qualitatively and quantitatively. Hemoglobin determinations were made by spectrophotometry using the oxyhemoglobin absorption spectrum wave length of 415 nm. The erythrocyte count (in a single microscope field) was made using a sample taken from the sediment after centrifugation. The erythrocyte count was considered elevated when the number of erythrocytes in the microscope field was more than three.

Results

The means of the ages, weights, heights and distances covered during training are shown in Table I. The midstream urine from all subjects was normal before the trials. Table II shows that in nine out of 25 athletes investigated (over one third) the daily excretion of protein in urine after training or competition was 0.2 to 3.3 gm. In the athletes who covered 25 km, no protein could be detected in the urine three to four hours after the training was over.

In two athletes participating in the Suomi-juoksu, hemoglobinuria occurred after the competition. One of these who had trained less discontinued after 26 km because of abdominal

Table I. The Means of Ages, Weights, Heights and Distances Covered
During Training in the Athletes Investigated

Distance km	N	Age Years	Weights kg	Height gm	Total Training km/yr
25	8	25 (20-29)	65 (57-80)	176 (170-186)	4357 (3500-6000)
26-80	8	35 (24-60)	64 (59-68)	175 (170-179)	4055 (1000-6500)
100	9	36 (29-43)	64 (56-72)	169 (158-175)	5062 (3000-10000)

Table II. Occurrence of Proteinuria, Hemoglobinuria and Hematuria
After Training or Competition Covering Various Distances

Distance km	N	kval	Proteinuria kvant gm/24 hr	Hemoglobinuria	Hematuria
25	8	4	0.2-1.2	0	0
26-80	8	2	1.8-3.5	1	1
100	9	3	0.3-1.6	1	0

discomfort, and his urinary samples contained large amounts of hemoglobin. The other runner completed the 100 km and had less hemoglobin in his urine. None of the urine samples taken after a training run of 25 km contained hemoglobin. Considerable hematuria was observed in only one athlete participating in the 100-km competition.

Strenuous training of long duration, or competition, did not result in glucosuria; neither were ketone body levels elevated after the training. The mean specific gravities of the urine before and after running were slightly different, but the difference was not statistically significant ($p > 0.5$).

Discussion

Since the beginning of the 1900s it has been known that proteinuria and hemoglobinuria occur in marathon runners after competition [2]. Later, several publications on the excretion of protein, hemoglobin and erythrocytes in urine in connection with endurance training and excessively long competitions have appeared [3-5, 7, 9, 10]. In these studies runners, football players and ice hockey players were investigated. In the present study the material comprised endurance athletes with extra long-distance running as their specialty, including one who was world champion at 100 km.

The sample collection and handling were hampered by the field conditions. The midstream urine samples collected before the training or competition proved normal, with no signs of proteinuria, hemoglobinuria or hematuria. During the trial and thereafter only one athlete experienced subjective symptoms. He complained of severe abdominal discomfort after 26 km, and a little later an abundance of hemoglobin was detected in his urine sample. A possible causative connection between the pain and the hemoglobinuria could not, however, be demonstrated. Extensive studies [3, 4, 10] have shown that only in extremely rare instances is hemoglobinuria connected with a clear pathological condition.

Bichler et al [1] have shown that it is not until after training of long duration that protein, mainly albumin, is excreted in the urine. According to Dancaster et al [3, 4] protein disappeared from urine within 24 hours of a 54-mile running competition. In the present study, however, no protein could be detected in urine after four hours had elapsed from the end of the exertion. In rare instances the amount of protein excreted in the urine was high, varying from 0.2 to 3.3 gm daily. This amount is so low, even if it occurred daily, that it does not need to be taken into consideration when planning the diet. According to Bichler [1] the protein excreted in the urine is mainly albumin.

Summary

The present study is an examination of the proportion of proteins, hemoglobin and erythrocytes in urine subsequent to nonstop training or competitive runs of 25 to 100 km. The material comprised 25 regularly training competition athletes of the endurance-type athletics. The measuring of proteins in urine was based on biuretic test and the measuring of hemoglobin on spectrophotometry. Erythrocytes were counted in Bürker's chamber. In one third (9) of the subjects, proteins in urine were found subsequent to the runs, the secretion of which varied during the times of measuring from 0.2 to 3.3 gm/liters/24 hours. The proportion of proteins was greater in the urine of athletes in poorer condition than in the urine of athletes in good condition. Hemoglobinuria occurred in two athletes and one had abundant erythrocytes in the urine. Proteins were secreted into the urine in shorter and longer distances in approximately as many cases. Hemoglobinuria and hematuria were found only in the runners of over 25 km. In the investigated cases secretion of proteins ceased one to four hours subsequent to the runs. Thus, the protein balance of the athletes is not affected by albumin lost in urine subsequent to even heavy performance of endurance running.

References

1. Bichler, K.H., Porzolt, F. and Naber, K.: Proteinuria unter körperlicher Belastung. Dtsch. Med. Wochenschr. 97:1229, 1972.
2. Collier, W.: Br. Med. J. 1:4, 1907.
3. Dancaster, C.P., Duckworth, W.C. and Roper, C.J.: S. Afr. Med. J. 43:758, 1969.

4. Dancaster, C.P. and Whereat, S.J.: S. Afr. Med. J. 45:147, 1971.
5. Davidson, R.J.L.: Exertional hemoglobinuria: A report on three cases with studies on the haemolytic mechanism. J. Clin. Path. 17:536, 1964.
6. Javitt, N.B. and Miller, A.T.: Mechanism of exercise proteinuria. J. Appl. Physiol. 4:834, 1952.
7. Lundquist, A.: Marschhemoglobinuri. Nord. Med. 73:536, 1965.
8. Nöcker, J.: Physiologie der Leibesübungen (Enke:Stuttgart -71).
9. Schlatter, Ch. and Foster, G.: Die Sporthämoglobinurie. Schweiz. Med. Wochenschr. 95:979, 1965.
10. Sidorowicz, W.: The changes in urine in the sportsmen. Pol. Tyg. Lek. 18:1057, 1963.

Evaluation of Lactic Acid Anaerobic Energy Contribution by Determination of Postexercise Lactic Acid Concentration of Ear Capillary Blood in Middle-Distance Runners and Swimmers

A. Mader, H. Heck and W. Hollmann

Introduction

It is generally accepted that the cellular and the general energetic metabolism or single components of it constitute limiting factors of performance under conditions of maximal dynamic work lasting between 30 seconds and six minutes (but also longer). One should try to examine the relationship between the mechanical dynamic work performed and the magnitude of isolated components of the energetic metabolism. This requires the elaboration of general and special mathematical models correlating the existing parameters.

Starting from a general metabolic formulation we tried to deduce a specific model describing the relationship between the dynamic work in running and swimming and the lactic acid energetic contribution.

Experimental support for this model is given. The equations can be used appropriately in practical sports.

General Model

The mechanical work expense in humans is based on three energetic sources, which can be represented by the following formula:

A. Mader, H. Heck and W. Hollmann, Institute for Sports-Medicine and Circulation Research, German Sports-University, Cologne, Federal Republic of Germany.

This study was supported by the Bundesinstitut für Sportwissenschaft, Cologne, Federal Republic of Germany.

A(mech. work) = E(mech. performance) · t(sec) =
B(creatinphosphate) + C(lactate) + D(oxygen uptake)

1) $A(mkp/kg) = E(mkp/sec \cdot kg) \cdot t \ (sec) = kCr \cdot B + kLa \cdot C +$

$$(k\dot{V}O_2 \cdot D/60 \cdot) \int_{t_o}^{t} (1 - e^{-(t - t_o)/T})dt$$

Each factor conforms to a proper equation which has to be described. In relation to the mechanical work performed at time t we define:

B = mobilizable part of the working muscle creatine phosphate (i.e., 80% of the total amount at rest) expressed as mmol/kg body weight (bw).

C = lactic acid concentration expressed in mmol/kg bw or mmol/l blood. (C mmol/kg bw = 0.75·C mmol/l blood).

D = max $\dot{V}O_2$ ml/min/kg of working muscle mass under steady-state conditions.

The integral $\int_{t_o}^{t} (1 - e^{-(t - t_o)/T}) \ dt$ considers the reduced

effective $\dot{V}O_2$ at the beginning of the exercise resulting from the delayed increase of $\dot{V}O_2$. It is supposed that the $\dot{V}O_2$ increase at the beginning of the exercise can be represented with sufficient accuracy by a differential equation of first order [7, 9, 12].

t = duration of the exercise in seconds.

t_o = delay time after the beginning of the exercise and the increase of the $\dot{V}O_2$ (t_o = 8 sec).

T = time constant of the $\dot{V}O_2$ increase of the whole organism.

The coefficients kCr, kLa and $k\dot{V}O_2$ represent, respectively, the amounts of work which can be obtained from 1 mmol creatinphosphate, 1 mmol blood lactic acid and 1 ml oxygen uptake.

The maximal amount of work which can be derived from B and C in a given period should be considered as being constant. On the other hand, the amount of work resulting from the oxygen uptake (the integral) is dependent upon the duration of the workloads.

For a given constant duration t ⩽ 4T and for an energy expense exceeding largely D the integral is assumed to be constant and independent from the anaerobic energy output. It can be further accepted that the amount of B (which is the mobilizable part of energy from the working muscle creatine phosphate) is completely exhausted above a certain work level leading to the production of lactic acid. Accordingly, this factor can also be considered as constant and the factor C remains as the only variable of the energy supply. During exercise there is primarily a consumption of creatine phosphate and a preponderance of the oxidative processes over the glycolytic processes (Pasteur effect). It follows that the amount of lactic acid formed at the exercise may be represented by:

2) $C = (1/kLa) \cdot (E \cdot t - (kCr \cdot B + (k\dot{V}O_2 \cdot D/60) \cdot$

$$\int_{t_o}^{t} (1 - e^{-(t - t_o)/T} dt))$$

This can be simplified for given durations but different mechanical workloads.

2a) $C = (1/kLa) \cdot t \cdot (E - A(B+F)/t) = (1/kLa) \cdot t \cdot \Delta E$

$$F = (k\dot{V}O_2 \cdot D/60) \cdot \int_{t_o}^{t} (1 - e^{-(t - t_o)/T} dt))$$

Where $A(B+F) = t \cdot \Delta E$ the amount of mechanical work which is derived from creatine phosphate and the integral is equal to the oxygen uptake.

Under submaximal anaerobic conditions, the produced lactic acid is directly proportional to the part of total mechanical work performed which is not supplied by the nonlactic and aerobic metabolism and the duration of work which we have postulated as constant.

It can be expected that for a given duration of exercise, during which a maximal tolerable amount of lactic acid can be formed, the produced acidosis may be the true limiting factor of maximal performance [2].

One has to consider the exponential increase of energy cost with increasing speed resulting from the higher resistance offered by air or water and the greater inertia following an increment of movement speed. Hence, the balance of energies in running and swimming should be expressed most simply by the exponential equations:

3) $E = b \cdot V^c$ 3a) $A = b \cdot t \cdot V^c$ V = speed m/sec or km/h

The coefficient b and the exponent c have to be determined experimentally.

From the work of Pugh [11] and Holmer [3] concerning the rise of $\dot{V}O_2$ with increasing speed in running and swimming the following equations can be derived:

Pugh [11] for running on a track.

4) $\dot{V}O_2$ (ml/min/kg) = 6.5 +1.75 $\cdot$ V^c (km/h) c = 1.2

Holmer [3] for freestyle swimming in a swimming flume.

5) $\dot{V}O_2$ (ml/min/kg) = 16 + 15 $\cdot$ V^c (m/sec) c = 3.2

These formulas are only valid if the energy of acceleration can be neglected in comparison to the total energy expense and if the energy expense in steady state can be covered by the oxygen uptake.

If in equation 1) the mechanical work performed during the time t_i and the speed V_i is replaced by the product

$$V_i^c \text{ (m/sec)} \cdot t_i = S_i' \ (V_i^c = S_i'/t_i \ ; t_i = S_i'/V_i^c)$$

where S_i' should also be regarded as an amount of work or a given distance, then the equation 1) can be reformulated as follows:

6) $V_i^c \cdot t_i = S_i' = B/\alpha Cr + C/\alpha La + (D/\alpha \dot{V}O_2 \cdot 60) \cdot$

$$\int_{t_o}^{t} (1 - e^{-(t - t_o)/T})dt)$$

When V_i or t_i is in the denumerator the durations of exercises for a given speed or the total speed for a given duration are calculated from B, C and D.

The coefficients αCr, αLa and $\alpha \dot{V}O_2$ correspond in the case of a linear relationship, i.e., exponent c = 1 within a limited range of velocity and time to the increments of energy expenses per velocity and time units by B, C and D. The solutions of the above equations require the evaluation of at least two components of the mobilizable energy (e.g., B and C) and the determination of the value of the coefficients and exponents. This includes also the evaluation of the lactic acid diffusion to the whole body and a determination of the lactic acid elimination within and after exercise to calculate the true amount of built up lactic acid from the blood lactic acid time curves (Figs. 1 and 2). This demands that a large number of measurements are made at different exercise times and for different intensities. The

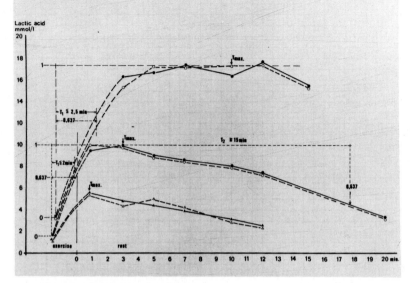

FIG. 1. Times curves of lactic acid measured simultaneously in both ears after 600-meter runs of different intensities.

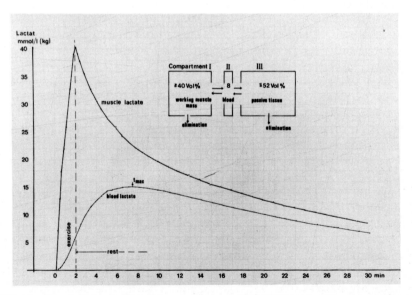

FIG. 2. Simulated computation of lactic acid build-up during a two-minute exercise performance in the muscle and its distribution in the blood during and after exercise, according to real measured curves.

mathematical computation is long and can only be realized by means of a digital computer. For practical purposes, however, simplified conditions and measurements with restricted terms of validity can be adopted.

Practical Useful Model

Under anaerobic working conditions, lasting between 30 seconds and approximately six minutes, a relation between the lactic acid level and the intensity and duration of the exercise load in running may be demonstrated according to a modification of the equation 2a) and 3a):

$$2b) \quad C = La_t \cdot t \cdot (V - V_o)^C \qquad 2c) \quad C = La_s \cdot a \cdot (V - V_o)^c$$

The lactic acid represents the integrated sum of the energy deficits. Hence, it cannot be measured during the exercise but only during a definite period afterwards, which remains to be evaluated. The lactic acid concentrations can be measured at the running track or at the swimming pool and utilized in the formula 2c). This presupposes that the measured lactic acid concentration at a certain moment is representative of the whole body production.

When the durations of the exercises are constant, the equation 2b) can be considered as accurate. However, when there are proportionally small variations of these exercise durations, the equation 2c) has only a relative validity.

In a limited range of velocities the exponential increase of the energy expenditure with the increase of speed may be simplified to a linear increase. It follows that it is sufficient to determine the inclination of a correlation axis in a diagram where on the ordinate y, one has the lactic acid concentration (mmol/l) and on the abscissa x the velocity V (m/sec). This can be done simply by measuring two points.

Within the mentioned restrictions the following test method on a determined running or swimming distance can be proposed. It will permit one to ascertain the individual axis or equation according to 2c). Two runs are performed. The first time the anaerobic contribution is moderate to intermediate, with a maximal postexercise lactic acid concentration situated between 5 and 8 mmol/l blood. In the second run an elevated to maximal anaerobic contribution should be reached with postexercise lactic acid concentrations (maximum) situated between 12 and 20 mmol/l. In order to evaluate the anaerobic metabolism the lactic acid concentration is measured from the hyperhemic ear lobule at 1, 3, 5, 7, 10, 12 and eventually 15 and 20 minutes after the end of the exercise (20 μl blood is collected in a calibrated microcapillary).

The immediate pre-exercise lactic acid concentration has also to be measured because its presence may lead to erroneous interpretations of the postexercise levels. Correct values can only be expected if the pre-exercise lactic acid concentration does not exceed 2.0 (3.0) mmol/l. The interval between both runs should be approximately between 20 and 25 minutes in order to allow the lactic acid levels to return to normal. One can also carry out both runs on different days at identical times. After the exercise it is further possible to study the acid base balance. There is a strong direct correlation (r = 0.95) in the same individual between its lactic acid and its base excess (−BE mval/l) which may be considered to reflect the work acidosis.

From two maximal postexercise lactic acid concentrations (La_1, La_2) and the corresponding running velocities (V_1, V_2) the rise in energy cost (αLa_s) on a given distance (100 meter) and for a determined speed increase in meters per second may be calculated.

7) $\alpha La_s = (La_2 - La_1)/(V_1 - V_2) \cdot a$ $a = S(meter)/100$
                                                      $S = $ running distance

Using given values (La_2) in the equation 2c) (c = 1), V_o may be calculated being equal to the sum of nonlactic anaerobic plus the aerobic energy supply.

8) $V_o = V_2 - La_2/\alpha La_s \cdot a$ $V_o = $ speed which corresponds to a lactic acid concentration of zero

Inserting various given values (La_i) the possible speeds for the test distance as well as for shorter and longer training distances may be calculated.

9) $V_i = V_o + La_i/\alpha La_s \cdot a'$ $a' = S'/100$
                                       $S' = $ training distances

This is valid also for the competition distance itself. These various velocities are tabulated with the corresponding times (Table I). Using an exponent (running c = 1.1 to 1.2; swimming c = 1.45 to 1.55) a greater range of distances and velocities with the restriction of minimal errors may be calculated. Theoretically, it is possible to derive an individual equation as in formula 1) and 2) or 6), which evaluate the total amount of supplied energy in a wide range of speeds and durations. However, time is insufficient here for the development of the theoretical aspects of this problem.

Table I. Computation of the Possible Maximal Competition Time From Two 600-M Runs From G.K. (Female)

1. RUN HB: 14

NBW	PH	PCO2	PO2	LA	BE	A.BIK	TOT.C	ST.BIK	SO2	BB
0	7.367	34.4	103.2	1.36	-4.84	19.43	20.46	20.74	97.6	42.7
3	7.306	29.2	116.3	5.64	-10.66	14.27	15.15	16.48	98.0	36.9
7	7.320	29.2	132.8	4.90	-9.88	14.75	15.63	17.02	98.6	37.7

2. RUN HB: 14

NBW	PH	PCO2	PO2	LA	BE	A.BIK	TOT.C	ST.BIK	SO2	BB
0	7.366	31.9	107.6	2.56	-6.08	17.98	18.93	19.79	97.9	41.5
3	7.049	28.9	131.2	14.47	-22.83	7.75	8.61	9.36	97.2	24.8
5	7.014	25.8	119.1	16.39	-25.07	6.38	7.15	8.31	96.1	22.5
10	7.023	23.7	113.1	16.19	-25.29	5.98	6.69	8.21	95.6	22.3
12	7.050	22.6	117.2	15.87	-24.55	6.07	6.75	8.54	96.3	23.0
15	7.104	23.0	113.6	15.03	-22.33	7.00	7.69	9.61	96.5	25.3

BE	LA
-4.84	1.36
-10.66	5.64
-9.88	4.90
-6.08	2.56
-22.83	14.47
-25.07	16.39
-25.29	16.19
-24.55	15.87
-22.33	15.03

N= 9   R= .998832
BE=-2.94788 -1.35259 *LA

TEST DISTANCE 600 METER

	1.LAUF	2.LAUF
TIME (SEC):	115.8	92.6
V (M/SEC):	5.181	6.479
LA MAX :	5.64	16.39

LAKTAT=0.5+ 6.4147 *(V- 4.34992)EXP 1.2
LAKTAT=0.5+ 8.28112 *(V- 4.56066)EXP 1
*LA: 1.38019
VO : 4.50028

DISTANCE(METER): 600

LAKTAT	BE	EXP M/SEC	M/SEC	EXP SEC	SEC	EXP MIN	MIN
2	-5.65	4.648	4.742	129.09	126.53	2: 9.09	2: 6.53
4	-8.36	4.954	4.983	121.13	120.40	2: 1.13	2: 0.40
6	-11.06	5.230	5.225	114.73	114.84	1: 54.73	1: 54.84
8	-13.77	5.489	5.466	109.31	109.76	1: 49.31	1: 49.76
10	-16.47	5.737	5.708	104.58	105.12	1: 44.58	1: 45.12
12	-19.18	5.976	5.949	100.39	100.85	1: 40.39	1: 40.85
14	-21.88	6.209	6.191	96.63	96.92	1: 36.63	1: 36.92
16	-24.59	6.436	6.432	93.23	93.28	1: 33.23	1: 33.28
18	-27.29	6.658	6.674	90.12	89.90	1: 30.12	1: 29.90
20	-30.00	6.876	6.915	87.26	86.76	1: 27.26	1: 26.76
22	-32.70	7.090	7.157	84.63	83.83	1: 24.63	1: 23.83

DISTANCE(METER): 800

LAKTAT	BE	EXP M/SEC	M/SEC	EXP SEC	SEC	EXP MIN	MIN
2	-5.65	4.584	4.697	174.51	170.34	2: 54.51	2: 50.34
4	-8.36	4.825	4.878	165.81	164.01	2: 45.81	2: 44.01
6	-11.06	5.042	5.059	158.67	158.14	2: 38.66	2: 38.14
8	-13.77	5.246	5.240	152.49	152.67	2: 32.49	2: 32.67
10	-16.47	5.441	5.421	147.02	147.57	2: 27.02	2: 27.57
12	-19.18	5.630	5.602	142.10	142.80	2: 22.10	2: 22.80
14	-21.88	5.813	5.783	137.63	138.33	2: 17.63	2: 18.33
16	-24.59	5.991	5.964	133.53	134.13	2: 13.53	2: 14.13
18	-27.29	6.166	6.146	129.75	130.18	2: 9.75	2: 10.17
20	-30.00	6.337	6.327	126.24	126.45	2: 6.24	2: 6.45
22	-32.70	6.506	6.508	122.97	122.93	2: 2.97	2: 2.93

Possible competition time is limited by a maximal acidosis (base excess − 30.0 mval/l). Correlation coefficient between simultaneous measurements of lactic acid and base excess is very high.

The application of our model in the practical and theoretical evaluation of the muscular metabolism in running and swimming raises the question of the representativity of the postexercise blood lactic acid concentration of the whole body lactic acid production. The existence of such a relationship has received negative [6] as well as positive [8] responses. The maximal postexercise blood lactic acid concentration has been taken as reflecting this whole body lactic acid production.

The dynamic of lactic acid changes in the ear capillary blood can be described as resulting from diffusion and transport processes in a three compartment model [1].

Within and after the end of exercise the lactic acid diffuses from compartment I (i.e., the working muscle mass) to compartment II (i.e., the vascular space) as long as a concentration gradient exists. Since blood volume is small in comparison with the cardiac output, a considerable mixing results and accordingly the concentration differences in the blood can be neglected. The transit of lactic acid into the compartment III (i.e., the extravascular tissue without working muscle mass) is also dependent upon the concentration difference and the rate of lactate elimination. It proceeds by diffusion and might possibly be changed by the importance of the perfusion (Fig. 2). The maximum blood lactic acid depends upon the relation of the distribution rate to the elimination rate of lactic acid [1]. The higher this lactic acid concentration is in the ear capillary blood, depending upon the intensity of exercise, the later it reaches a peak value (Fig. 1). This is particularly true for short running periods between 35 seconds and two minutes and this does not agree with general acceptance of a constant lactic acid elimination rate. Further, it can be demonstrated that the distribution of lactic acid proceeds seven to eight times faster than the elimination. For this reason it is probable that the postexercise dynamic distribution equilibrium (represented by the postexercise maximum on blood lactate) is closely related to the static distribution equilibrium in the whole body. However, the requirement of an equal distribution of lactic acid for the calculation of the anaerobic energy participation is not absolutely necessary. It is sufficient that the maximal postexercise lactic acid concentration demonstrates a close linear correlation with the whole body lactic acid production. The following experimental data support the existence of such a relationship particularly for exercise lasting between 35 seconds and six minutes.

1. In most of the accurately performed studies, almost identical values for lactic acid have been found when simultaneous determinations from both ears were made (Fig. 1).

2. By the repetition of running or swimming tests on identical distances but with different speeds very similar individual curves are found, taking into consideration the possible technical sources of error (Fig. 3).

From Figures 3 and 4 it can be seen that the inclination of the individual axis (= αLa_s) is dependent upon the covered distance and as a consequence on the exercise duration but not on the individual performance capacity. This is true for running as well as for swimming. There is an increase of the coefficient αLa_s with increasing running speed and decreasing duration. This results from the exponential rise of the energy cost with higher speed (Equation 3) and the decline of the aerobic energy contribution with the reduction of exercise duration (Equation 1).

The coefficient αLa_s deviates from a mean value recorded for a given distance when the speed is changing considerably during the running itself or when pronounced pre-exercise lactic acid values are present. These do not add linearly to the postexercise lactic acid values.

It is indicated to carry out in the same athlete two tests with different distances and durations because of the time dependence of the aerobic energy supply. A first test is performed for a duration of

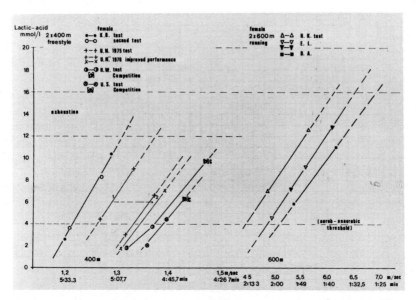

FIG. 3. Results from 400-meter swimming and 600-meter running tests in female, including results of repeated tests and results from competitions.

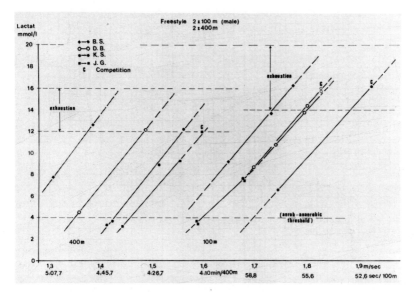

FIG. 4. Comparison of 100- and 400-meter freestyle swimming tests in man. There is dependence between the results from the endurance tests (400 m) and the sprint tests (100 m). The maximal lactic acid values after competition agree with the individual curve obtained from the tests.

work which requires mainly the anaerobic metabolism but is situated within the dynamic increase of the oxygen uptake (t_1, t_2 ≤ 2 minutes or running distances of 300, 400, 600 or 800 meters and a swimming distance of 100 meters).

A second test should last longer and mainly require the participation of the aerobic metabolism with nearly constant oxygen consumptions (t_1, t_2 = 4 to 10 minutes or running distances of 2000 and 3000 meters and a swimming distance of 400 meters). This test should permit the evaluation of the endurance capacity. The results of similar tests for 100- and 400-meter freestyle are represented in Figure 4.

Practical Application

As a preliminary hypothesis we consider that for exercises lasting between 30 seconds and six minutes the acidosis resulting from the lactic acid production is the true limiting factor of performance. We calculate the possible performance during the competition race by extrapolating the values of the individual axis or equation elaborated for this competition distance. This maximal performance can be predetermined particularly when the maximal acidosis is calculated from a regression line between the lactic acid concentrations and the simultaneously measured base excess values. Two general methods should be considered. The test may be performed on a distance which is shorter than the competition distance and the speed of the second of the two runs corresponds to the speed wanted for the competition. This prevents the occurrence of a maximal acidosis. One calculates if, for the desired competition speed, the theoretical possible acidosis is not exceeded.

The test may also be performed on the same distance as in the competition. The speed is lower than in competition in order to prevent the formation of an extremely high acidosis.

With the first method the linearity of the model is sufficiently high to permit an extrapolation and a maximal acidosis can be calculated.

With the second method the calculated competition speeds are too high. In this case the elaboration of equations with empirically determined exponents allows better predictions.

The maximal tolerable acidosis in competition can be estimated by two methods: (1) The range of attainable acidosis levels for each discipline can be derived from the postexercise lactic acid levels in top athletes during major competitions and (2) from theoretical maximal permitted intracellular acidosis, maximal values for specific sport performances may be predicted.

This possibility to forecast the maximal acidosis tolerated in competition becomes more difficult when this maximal limit is approached. The fact that with a decline of intracellular pH of 0.6 to 0.7 units, the glycolytic processes are arrested within a few seconds by the inhibition of the phosphofructokinase, constitutes a theoretical argument for the performance limiting effect of the intracellular acidosis [2]. This pH decline may produce a sudden performance breakdown which can frequently be observed during 400- and 800-meter running competitions. Calculating the distribution of the buffer capacity between the working muscle mass and the rest of the organism the general decrease of pH can be evaluated. It should be expressed by a base excess of -28.0 to -30.0 mval/l. This corresponds to the values found in the literature [2, 5, 6, 10] and by ourselves.

In swimming, however, the maximal acidosis levels found at the end of competition races are lower than in running (between -16.0 and -26.0 mval/l base excess). But again the values found in top athletes are higher than those found in less successful athletes. There is a good correlation between the acidosis values calculated from the measurements made during tests in running and swimming and the acidosis values recorded during competitions. Some examples are shown in Figures 3 and 4.

From the following points of view the presented methods can be interestingly used to follow up athletes:

1. The results of the tests in running and swimming can be used to select identical training intensities for athletes of different performance capacities. This is valid for anaerobic as well as for aerobic training. As a limit between a prevalent anaerobic and a prevalent aerobic energy supply, a blood lactic acid level of 4.0 mmol/l can be accepted.

2. It is possible to examine the metabolic adaptation to a training program in an objective way independently of subjective feelings and motivation. Similarly, one can study accurately the efficiency of a certain type of training and can also verify hypotheses concerning modes of action of certain means intended to enhance the effects of training.

3. The proportion of aerobic and anaerobic performance capacity optimal for a determined competition race can be deduced theoretically and compared with the actually measured metabolic capacities. This may lead to the accentuation of training of a certain component of the metabolic adaptation.

4. The results of these tests make it possible to detect particularly talented young athletes (regarding their metabolism), and whose training could be individually followed.

References

1. Dost, F.H.: Grundlagen der Pharmakokinetik. Stuttgart:Georg Thieme Verlag, 1968.
2. Hermansen, L. and Osnes, J.B.: Blood and muscle pH after maximal exercise in man. J. Appl. Physiol. 32(3):304-308, 1972.
3. Hólmer, I.: Physiology of swimming man. Acta Physiol. Scand. Suppl. 407, 1974.
4. Kindermann, W., Fürsterling, D. und Keul, J.: Anoxidative Energiebereitstellung beim Laufen und Schwimmen in Abhängigkeit vom Geschlecht. Med. Sport 15:353, 1975.
5. Kindermann, W., Huber, G. and Keul, J.: Anaerobe Energiebereitstellung und Herzfrequenz während und nach verschiedenen Trainingsmethoden des Mittelstrecklers. Leistungssport 1:66-70, 1975.
6. Klausen, K., Rasmussen, B., Clausen, J.P. and Trap-Jensen, J.: Blood lactate from exercising extremities before and after arm or leg training. Am. J. Physiol. 227(1):67-72, 1974.
7. Linnarson, D.: Dynamics of pulmonary gas exchange and heart rate changes at start and end of exercise. Acta Physiol. Scand. Suppl. 415:5-67, 1974.

8. Margaria, R., Cerretelli, P. and Mangili, F.: Balance and kinetics of anaerobic energy release during strenuous exercise in man. J. Appl. Physiol. 19(4):623-628, 1964.

9. Margaria, R., Mangili, F., Cuttica, F. and Cerretelli, P.: The kinetics of oxygen consumption at the onset of muscular exercise in man. Ergonomics 8:49-54, 1964.

10. Osnes, J.B. and Hermansen, L.: Acid-base balance after maximal exercise of short duration. J. Appl. Physiol. 32:59-63, 1972.

11. Pugh, L.G.C.E.: Oxygen intake in track and treadmill running with observations on the effect of air resistance. J. Physiol. 207:823-835, 1970.

12. Whipp, B.J. and Wasserman, K.: Oxygen uptake kinetics for various intensities of constant-load work. J. Appl. Physiol. 33(3):351-356, 1972.

Investigation of Pretraining and Posttraining Blood Clotting, Viscosity and Acid-Base Parameters in Adolescent Swimmers and Adult Weightlifters

Kálmán Lissák, Kornél Fendler,
Gábor L. Kovács and Arpád Mátrai

The experiments, carried out by Barclay in 1974 [1] on dog gastrocnemius plantaris, proved convincingly that the blood flow is the limiting factor for muscle contraction above certain limits. This observation has been usefully complemented by studies on heart, circulation and breathing. However, such factors as flow resistance of the blood itself are poorly understood. It is known that acidosis increases the blood viscosity [2] and muscle work alters the blood pH in acidic direction. It is necessary to extend the investigation of the muscle work during adaptation to viscosity and clotting of the blood and plasma. This way one may expect to obtain new data on basic regulative processes.

Our observations were done on childhood and adolescent swimmers' yearly preparatory and racing period, on weightlifters in competition period and nontrained volunteer medical students. The two kinds of sports represent the competitive and athletic sports and the population investigated gave an opportunity to study the adaptative characteristics of the juvenile organism during heavy exercise.

For the laboratory investigation blood was taken prior to training in the laboratory and after training at the place of the exercise. The swimmers had their training twice daily in the morning and early evening. In each case the later training was studied. The weightlifters had their training once daily in the afternoon. The time between lunch and the first blood sample taken was at least three hours. The

Kálmán Lissák, Kornél Fendler, Gábor L. Kovács and Arpád Mátrai, Department of Physiology, University Medical School, Pécs, and Central Laboratories of County Hospital, Baranya, Pécs, Hungary.

acid-base parameters were measured by Astrup microanalyzator, fibrinogen determination by thrombin clotting effect of the fibrinogen and the biuret method, plasma ammonia level following ion-exchange purification by Berthelot reaction with photometric measurement. For the measurement of blood and plasma viscosity a capillary viscosimeter was developed which was constructed for series of measurements simultaneously [3] which can be used for measurement between 10 and 120 shear rate with 250 μl volume. The results of viscosity were calculated on ideal 45% hematocrit because in our experiment we wanted to insure that the viscosity of the subject was not due to possible hemoconcentration. However, in the experiments marked hemoconcentration did not occur.

Data of nontrained medical students are given following 90-minute running (Fig. 1). The level of fibrinogen increased as well as the blood and plasma viscosity. The decrease in pH and base excess is in agreement with the literature. The plasma ammonia level from the starting 30 to 50 μg/100 ml plasma in some cases showed a slight increase. However, it never exceeded 70 μg/100 ml level.

Data of swimmers aged 10 to 15 in the yearly preparatory training period are summarized in Figure 2. Starting fibrinogen level

CHANGES IN BLOOD VISCOSITY, FIBRINOGEN AND
ACID-BASE PARAMETERS OF VOLUNTEERS

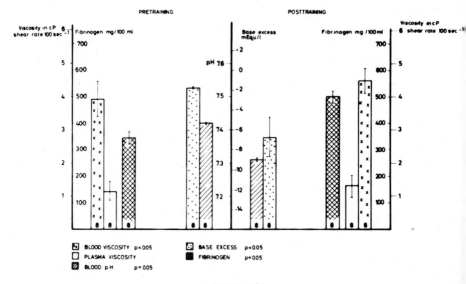

FIGURE 1.

CHANGES IN BLOOD VISCOSITY, FIBRINOGEN AND
ACID-BASE PARARAMETERS OF SWIMMERS IN YEARLY PREPARATORY PERIOD

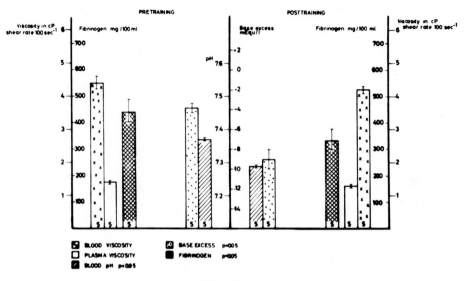

FIGURE 2.

was high possibly due to morning training which decreased considerably at the end of the training. The lysis time of the euglobulin decreased most remarkably. The values of viscosity did not increase. On the contrary, they decreased and acidosis as can be seen is very expressive. The changes in ammonia level are similar to medical students. It should be mentioned that in the racers remarkable platelet spreading can be observed in the peripheral blood smears.

Data of swimmers in the racing period are summarized in Figure 3. Before training the fibrinogen level was not increased and after training did not show a decrease versus the starting period. On the contrary, a slight increase was observed. The value of viscosity after training showed a slight but not significant increase. It is interesting that the acidosis was very small. However, the plasma ammonia level increased from 44 μg/100 ml to 90 μl/100 ml.

Data of weightlifters prior to and after training are shown in Figure 4. The viscosity of the plasma and blood did not increase; fibrinogen level and pH did not change. Ammonia level after training increased considerably from the average 45 μg/100 ml to 150 μg/100 ml. In some cases values above 300 μg/100 ml could also be seen.

From our data we conclude that in trained individuals physical exercise, especially in children who have a tendency against acidosis a

CHANGES IN BLOOD VISCOSITY, FIBRINOGEN AND
ACID-BASE PARAMETERS OF SWIMMERS IN YEARLY RACING PERIOD

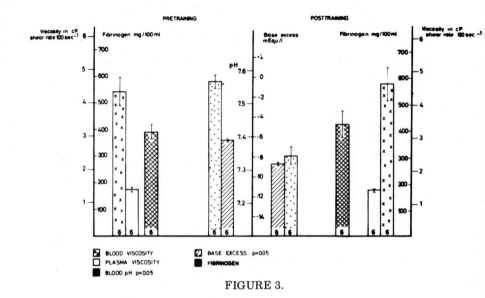

FIGURE 3.

CHANGES IN BLOOD VISCOSITY, FIBRINOGEN AND
ACID- BASE PARAMETERS OF WEIGHT LIFTERS

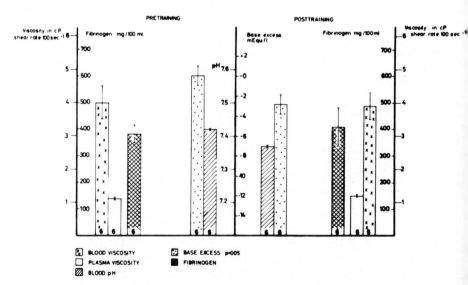

FIGURE 4.

viscosity decreasing mechanism is operating. Our data suggest that in trained individuals beside or instead of the well-known hemoglobin saturation-inhibiting bicarbonate-pH shift an increased ammonia genesis is induced which presumably serves the acid-base regulation of the trained person. The increased ammonia level cannot be explained by malfunction of the liver because in some cases especially in weightlifters, the high level of ammonia exceeds the level observed in severe hepatergic coma.

The changes in blood viscosity in a non-Newtonian fluid system are determined mainly by two factors: number of corpuscles and the distance between them. The number of particles in our experiment, because the calculation was on the basis of ideal hematocrit, does not play a role. The distance between the particles depends upon the molecule of fibrinogen which in intact stage increases the rouloux and sludge formation of the erythrocyte and platelet aggregation. From the data of Rampling and Gaffney [4] it is known that Y fragment coming from fibrinogenolysis inhibits aggregation. In our observation a facilitated lysis can be obtained which in some child swimmer was associated with decreased fibrinogen. We suppose that during muscle work a strong fibrinogenolysis is induced from the wall of the blood vessels by the gradually deliberating plasminogen activators which increases the formation of Y fragments, the dispersion of the particles, which eventually decreases the viscosity. In order to prove our supposition animal experiments were carried out on rats made to swim until exhaustion. In these experiments in double-blind controls were used with Syncumar (Acenocoumarolum, Alkaloida Budapest) treatment which drug is known to inhibit aggregation. The experiments were carried out in 26 C water without weightloading. The experimental animals were divided into two groups: one swimming 40 minutes until exhaustion and the second swimming longer than 100 minutes. The experiments were carried out on the first group, because one may suppose this group similar to humans may reach the "dead-point" phenomenon. Daily swimming lengthened the swimming time which showed some sort of adaptation. The experiments were carried out according to the following scheme: Following the first session in which the animals were made to swim until exhaustion, the animals being exhausted below 40 minutes were not trained for 20 days in order to eliminate the effects of training. On day 20 and 21, 0.6 mg/100 g b.w. Syncumar was given to the animals via stomach tubing which was followed with a half dose on day 22 and 23. Half of the animals according to the rule of double-blind experiments received placebo treatment. On fourth

CHANGES OF EXHAUSTION TIME BY RATS

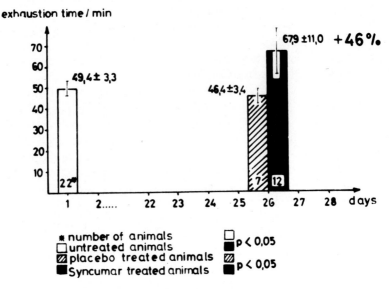

FIGURE 5.

day, on the day 23, the animals swam until exhaustion. The results are summarized in Figure 5.

The swimming time in the Syncumar-treated animals, the time necessary until exhaustion, increased about 40% versus placebo control. From our other experiments it is known that the Syncumar treatment decreases the viscosity, so it is possible that for the effect observed here of the aggregation decreasing influence, decreased viscosity is responsible. However to prove this supposition in further experiments the degradation products of the fibrinogen must be studied.

References

1. Barclay, J.K. and Stainsby, W.N.: Med. Sci. Sports 6:77, 1974.
2. Copley, A.L.: Hemorrheology. Oxford:Pergamon Press, 1968.
3. Mátrai, A., Fendler, K. and Lissák, K.: Kisérletes Orvostudomány. Budapest, 1976. (In press.)
4. Rampling, M.W. and Gaffney, P.J.: Clin. Chim. Acta 67:43, 1976.

Inotropic and Metabolic Effects of Potassium Infusion in Contracting Skeletal Muscle in Situ

J. K. Barclay, E. L. Price
and J. K. Thompson

Introduction

Fatigue in skeletal muscle in situ can be defined operationally as a decrease in developed isometric tension at a constant contraction rate. The causes of this decrease are controversial. Two possibilities are interstitial potassium concentration and the availability of inorganic phosphate. These substances are necessary for normal function, but a net efflux has been demonstrated during contractions. Is this efflux large enough to alter function? The purpose of these experiments was to identify if changes in the extracellular concentration of these substances would alter the amount of tension developed by fatigued and nonfatigued skeletal muscle in situ.

Methods

Mongrel dogs of either sex (N = 15) were anesthetized with sodium pentobarbital, 30 mg/kg intravenously. Additional 30-mg doses were given as required.

The circulation to the gastrocnemius plantaris muscle group was isolated by tying off all arterial and venous branches that did not feed or drain the muscle. The artery feeding the distal area of the gracilis muscle was cannulated and used for infusions. The artery feeding the distal semitendinosis muscle was cannulated and used for sampling and monitoring blood pressure. Venous return was via a catheter in the femoral vein to the jugular vein. All animals were heparinized, 2370 units/kg, prior to cannulation.

Blood flow was measured with an electromagnetic flow probe placed in the venous outflow tubing. The probe was calibrated during the experiment using a timed collection of blood.

J. K. Barclay, E. L. Price and J. K. Thompson, Department of Biomedical Sciences, University of Guelph, Guelph, Ontario, Canada.

　　　　　　　　　　　　　　J. K. BARCLAY ET AL

The distal stump of the sciatic nerve was stimulated with supramaximal square wave DC impulses of .2 msec duration and 4 volts. Frequencies of two and four contractions per second were used. The isometric developed tension was monitored with a pneumatic lever. The lever was calibrated with weights at the end of each experiment.

The general experimental protocol consisted of a five-minute blood perfusion or control period followed by a three-minute period of infusion of various salt solutions into the arterial supply. This procedure was repeated several times during an experiment. All infusion solutions were at pH 7.4 and isosmotic with dog plasma. In each experiment, .85M sodium chloride was used as a control. Solutions of potassium phosphate, potassium chloride and sodium phosphate were used. Verapamil, 1 mg/ml (Knoll), was used to induce maximal vasodilation. Two milliliters arterial and venous samples were drawn at two minutes during infusion and four minutes during control, centrifuged and analyzed for osmolality (freezing point depression), sodium and potassium concentration (flame photometer) and inorganic phosphate concentration [2]. Arterial and venous samples of 0.6 ml were drawn anaerobically at 2 to 5 minutes during infusion and 4.5 min of control, capped and stored on ice. These were then analyzed for oxygen content (Lex-O_2-Con).

Results

Control values (N = 7) for arterial and venous potassium concentrations were 3.2 ± .2 and 3.5 ± .1 mEq/l, respectively. The values (N = 3) for inorganic phosphate were 5.5 ± 1.2 and 5.8 ± 1.3 mg/100 ml. With maximum infusion the potassium values (N = 4) reached 16.0 ± 1.9 and 22.6 ± 6.4 mEq/l for arterial and venous samples. The arterial inorganic phosphate content reached values between 30 and 40 mg/100 ml in the two experiments where this was determined. The arterial osmolality did not vary appreciably from control in studies comparing the response to different salt solutions.

Figure 1 depicts the effect of increasing amounts of potassium, infused as potassium phosphate, on the amount of isometric developed tension above the preinfusion control. These data are almost linear over the range shown and take the same form if plotted against phosphate infused. However, if the amount of potassium infused is greater than 15 nM/gm wet weight a very characteristic response is seen. This is an initial increase in developed tension followed by a steady decrease in the developed tension until, if the

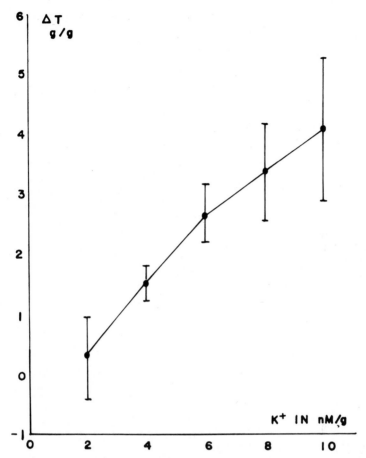

FIG. 1. Effect of increasing amounts of infused potassium on changes in developed tension. Values are means ± SEM.

stimulation is continued, there is little or no tension developed. This process is reversible, with a slightly slower time course if the infusion is stopped. The infusion of potassium phosphate over the above range into a noncontracting muscle resulted in no change in the resting tension or in the development of tension.

Potassium chloride was infused into the system to see if the effect was a function of the potassium content. As can be seen in Table I, potassium phosphate infusion resulted in an increase above control in both flow and developed tension. Potassium chloride had only slight effects although in the same direction as the potassium phosphate. The decrease in tension at high potassium chloride concentrations was also seen.

Table I. Changes in Blood Flow and Tension Resulting From
Infusion of Equimolar Amounts of Potassium Salts

	N	$\Delta \dot{Q}$ ml/min × 100 g	ΔT g/g
Potassium phosphate	7	+10.4 ± 3.7	+4.5 ± 3.1
Potassium chloride	7	+ .6 ± 3.4	+ .1 ± .7

Values are means ± SEM.

Since the changes in tension with potassium chloride and potassium phosphate were in the same direction as the change in flow, the flow response to increasing amounts of infused potassium was plotted. This is presented in Figure 2. The resulting curve is almost parallel to the curve in Figure 1.

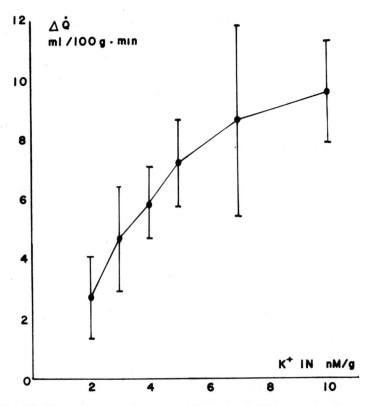

FIG. 2. Effect of increasing amounts of infused potassium on changes in blood flow. Values are means ± SEM.

In an attempt to separate direct potassium effects from other flow-related effects, verapamil was injected into the arterial system to obtain maximal vasodilation. At the peak of the effect, potassium phosphate was infused. This infusion resulted in a slight increase in the amount of developed tension (less than 1 g/g) when there was no additional increase in flow.

The metabolic effects of the different potassium and phosphate infusions are presented in Table II. Generally it appears that the observed effects of potassium phosphate cannot be duplicated by solutions containing either potassium or phosphate.

Discussion

These data indicate an inotropic effect with potassium phosphate infusion. This effect appears to be on the skeletal muscle system itself and could involve changes in several aspects of cell function. One of these could be changes in membrane potential. Using the Nernst equation and assuming that venous potassium concentration sets a lower limit for the interstitial or extracellular potassium concentration and that the intracellular potassium concentration is constant at 150 mEq/l. The range of membrane potentials seen in these experiments would be -96 to -40 mv. Values over the range could have effects on the timing and possibly the size of the calcium flux. This would alter the amount of tension developed. Changes in membrane potential could account for the decrease in tension that was seen at very high potassium concentrations. The flow to the muscle also decreases at the high potassium levels, but it is not possible to separate cause and effect. The consistent inotropic effect

Table II. Changes in Blood Flow and Oxygen Uptake Resulting From Infusion of Potassium and Phosphate Containing Salts

	N	$\Delta a\text{-}v\ O_2\ diff$ $mlO_2/100\ ml$	$\Delta \dot{Q}$ $ml/min \times 100\ g$	ΔVO_2 $ml/min \times 100\ g$
a) Potassium phosphate	7	+ .33 ± .21	+10.4 ± 3.7	+ .87 ± .36
Potassium chloride	8	+ .34 ± .38	+ .6 ± 3.4	0 ± .18
b) Sodium phosphate	3	− .5 ± .55	−10.7 ± 5.6	−1.78 ± .93
Potassium phosphate	3	+1.07 ± .52	+ 6.6 ± 8.0	+1.47 ± .76

Values are means ± SEM.

of potassium phosphate did not appear to be due to a potassium contracture, since the same range of concentrations had no effect in noncontracting muscle. A role for the phosphate component is also possible as are alternative roles for potassium.

The increases in oxygen uptake parallel the increase in developed tension in which there appears to be a consistent relationship, i.e., that as developed tension changes at a given contraction rate, the oxygen uptake changes in the same direction. At 4/sec, the correlation coefficient was .84 for this relationship. This relationship held in both fresh and fatiguing muscles. The increase in oxygen uptake of the potassium phosphate-infused muscles was the result of an increased arteriovenous oxygen concentration difference and an increased flow. Usually with increased flow, the arteriovenous concentration difference decreases. Thus both utilization and supply have increased in these experiments. Inorganic phosphate could play a role in the increased demand by increasing the amount of inorganic phosphate available to serve as a coupler to link cytoplasmic and mitochondrial ATP producing and utilizing systems.

The majority of the potassium phosphate inotropic effect appears to be related to the increases in flow resulting from vasodilatory effects on the vascular smooth muscle. This flow-related increase in developed tension has been reported previously [1]. In the present experiments, the increase in flow took from 10 to 20 seconds to reach the new steady level while the tension increase was over one to two minutes. This argues against a direct physical effect of the flow increase, but does not identify the component involved.

Therefore, the oxygen uptake at a given contraction frequency follows the developed tension and the developed tension appears to follow changes in the blood flow. Although potassium phosphate has a direct effect, these experiments appear to support the flow limiting hypothesis. The results still leave the limiting component or components of the flow unidentified.

References

1. Barclay, J. K. and Stainsby, W.N.: The role of blood flow in limiting maximal metabolic rate in muscle. Med. Sci. Sports 7:116-119, 1975.
2. Goldenberg, H. and Fernandez, A.: Simplified method for the estimation of inorganic phosphorus in body fluids. Clin. Chem. 12:871-882, 1966.

Effects of Different Initial Muscle Glycogen Levels on Prolonged Severe Exercise

P. L. Jooste and N. B. Strydom

Introduction

The capacity for prolonged heavy exercise in well-trained individuals is strongly affected by the initial glycogen content of the working muscles [3, 12]. High initial glycogen content of the muscles can be attained through the manipulation of diet and exercise sessions [3]. However, it is neither advisable nor practical to change the nutritional routine weekly or biweekly in order to elevate the muscle glycogen levels. Thus, there was a need for research which could suggest a more practical alternative or substitution for the elevation of muscle glycogen through a diet-exercise regime.

This study was designed to demonstrate the physiological and metabolic effects of a high or a low initial glycogen level during prolonged heavy exercise. Conditions of high or low initial glycogen levels were to be attained through manipulation of the exercise sessions without an alteration to the diet. This approach was considered in order to ease the implementation of the results in practice.

Methods

The following experimental design was employed in order to achieve the required initial muscle glycogen levels. Six well-trained male subjects exercised at 80% $\dot{V}O_2$ max for two hours on each of three consecutive days. Thereafter a rest period of three consecutive days was allowed during which no hard physical work was done and it was assumed that the glycogen stores were repleted on the first morning following the three-day rest period. Again three consecutive days of heavy prolonged exercise were performed with the first and last sessions of this three-day period being the test days. On the third

P. L. Jooste and N. B. Strydom, Industrial Hygiene Division, Chamber of Mines of South Africa, Johannesburg, Republic of South Africa.

day it was assumed that the initial glycogen stores were relatively depleted because of the heavy prolonged exercise on the previous two consecutive days.

On the test day the subjects first warmed up on the treadmill for ten minutes at approximately 60% $\dot{V}O_2$ max. Thereafter a siliconed needle with a resealing injection site was inserted into a forearm vein. The dead space of the needle was filled with a 3.8% w/v sterile solution of sodium citrate. Rectal temperatures were obtained immediately before the experiment commenced.

The subjects ran on the treadmill at a predetermined workload requiring 80% $\dot{V}O_2$max for two hours. Expired air was sampled, heart rate monitored and blood samples collected after four minutes and half-hourly thereafter until termination of exercise. Half-hour observations included rectal temperature measurements. Body mass was also determined prior to and after completion of the experiment. The subjects were encouraged to drink adequate amounts of water in order to remain in water balance. Approximately 1140 ml of water was taken by each subject on each of the two test days.

Expired air was sampled according to the conventional Douglas bag method and analyzed for volume in a chain compensated spirometer. Duplicate air samples were collected in butyl rubber bags and analyzed for carbon dioxide content on a Beckman LB-1 infrared medical gas analyzer. The remainder of the air in the rubber bags was then analyzed for oxygen concentration on two Beckman Model E2 paramagnetic oxygen analyzers according to the method described by Strydom et al [13]. Gross oxygen uptake was then calculated at STPD.

Analytical Procedures

The concentrations of lactate, glucose and glycerol in the blood samples were determined by means of enzymatic spectrophotometric methods using the Biochemica Test Combination according to the instructions of Boehringer Mannheim GmbH. Plasma free fatty acids (FFA) were determined with a gas chromatographic method described by Hagenfeldt [5].

A two-sided dependent t-test with a 5% level of significance was used to test for differences between the two series of experiments at each of the sampling times.

Results

The means and standard error of the means for the variables studied are given in Figures 1 and 2. Table I presents the

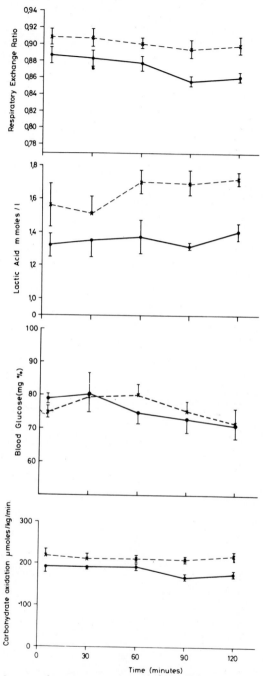

FIG. 1. Respiratory exchange ratio, lactic acid, blood glucose and carbohydrate oxidation relative to time (x----x: HIG experiments; ●———●: LIG experiments; ⊥: standard error of the mean).

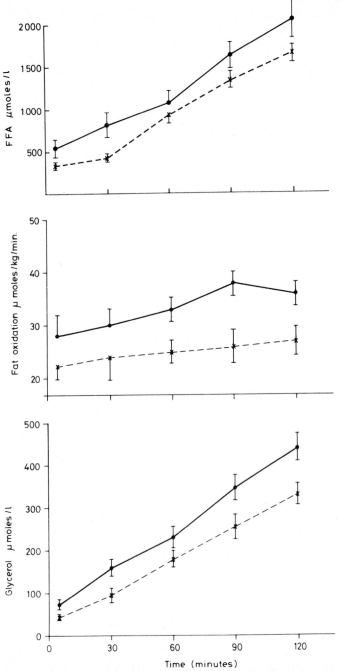

FIG. 2. Plasma free fatty acid, fat oxidation and glycerol relative to time (x----x: HIG experiments; •———•: LIG experiments; $\top$: standard error of the mean).

Table I. Significant Changes With Different
Initial Glycogen Levels

| Parameter | Time (Minutes) | | | | |
	5	30	60	90	120
Lactate				S	S
Glucose	S		S		
Carbohydrate oxidation			S	S	S
FFA		S			
Fat oxidation			S	S	S
Glycerol	S	S			S
RQ			S	S	S

S denotes a significant (P < 0.05) difference.

"significant" and "not significant" differences between the two series of experiments for the studied variables at the different sampling times.

For ease of reference the series of high initial glycogen experiments will be described as HIG and the low initial glycogen as LIG.

Oxygen uptake ($\dot{V}O_2$). A slight increase in $\dot{V}O_2$ with time from 2.7 to 2.85 l/min was observed in both series of experiments with no significant difference between them.

Respiratory quotient (RQ). RQ values observed during the LIG experiments (0.88 to 0.86) were lower than those observed during HIG experiments (0.90), significantly so from 60 to 120 minutes (Fig. 1).

Heart rate, rectal temperature and sweat rate. The mean heart rate increased steadily during both series of experiments from 158 to 171 beats per minute.

The mean rectal temperature increased from 37.4 to 38.7 C during both conditions with no significant difference between them. Neither did the delta values between resting and 120 minutes differ significantly. There was also no difference observed in sweat rate between the HIG and LIG conditions.

Metabolic Responses

Blood lactic acid. During the HIG experiments blood lactic acid increased slightly with time from 1.5 to 1.7 m moles/l. The lactic acid concentration remained relatively constant between 1.3 and 1.4 m moles/l (Fig. 1) during the LIG experiments. Observations on the 90th and 120th minute of exercise were significantly lower during the LIG experiments when compared to the HIG experiments.

Blood glucose. The mean blood glucose increased from 75 to 80 mg/100 ml during the first hour of the HIG experiments whereafter it decreased steadily until termination of exercise (Fig. 1). During the LIG experiments the mean blood glucose was initially significantly higher than in the HIG experiments, but decreased after approximately 30 minutes of exercise and remained lower than values observed during the HIG experiments.

Calculated carbohydrate oxidation. The mean carbohydrate oxidation remained fairly constant between 210 and 212 μmoles/kg/min during the HIG experiments (Fig. 1). During the LIG experiments carbohydrate oxidation was significantly lower from 60 to 120 minutes when compared to the HIG experiments.

Plasma FFA. The mean plasma FFA increased from 344 μmoles/l to 1650 μmoles/l during the HIG experiments and from 531 to 2048 μmoles/l during the LIG experiments (Fig. 2). The FFA concentration during the HIG experiments was lower than the FFA concentration during the LIG experiments, although only significantly so at the 30th minute of exercise.

Calculated fat oxidation. A slight increase in mean FFA oxidation from 22.5 to 26.9 μmoles/kg/min was observed during HIG experiments. The mean fat oxidation during the LIG experiments was higher than during the HIG experiments, significantly so from 60 to 120 minutes.

The rate of increase in FFA oxidation was also higher during the LIG experiments than during the HIG experiments as is shown by the significant difference between values obtained on the 5th and 90th minutes of LIG exercise. The difference between values obtained on the 5th and 90th minutes of HIG exercise was not significant.

Glycerol. The serum glycerol increased at least sixfold during both series of experiments. However, the glycerol was significantly lower during the HIG experiments than during the LIG experiments at 5, 30 and 120 minutes of exercise (Fig. 2).

Discussion

It has been shown previously that an exercise-diet program can be used to elevate initial muscle glycogen levels [3, 9]. It was reported that hard prolonged exercise on successive days depletes the muscle glycogen stores [4] and that a three-day rest period would allow the glycogen stores to replete. An overshooting effect of glycogen is likely to occur resulting in elevated muscle glycogen stores.

In the present study the physiological and metabolic effects after exercise-induced repletion and depletion of glycogen stores were studied. Although not measured, it could be assumed that the initial glycogen stores differed on the two test days. The subjects did not exercise until complete exhaustion but performed exactly similar exercise tests under similar conditions on the two test days. The differences obtained are thus related to the effects of the variation in the pre-test exercise sessions and not subjective in nature.

The physiological stress indicated by oxygen uptake, heart rate, rectal temperature and sweat rate was the same during the two series of experiments. Also, there was no difference in energy expenditure or mechanical efficiency between the two experiments as was indicated by the oxygen uptake.

However, the respiratory quotient (RQ), as an indicator of substrate which was utilized predominantly [1], remained remarkably constant during the HIG experiments and was significantly lower from 60 to 120 minutes during the LIG experiments. The lower RQ indicates a relatively higher utilization of FFA as fuel for muscular activity.

During cross-country skiing at a high intensity (82% of $\dot{V}O_2$ max) Hedman [6] recorded an essentially constant RQ over a three-hour period. Hermansen et al [7] also reported constant RQs during exercise at 76% or higher of $\dot{V}O_2$ max and concluded that the muscles are not able to substitute carbohydrate with fat even when the available glycogen stores are emptied. Bergström et al [3] supported this view but added that the carbohydrate supply must be limited for some time before exercise to permit the adaptation to fat combustion to take place. The difference in RQ between the HIG and LIG experiments in the present study indicates that a certain degree of fat substitution and/or adaptation to fat oxidation had occurred when carbohydrate stores were previously depleted through exercise. Furthermore, the RQ was lower from the onset of the LIG experiment and decreased during the exercise indicating a gradual increased fat metabolism and decreased carbohydrate metabolism.

The significantly lower RQ from 60 to 120 minutes of LIG exercise corresponds with the significantly lower carbohydrate oxidation and higher fat oxidation during the same time period. These observations might be somewhat biased because the RQ is used in the calculation of the carbohydrate and fat oxidation. However, the striking similarity between the graphs of RQ and that of carbohydrate oxidation suggests that carbohydrates are predominantly utilized during hard prolonged exercise provided that enough glycogen is available. If a shortage of glycogen exists, as was assumed during the LIG experiments, the body is forced to utilize a comparatively larger percentage of fats as fuel, even for high intensity exercises. More evidence supporting this view can be found when comparing the correlations of FFA concentration and FFA oxidation of the two experimental conditions (Fig. 3). Over the FFA concentration range of 900 to 2,100 m moles/l significantly more FFA were oxidized during the LIG experiments.

Hermansen et al [7] also reported that prolonged heavy exercise over a 90-minute period depletes the glycogen stores exponentially. Comparing this observation to the results of RQ and carbohydrate

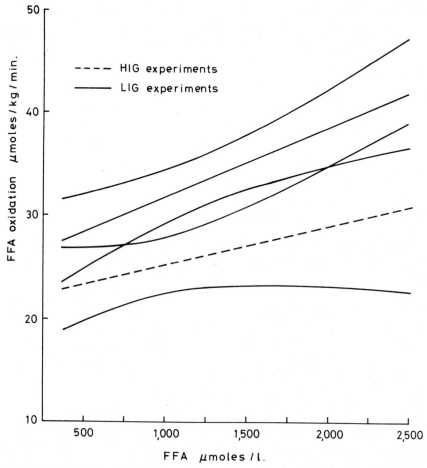

FIG. 3. Interrelationship between plasma FFA concentration and FFA oxidation during the HIG and LIG experiments.

oxidation of the HIG experiments obtained in the present study, it seems as if a discrepancy in carbohydrate supply to the working muscles existed. If the muscle glycogen stores decrease exponentially [7] and the RQ and carbohydrate oxidation remains constant, there must be a carbohydrate supply to the cellular oxidative processes other than that originating from glycogen. It is believed that blood glucose plays a very important role in this respect.

The blood glucose concentration is maintained through glucogenesis and gluconeogenesis in the liver in such a way that hepatic glucose production almost balances the utilization by the muscles. The reported initial decrease of insulin during exercise [2, 11, 14] explains the initial increase in blood glucose in the present study. The eventual decrease in blood glucose may reflect the increasing contribution of blood glucose to the total carbohydrate utilization during prolonged exercise despite a reduction in insulin levels [2, 14].

The lactic acid concentration provides further support for the view of a higher carbohydrate metabolism during the HIG experiments. Higher lactic acid concentrations during the HIG experiments indicate that the working muscles rely probably to a greater extent on enhanced glycogen stores and the production of energy by glycolysis [11]. Depletion of glycogen stores prior to the LIG experiments limited the availability of glycogen and consequently the alternative energy source was that of fat utilization. Evidence for this view can be found in the low lactate levels (1.3 to 1.4 m moles/l) during the LIG experiments. These low lactate levels suggest that the muscle cells have an ability to adapt to oxidizing more fat at extremely high workloads, provided that the intramuscular carbohydrate availability is limited at the onset of exercise.

During the LIG experiments the intramuscular carbohydrate stores were indeed limited at the onset of exercise because of the exercise on the preceding three successive days. Thus, the muscles were more dependent upon fat oxidation for energy supply and the increase in FFA was expected. In fact, the increase in plasma FFA during prolonged exercise is a well-known phenomenon and is also considered to be a good indication of fat oxidation [10]. However, it is interesting to note the increase in FFA concentration during both HIG and LIG experiments whereas Figure 2 illustrates the difference in oxidation of the available plasma FFA. Under these conditions of high and low initial glycogen levels during prolonged exercise at a high intensity there seemed to be a lower fat oxidation associated with a high initial glycogen despite the increased FFA concentration. A higher FFA/glycerol ratio from 60 to 120 minutes during the HIG experiments provides further evidence for a relative decrease in FFA utilization [11].

Issekutz et al [8] reported that the FFA do not seem to inhibit the glucose turnover or interfere with glycolysis in exercising dogs. Likewise, the increased FFA concentration in the present study did not seem to affect the carbohydrate oxidation when carbohydrates were available.

It seems as if a difference in initial carbohydrate stores does not cause a difference in physiological responses during prolonged severe exercise. However, marked and significant differences in the metabolic responses were observed which could influence the performance and/or ability during hard exercise.

References

1. Benade, A.J.S., Jansen, C.R., Rogers, G.G. et al: The significance of an increased RQ after sucrose ingestion during prolonged aerobic exercise. Pflügers Arch. 342:199-206, 1973.
2. Benade, A.J.S., Wyndham, C.H., Jansen, C.R. et al: Plasma insulin and carbohydrate metabolism after sucrose ingestion during rest and prolonged aerobic exercise. Pflügers Arch. 342:207-218, 1973.
3. Bergström, J., Hermansen, L., Hultmar E. and Saltin, B.: Diet, muscle glycogen and physical performance. Acta Physiol. Scand. 71:140-150, 1967.
4. Costill, D.L., Bowers, R., Branam, G. and Sparks, K.: Muscle glycogen utilization during prolonged exercise on successive days. J. Appl. Physiol. 31:834-838, 1971.
5. Hagenfeldt, L.: A gas chromatographic method for the determination of individual free fatty acids in plasma. Clin. Chim. Acta 13:266, 1966.
6. Hedman, R.: The available glycogen in man and the connection between rate of oxygen intake and carbohydrate usage. Acta Physiol. Scand. 40:305-321, 1957.
7. Hermansen, L., Hultman, E. and Saltin, B.: Muscle glycogen during prolonged severe exercise. Acta Physiol. Scand. 71:129-139, 1967.
8. Issekutz, B., Jr., Issekutz, A.C. and Nash, D.: Mobilization of energy sources in exercising dogs. J. Appl. Physiol. 29:691-697, 1970.
9. Karlsson, J. and Saltin, B.: Diet, muscle glycogen, and endurance performance. J. Appl. Physiol. 31(2):203-206, 1971.
10. Paul, P.: FFA metabolism of normal dogs during steady-state exercise at different work loads. J. Appl. Physiol. 28:127-132, 1970.
11. Rennie, M.J. and Johnson, R.H.: Effects of an exercise-diet program on metabolic changes with exercise in runners. J. Appl. Physiol. 37(6):821-825, 1974.
12. Saltin, B. and Hermansen, L.: Glycogen stores and prolonged severe exercise. In Blix, G. (ed.): Symposia of the Swedish Nutrition Foundation V Nutrition and Physical Activity. Uppsala:Almqvist and Wiksells, 1967.
13. Strydom, N.B., Cooke, H.M., Miller, H.D. and Winer, P.: Errors in respiratory gas analysis. A comparison of the Haldane and Pauling gas analysers. Int. Z. Angew. Physiol. Eishchl. Arbeitsphysiol. 21:13-26, 1965.
14. Wahren, J., Felig, P., Ahlborg, G. and Jorfeldt, L.: Glucose metabolism during leg exercise in man. J. Clin. Invest. 50:2715-2725, 1971.

The Effect of Bee Pollen Tablets on the Improvement of Certain Blood Factors and Performance of Male Collegiate Swimmers

Ralph E. Steben, John C. Wells and Ivan L. Harless

Introduction

Newspaper reports [3, 5, 17] have extolled the rejuvenating quality of bee pollen tablets on the body with attendant testimonials of "how the athlete and trainer feel" about the product. However, there has been very little, if any, support for such claims in scientific literature. Athletes may be using them, but supporting evidence of the possible value of ingesting bee pollen tablets for improvement of athletic performance has been difficult to obtain in the United States because of the recency of the practice and the expense of the product.

To quote Seppo Nuutilla [3], head trainer of Finland: "To train 25 miles a day, Lasse (Virin) needs a food intake equivalent to 5,000 calories a day — and there are not enough hours in the day to digest ordinary food and run at that (a demanding) pace. Pollen (Pollitabs*) helps break down food taken in to build red cells to transport oxygen." Millar [15] reported that while average hemoglobin concentration of the Finnish runners increased from 12 gm/100 ml of blood in 1968 to 16.25 in 1972, no direct correlations between pollen ingestion and hemoglobin increase were established.

A symposium conducted by Cernelle [12] in 1972 reported that Finnish runners using a Swedish pollen product and running the prescribed daily 25 miles also experienced resistance to colds and

Ralph E. Steben, John C. Wells and Ivan L. Harless, Department of Health, Physical and Recreation Education, Louisiana State University, Baton Rouge, La., U.S.A.

*The pollen preparations in this case were supplied by A. B. Cernelle, Vegeholm, Sweden.

influenza, as well as showed weight gains. Binding and Donadieu [4, 7] continue the questionable endorsement by describing pollen "as a wonderful, perfect natural food, capable of restoring zest for living; a tonic aiding in either the increase or decrease of weight; as well as containing an antibiotic capable of controlling dangerous bacteria in the intestines."

For some time, less conservative Europeans have been using bee pollen tablets made from pollen residue mixed with vitamins (Cernilton*) for successful treatment of prostatitis [1, 2, 6, 19], bleeding stomach ulcers [9] and for reduction of respiratory infections and allergen reactions [10, 11, 14]. Fijalkowski [8] reported improved working capacity of Polish national team weight-lifters receiving bee pollen tablets (Pollitabs and Stark protein*) as evidenced by higher increases in stroke volume, systolic pressure and more distinct changes in diastolic pressure. Specific EKG and respiratory parameters also improved and lactate levels decreased significantly.

Of further interest is the recent work of Rose [18] relating to hypokalemia in varsity distance runners. Since potassium is the principal mineral in bee pollen, it is suggested that pollen may be taken to alleviate or prevent this condition, which manifests itself in muscle weakness and lethargy, despite otherwise good aerobic condition. Severe cases, not apt to be seen in athletics, are characterized by decreased smooth muscle contractility and attendant gastrointestinal conditions, cardiac arrhythmias and renal disturbances [13, 16].

Since athletes, in particular, have shown considerable interest in any potential psychological or physiological advantage over an opponent, the purpose of this study was to investigate certain claims that have been made for the recently adopted practice of ingesting bee pollen tablets for improved athletic performance. A question of interest is whether considerable mileage per day along with adequate nutrition, or mileage, proper nutrition, plus the pollen tablets is responsible for success in endurance events. Analysis of specific biochemical parameters, especially hemoglobin content and hematocrit, could authenticate suggested improvement of oxygen carrying ability of the blood and test the hypothesis that ingestion of pollen may prevent the hypokalemia that may accompany prolonged vigorous aerobic training.

---

*Also from A. B. Cernelle, Vegeholm, Sweden.

Procedures

The placebo double-blind experiment was undertaken at Louisiana State University for eight weeks during the Fall Semester, 1975, with 27 volunteer male collegiate swimmers, randomly subdivided into three groups. Each of the eight individuals in group 1 (placebo group) orally ingested ten placebo tablets* daily, after practice and before the evening meal on nonactivity days. A similar procedure prescribing ten pollen tablets* was followed by the nine individuals in group 2 (pollen group), while the ten individuals of group 3 (combination group) took five bee pollen and five placebo tablets to help determine whether half the number of bee pollen tablets were as effective as the ten-tablet prescription of group 2.

At the beginning and the conclusion of the experiment, blood samples were drawn† from each individual for three consecutive days before practice. Extracellular sodium and serum potassium levels were analyzed by an Instrument Lab (IL) flame photometer. Hemoglobin and hematocrit levels were determined by a Cotter S Automatic Counter. All the participants dined at the L.S.U. athletic training table, and diet was assumed to be basically the same for all. Training consisted of a repetition program at the beginning of the season, gradually evolving into an interval program as condition of the swimmers improved. Each individual, regardless of specialty, swam a total of three to four miles per day.

Performance data were collected for each swimmer just prior to the beginning of, and again at the termination of, the experiment. Pre-experiment work bouts consisted of a set of 12×200 yard freestyle swims, developed for each swimmer so that the starting time for each of the 200's was held constant. Times were recorded for each of the swims and an average time determined and converted into velocity in yards per second for statistical analysis. The postexperiment performance data were collected in an identical manner two days after completion of the experiment. The data — potassium (K) mEq/l; sodium (Na) mEq/l; hemoglobin (Hgb) gm; hematocrit (Hct) %; and performance, yards per second for average 200-yard freestyle velocity — were statistically examined with the t test for correlated means and analysis of covariance.

---

*The 500 mg pure natural bee pollen tablets and the placebos used in this study were obtained from Les Ruchers de la Côte d'Azur, Inc., 60 East 42nd St., New York, N.Y.

† Laboratory blood analysis was completed by The Pathology Laboratory of Baton Rouge, La.

Results

The t test revealed a significant improvement in the quantity of extracellular potassium and Hct values in the subjects of the combination and pollen groups, respectively (Table I), but an ANCOVA did not detect any significant improvement over that of the other groups (Tables II and III). None of the other groups made significant gains in extracellular sodium or Hgb values (Table I). Therefore, no further analysis was done. The t tests for improvement in performance were all significant (Table I); however, ANCOVA failed to establish any difference in performance values among the three groups (Table IV).

Table I. T-Tests of Significance for Five Variables
After Eight Weeks of Training

Group	n	Mean Gain	SE Gain	t	P
Potassium (K)					
Placebo	8	-.11	.14	.79	N.S.
Pollen	9	.13	.08	1.63	N.S.
Combination	10	.36	.11	3.27	.05
Sodium (Na)					
Placebo	8	-1.19	.52	2.29	N.S.
Pollen	8	.97	.58	1.67	N.S.
Combination	9	.64	.60	1.07	N.S.
Hemoglobin (Hgb)					
Placebo	8	.02	.19	.11	N.S.
Pollen	8	.15	.13	1.15	N.S.
Combination	10	.18	.22	.82	N.S.
Hematocrit (Hct)					
Placebo	8	.29	.49	.59	N.S.
Pollen	8	1.03	.33	3.12	.05
Combination	10	1.19	.61	1.95	N.S.
Performance					
Placebo	8	.11	.02	5.5	.05
Pollen	9	.12	.01	12.0	.05
Combination	10	.13	.01	13.0	.05

n 8, needed for significance at .05 level, 2.36.
n 9, needed for significance at .05 level, 2.31.
n 10, needed for significance at .05 level, 2.26.

Table II. ANCOVA for Levels of Serum Potassium
in Three Sample Groups

SOV	Adj SS	df	M^2	F	P
Between	0.42	2	.21	2.10	N.S.
Within	2.25	23	.10		
Total	2.67				

F needed for significance at .05 level, 3.42.

Table III. ANCOVA for Blood Hematocrit in Three Sample Groups

SOV	Adj SS	df	M^2	F	P
Between	3.72	2	1.86	.87	N.S.
Within	46.81	22	2.13		
Total	50.53				

F needed for significance at .05 level, 3.44.

Table IV. ANCOVA of Improvement in Performance
of Three Sample Groups

SOV	Adj SS	df	M^2	F	P
Between	.01	2	.005	1.67	N.S.
Within	.07	23	.003		
Total	.08	25			

F needed for significance at .05 level, 3.42.

Discussion

There is apparently no advantage in taking bee pollen tablets for postulated maintenance of normal extracellular potassium levels for prevention of hypokalemia. It is possible, however, that a longer experiment, e.g. Rose [18], impossible in this study, would reveal more information. It is of interest here that while Finnish runners did not include pollen in their high protein diets to prevent hypokalemia, physiologically these diets actually enhance renal potassium excretion. Biochemically, sulfates formed during high nitrogen intake are excreted with their full base equivalents, increasing prospects for potassium depletion. The 1972 Olympic Games efforts of Finnish endurance runners, however, were not only conspicuously marked by excellent aerobic condition, but also by apparent neuromuscular zest for running. The fact remains, however, that there is no substitute for a regular diet, supplemented with potassium-rich citrus and bananas, for maintenance of normal serum potassium levels.

Extracellular sodium values were included as a variable in the study because the blood analysis procedures employed allowed computation of both potassium and sodium values in one operation. Sodium levels could diminish if taking too many pollen tablets increased potassium levels inordinately, producing a hyperkalemia.* However, this did not occur with the dosages used. There have been reports of far greater amounts of pollen taken on a daily basis without ill effects [7, 10, 18]. Clinically, hypokalemia is treated by administering as much as 40 mEq of potassium chloride three to four times daily, usually not to exceed a total of 160 mEq during the first 24 hours in more severe cases. A flame photometer assay of the product used in this experiment did not exceed 0.088 mEq of potassium per 500 mg tablet.

Millar [15] reported no direct correlation between ingested pollen and hemoglobin increase among Finnish runners. Similarly, no beneficial effects for increased hemoglobin from taking bee pollen were obtained in this study. It is conceivable that the high protein diet followed by Finnish runners for several years (1968-1972), alternated with a high carbohydrate diet a few days prior to competition, may have accounted for the improvement in the average hemoglobin levels of the runners.

Although a significant gain in Hct was evidenced by the combination group, no differences among groups were detected. An increase in hematocrit as a result of physical activity is normal, however. The degree of physical activity of an individual largely determines the rate at which red blood cells are produced. The fact that exercise increases the rate of red blood cell production is an indication that tissue anoxia causes extra red cell production because the supply of oxygen becomes depleted during exercise. Any theorizing that an increase in either Hgb or Hct can enhance endurance capabilities of athletes does not consider that the rate of oxygen transport to tissues is actually reduced by an excessive rise in hematocrit. Nuuttila's [3, 5, 17] opinion that pollen can somehow improve the transportation of oxygen by the blood is questionable. Even in the compensatory increases during anemia, there is an overall

---

*Personal interview with Albert McQuown, M.D., January 8, 1976.

reduction in the rate of oxygen transport to the tissues. One conclusion can be reached here: either the training program for the swimmers was not sufficiently stressful, or they were in good condition before the season started.

There does not seem to be any advantage in taking ten pollen tablets as opposed to half that amount. The prescribed dosage (three to six tablets daily) should be sufficient for advertised results. Finally, although performance improved in all three groups, it would seem to be the result of training rather than due to the real or imagined advantage of ingesting bee pollen.

References

.1 Ask-Upmark, E.: Treatment of prostatitis. Z. Urol. Nephrol. 56:113-116, 1963.

2. Ask-Upmark, E.: Prostatitis and its treatment. Acta Med. Scand. 181:355-357, 1967.

3. Bee prepared. Track and Field News 28:48, 1975.

4. Binding, C.J.: About Pollen. London:Thorsons Publishers Limited, 1971.

5. A body builder from the bee's knees. The San Francisco Chronicle, February 28, 1975, p. 22.

6. Denis, L.J.: Chronic prostatitis. Acta Urol. Belg. 34:49-56, 1966.

7. Donadieu, Y.: Le Pollen. Paris:Maloine, 1973.

8. Fijalkowski, A. et al: Results of studies on effects of taking "pollitabs" and "stark protein" drugs on improvement of working capacity of weight lifters. A. B. Cernelle Symposium for Sportsmen. London, November 1973.

9. Georgieva, E. and Vasilex, V.: Symposium on use of bee products in human and veterinary medicine. International Beekeeping Congress 23, 1971.

10. Helander, E.: Hay fever and pollen tablets. Grana Palynologia 2:119-123, 1960.

11. Klapsch, H.: Experiences of fluaxin, an anti-influenza medicine in tablet form. A. B. Cernelle Symposium for Sportsmen. Helsingborg, July 1972.

12. Kvante, E.: The effects of nutritive supplement substances on athletes. A. B. Cernelle Symposium for Sportsmen. Helsingborg, July 1972.

13. Lowenstein, J.: Hypokalemia and hyperkalemia. Med. Clinics N. Am. 57:1435-1439, 1973.

14. Malmström, S. et al: Pollen as a prophylactic against the common cold. A. B. Cernelle Symposium for Sportsmen. Helsingborg, July 1972.

15. Millar, S.L.: Flower power pills. Track Technique 54:1706-1708, 1973.

16. Newmark, S.R. and Dluhy, R.G.: Hyperkalemia and hypokalemia. JAMA 231:631-633, 1975.

17. Nuuttila, S.: Nutrition programme for athletes. London Sunday Times, August 5, 1973, p. 21.

18. Rose, K.: Warning for millions: Intense exercise can deplete potassium. Physician and Sportsmed. 3:67-70, 1975.

19. Saito, Y.: Diagnosis and treatment of chronic prostatitis. Clin. Exp. Med. 44:614-629, 1967.

Changes in Lipid Metabolism After Exercise or Hypokinesia During Pre- or Postnatal Ontogeny

J. Parízková, T. Petrásek and R. Poledne

Metabolic consequences of adaptation to exercise (three hours run daily on a treadmill, at a speed of 16 to 18 meters/min for 60 to 120 days) characterized as an aerobic workload of mild or medium intensity are manifested not only during the actual load, but also at rest. Exercised animals (male rats) are characterized by increased oxygen uptake and/or increased caloric intake/100 gm weight/day, i.e., an increased level of energy turnover per unit of time. Simultaneously, they display a different transfer of fatty acids to individual tissues as ascertained by the increased inflow rate of injected palmitate $^{-14}$C, even 24 hours after the last exercise, to the heart and soleus muscles, and a reduced inflow rate to adipose tissue. This was paralleled in the exercised animals by a decreased body weight and fat ratio. Increased output of ^{14}C during 30-minute infusion of palmitate $^{-14}$C into the femoral vein under pentothal anesthesia was also found in regularly exercised animals, again 24 hours after the last run on the treadmill, indicating persistence of greater fatty acid utilization even under conditions of muscular rest.

On the other hand, adaptation to restricted physical activity — hypokinesia (i.e., confinement to spaces $8 \times 12 \times 20$ cm since weaning) resulted in a reduced outflow rate of injected palmitate $^{-14}$C from plasma, its reduced inflow rate to the heart and soleus muscles, and increased inflow rate to adipose tissue. Body fat ratio and weight were highest in the hypokinetic animals despite a spontaneously reduced caloric intake. These differences were obvious, not only when comparing the hypokinetic animals to exercised ones, but also to control animals living in normal cages. Apparently, adequate motor stimulation which plays a key role in the lipid metabolism cannot be compensated by decreased caloric intake [7, 9, 10, 12] (Figs. 1 and 2; Table I).

J. Parízkova, R. Petrásek and R. Poledne, Res. Inst. FTVS, Charles University; Institute of Clinical Experimental Medicine, Prague, Czechoslovakia.

CALORIC INPUT

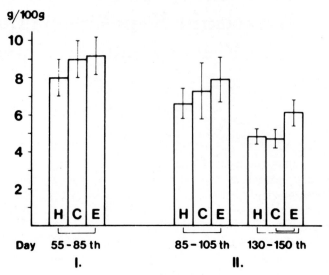

FIGURE 1.

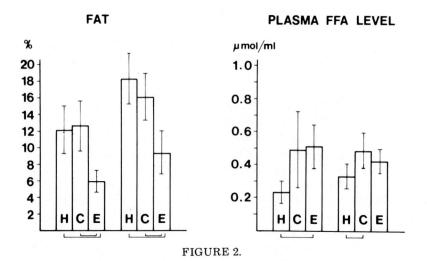

FIGURE 2.

   The mentioned changes in lipid metabolism, body composition, weight, etc., resulted from different physical activity regimens induced during postnatal ontogeny, starting at very early periods of life (18th to 30th day of life). Oscai et al [6] also demonstrated important delayed effects of daily swimming starting on the fifth day

Table I. Inflow Rate of Free Fatty Acids Into Different
Tissues of Male Rats Adapted to Different Physical Activity
Regimens (in m μmol/min)

		Control	Exercised	Hypokinetic
Soleus muscle	I	1.19	2.39	1.38
	II	4.35	6.96	2.08
Adipose tissue	I	4.15	1.96	1.86
	II	6.46	3.11	3.86
Heart	I	–	–	–
	II	145.1	191.1	73.3

I = 90 days old; II = 150 days old.

of life, manifested in different weight curves, weight and cellularity of the epididymal fat pad during adult life. But already during prenatal ontogeny it is possible to interfere with later development of the offspring by changes in the physical activity regimen of the pregnant mother. In a previous study a significant increase in capillary density of the heart muscle in the offspring of mothers exercised during pregnancy was demonstrated [8]. Regular workloads change significantly the level of various metabolites in the blood (glycemia, free fatty acids, pyruvate, lactate, etc.) and increase the release of catecholamines and their synthesis in the adrenals [5]. This modifies the milieu interieur of the mother with possible impact on the fetus. Therefore, selected parameters of lipid metabolism in the liver were studied in addition in another series of experiments where the offspring of both sexes of rat mothers exercised during pregnancy were followed. Total lipids and fatty acid concentration (assessed gravimetrically) in the liver of female offspring of the exercised mothers at the age of 35 and 90 days were significantly higher than in the liver of female offspring of control mothers. In 35-day-old female and male offspring in which also cholesterol concentration was ascertained (by a chemical method according to Abell [1]), the concentration was also significantly higher in the liver of the offspring of exercised mothers compared to those from control mothers. Total lipid and fatty acid concentrations in the liver of male offspring either did not differ, or the differences were reversed (Fig. 3).

The synthesis of total lipids and fatty acids was significantly reduced in female offspring of exercised mothers at the age of 35 days. In the following series when measuring female offspring of the same age no significant differences were found, but at the age of 90

CONCENTRATION OF LIPIDS, FATTY ACIDS AND CHOLESTEROL
IN THE LIVER OF THE OFFSPRING OF EXERCISED AND
CONTROL RAT MOTHERS   (IN VIVO STUDY)

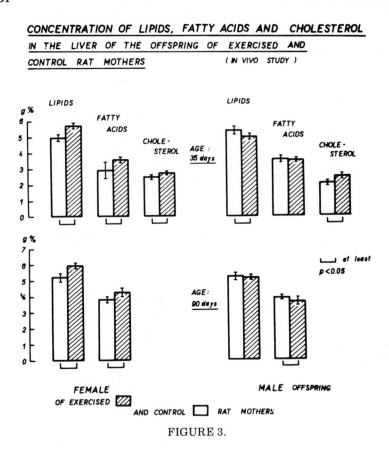

FIGURE 3.

days the total lipid and fatty acid synthesis (investigated in vivo, based on ^{14}C incorporation from injected Na acetate) was significantly lower, too. The synthesis of fatty acids in the liver of the male offspring of exercised mothers at the age of 35 days was increased, but that of total lipids was decreased. In 90-day-old male offspring there were no differences, with the exception of cholesterol synthesis which was higher in male offspring of exercised mothers, similarly as in female offspring of exercised mothers (Fig. 4).

Another experiment in 108-day-old male offspring (in vitro study — incubation of liver slices using Na-acetate-1^{14}C, as described by Avoye [2]) showed also lowered concentrations of lipids in the liver of the offspring of exercised mothers, and in this case also lowered concentrations of fatty acids; the cholesterol concentration did not differ. The serum level of free fatty acids was significantly higher in the offspring of exercised mothers. Lipid synthesis in the liver of the

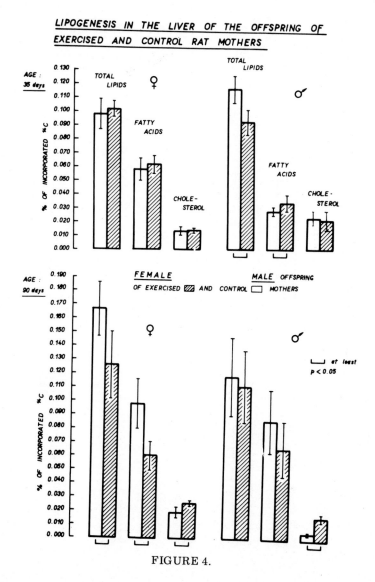

FIGURE 4.

offspring did not differ in relation to the physical activity regimen of the pregnant mother (Fig. 5).

The mentioned results indicate that regular exercise has a profound impact on lipid metabolism not only during postnatal ontogeny, but also during intrauterine life, i.e., due to the exercise of the pregnant mother. More marked impact in female offspring of exercised mothers, manifested, e.g., in increased concentration of

CONCENTRATION OF LIPIDS AND LIPOGENESIS IN
THE LIVER AND SERUM NEMK IN MALE OFFSPRING
OF EXERCISED AND CONTROL RAT MOTHERS
(IN VITRO STUDY)

CONCENTRATION OF LIVER:

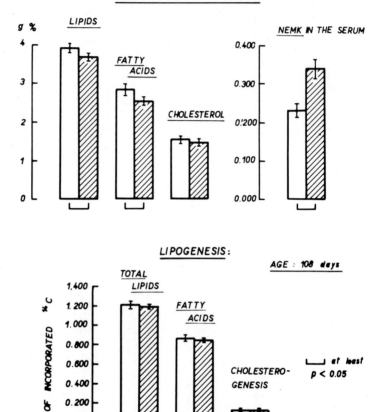

FIGURE 5.

total lipids, fatty acids, etc., as well as in a changed lipogenesis may
be related to sexual dimorphism in fatness and lipid metabolism due
to the action of female sex hormones (about which very little is
known until now) and a different role of lipids in future life of a
female, considering especially pregnancy and lactation, which may
cause greater sensitivity of the lipid metabolism to various stimuli
including exercise also during prenatal period. During postnatal

ontogenesis Fröberg [4] found in an exercised group increased liver triglycerides. Lipogenetic processes in the liver did not display the same homogeneity as the changes in the lipid concentration obviously due to their more dynamic character and variability. More detailed studies are needed for their definition. The mechanisms of changes mentioned above could be caused by an increase in free fatty acids serum levels: it is known that during long-lasting aerobic work mobilization of lipid metabolites occurs [11] especially when such a load is regularly repeated. An increased free fatty acid level was also found in male offspring of exercised mothers. The increase of the blood level could concern also other lipid metabolites of the mother. It was shown that free fatty acids could be transferred through the placenta [3] and thus influence lipid metabolism of the fetus. This might also persist even in later periods of postnatal life. The importance of the mentioned findings as well as their mechanism is still obscure and is being studied in subsequent experiments. Nevertheless, the importance of the physical activity regimen seems to be obvious even during the prenatal period of life and is relevant for future metabolic development of the offspring in the physiological and possibly the pathological sphere.

References

1. Abell, L.L., Levy, B.B. and Kendall, E.F.: J. Biol. Chem. 195:357, 1951.
2. Avoye, D.R., Swyryd, E.A. and Gould, R.G.: J. Lipid Res. 6:368, 1965.
3. Dancis, J.: In Camerini-Davalos, R.A. and Cole, H.S. (eds.): Early Diabetes in Early Life. New York:Academic Press, 1975, p. 233.
4. Fröberg, S.O.: Metabolism 20:1044, 1971.
5. Kvetnanský, R., Parízková, J., Mikulaj, L. et al: Physiol. Bohemoslov. 24:66, 1975.
6. Oscai, L.B., Babirak, S.P., McGarr, J.A. and Spirakis, C.N.: Fed. Prod. 33:1956, 1974.
7. Parízková, J.: In Nijnhoff, M. (ed.): Body Fat and Physical Activity. The Hague, The Netherlands. (In press, 1976.)
8. Parízková, J.: Eur. J. Appl. Physiol. 34:1, 1975.
9. Parízková, J. and Poledne, R.: Eur. J. Appl. Physiol. 33:1, 1974.
10. Parízková, J. and Stanková, L.: Br. J. Nutr. 18:325, 1969.
11. Paul, P.: In Howald, H. and Poortmans, J.R. (eds.): Metabolic Adaptation to Prolonged Physical Exercise. Basel:Birkhäuser Verlag, 1975, p. 156.

Utilisation de certains métabolites pour stimuler la capacité d'effort et la récupération lors d'efforts physiques chez les rats blancs

Y. Afar

L'un des principaux indices d'un haut degré d'entraînement et d'une grande capacité d'effort est la tolérance de l'organisme à de grands efforts physiques et neuropsychiques, ainsi que la vitesse avec laquelle il récupère après l'effort. Le maintien d'un haut degré d'entraînement n'est possible que si l'effort physique et le repos se trouvent judicieusement combinés. Cela est possible également si on aide à accélérer les processus de récupération dans l'organisme du sportif.

On peut recourir et on recourt à divers moyens pour accélérer la récupération. L'utilisation de tels moyens permet à l'organisme, dans des délais réduits, de fournir un nouvel effort physique, et cela sur la base de plus grandes possibilités fonctionnelles. De telle sorte, on parvient indirectement à accroître la capacité d'effort.

L'utilisation de substances biologiquement actives, notamment des métabolites, a été suscitée par le désir d'éviter les facteurs nuisibles et les changements fonctionnels inhérents à la fatigue ou bien de les réduire au minimum possible. D'autre part, on cherche ainsi à introduire dans l'organisme des produits qui interviennent rapidement dans les processus de synthèse intensifiée dans la période de repos.

La force et la vitesse, qui sont des qualités essentielles et obligatoires pour la capacité d'effort sportif, reposent sur la caractéristique qualitative et quantitative de l'échange protéique.

Sur la base d'un hydrolysat protéique, nous avons élaboré un produit enrichi de certains métabolites et dont nous avons expérimentalement vérifié l'effet physiologique sur des animaux et, plus tard, éprouvé sur des sportifs.

Yakov Afar, Chargé de cours, agrégé en médecine, Sofia, Bulgarie.

Les recherches avec des animaux ont été effectuées sur six groupes de rats blancs, mâles, et pesant chacun en moyenne 200 grammes. Le mélange alimentaire stimulant était composé de: 200 mg d'hydrolysat de caséine (1 gramme par kilogramme poids du corps); 50 mg de glycérinoaldéhydephosphate de sodium; 50 mg de succinate de sodium; 50 mg d'acide fumarique; 50 mg d'acide ascorbique et 2 mg de créatine.

En tant que modèle d'effort physique chez les animaux, nous avons appliqué la nage: nous faisions nager les rats jusqu'à bout de forces, dans l'eau à une température de 28-30°, avec une charge supplémentaire représentant 10% du poids de leur corps.

Le mélange alimentaire était introduit par la bouche à l'aide d'une sonde: dans une des séries (groupe II) — 30 minutes avant l'effort, dans une autre — après la fin de l'effort. Dans ce dernier cas, les animaux étaient examinés soit après 3 heures de repos (groupe IV), soit après un deuxième effort poussé à l'extrême et appliqué 3 heures après le premier (groupe VI).

Dans tous les cas, parallèlement aux groupes expérimentés, on procédait à des examens sur des animaux témoins auxquels on n'administrait pas de mélange alimentaire (groupes I, III et V).

Les animaux étaient décapités et on déterminait dans le tissu musculaire la teneur en créatine-phosphate, glycogène et lactate. Parallèlement, on déterminait aussi le niveau de lactate dans le sang. En outre, en tant qu'indice de la capacité d'effort, on mesurait la durée de nage des animaux.

Analyse des résultats

Conformément aux données obtenues et représentées sur le tableau I et la figure 1, l'absorption du mélange alimentaire 30 minutes avant l'effort physique n'influe pas sur la durée de la nage, c'est-à-dire sur la capacité d'effort (172.00 sec contre 161.70 sec; statistiquement, la différence n'a pas le niveau de confiance requis). Le niveau de créatine-phosphate dans le tissu musculaire des rats ayant absorbé le mélange alimentaire (D) après la nage est supérieur à cèlui chez les rats n'ayant pas absorbé de mélange alimentaire. La consommation de glycogène (E) qui est de 278.75 mg%, ainsi que l'accumulation d'acide lactique dans les muscles (B) de 90.67 mg% et dans le sang (C) de 163.00 mg% chez les animaux témoins avait été inférieure à celle des animaux expérimentés, respectivement 213.75 mg%, 145.90 mg% et 221.30 mg%. Cela nous incite à considérer que l'effort fourni par les animaux ayant absorbé le mélange alimentaire a

Tableau I. Valeurs des paramètres étudiés chez des rats blancs
immédiatement après la nage

Paramètres étudiés	Durée de la nage en sec. M	Lactate en mg% Tissu m M	Lactate en mg% Sang M	Cr-P en mg% M	Glycogène en mg% M
1(e) groupe sans mixture nutritive	172.0 ± 2.5	90.7 ±15.6	163.0 ± 9.2	219.4 ±32.8	278.7 ±17.3
2(e) gróupe avec mixture nutritive	161.7 ±18.5	145.9 ±11.9	221.3 ±20.4	314.6 ±24.5	213.7 ±16.3

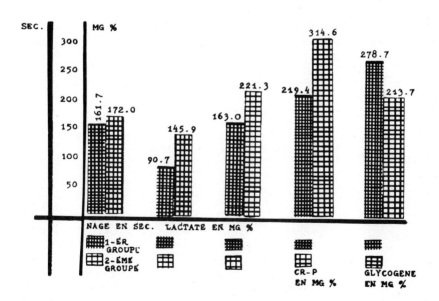

FIGURE 1.

été énergétiquement assuré pour le compte surtout de l'oxydation des hydrocarbures par la voie d'activisation de la glycolyse.

Il était particulièrement intéressant pour nous d'élucider le rôle du mélange alimentaire utilisé sur les processus de récupération. A cet effet, un groupe d'animaux (groupe III) fut soumis à la nage jusqu'à abandon sans qu'on lui ait administré le mélange alimentaire ou quelque autre (groupe IV) et en lui faisant prendre ce mélange dès la fin de l'effort. L'examen fut effectué après un repos de 3 heures. Comme on peut le voir des données consignées au tableau II et à la figure 2, le niveau de l'acide lactique dans le sang (C) de 18.83 mg% et dans le tissu musculaire (B) de 91.67 mg% des animaux recevant le mélange alimentaire se rétablit beaucoup plus vite que chez les animaux servant de témoins, respectivement 45.83 mg% et 292.65 mg%.

Le créatine-phosphate (D) après 3 heures de repos se rétablit également — 400 mg%, voire même elle se surrétablit dans les cas d'absorption du mélange alimentaire, tandis que le glycogène (E) dénote une tendance marquée à se maintenir haut et à se rétablir — 415.00 mg%.

Afin de s'assurer et de confirmer l'effet du mélange alimentaire sur les processus de récupération, nous recourûmes à un modèle où l'effort physique devait être exécuté deux fois.

Les animaux étaient soumis au deuxième effort 3 heures après le premier, tout aussi bien dans les conditions d'absorption d'un mélange alimentaire (groupe VI) que non (Groupe V).

Tableau II. Valeurs des paramètres étudiés chez des rats blancs à la troisième heure du repos après l'effort physique

Paramètres étudiés	Durée de la nage en sec. M	Lactate en mg% Tissu m. M	Sang M	Cr-P en mg% M	Glycogène en mg% M
3(e) groupe sans mixture nutritive	168.0 ±37.1	292.6 ±62.9	45.8 ±9.8	234.2 ±14.9	340.0 ±60.6
4(e) groupe avec mixture nutritive	123.0 ±16.0	91.7 ±7.8	18.8 ±5.2	400.0 ±24.3	415.0 ±44.2

VALEURS DES PARAMETRES ETUDIES CHEZ DES RATS BLANCS
A LA 3-EME HEURE DU REPOS APRES L'EFFOT PHYSIQUE

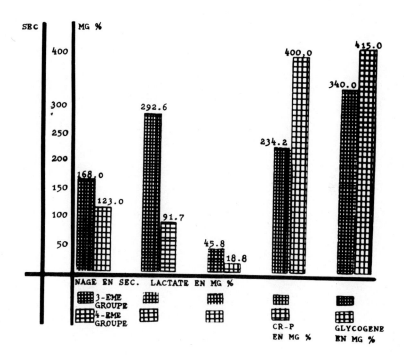

FIGURE 2.

Outre les paramètres biochimiques, on mesura la durée de la première et de la deuxième nages. Les résultats obtenus et présentés sur le tableau III et la figure 3 montrent que les animaux auxquels on avait fait prendre le mélange alimentaire avaient nagé plus longtemps, ce qui témoigne d'une capacité d'effort plus élevée (A).

Si les résultats chez les animaux n'ayant pas absorbé de mélange alimentaire lors du deuxième effort marquent une baisse (179.00 sec contre 156.00 sec), il n'en est pas de même pour les animaux ayant absorbé ce mélange: ici la durée de la deuxième nage augmente considérablement (252.00 sec contre 542.00 sec). En outre, on constate un moindre accroissement du lactate dans le sang (C) et

Table III. Valeurs des paramètres étudiés chez des rats blancs
après un effort physique réitéré

Paramètres étudiés	Durée de la nage en sec. M	Lactate en mg% Tissu m. M	Sang M	Cr-P en mg% M	Glycogène en mg% M
5(e) groupe 1(e) effort sans mixture nutritive	179.0 ±13.0				
5(e) groupe 2(e) effort sans mixture nutritive	156.0 ± 8.0	272.5 ±30.5	184.1 ± 3.5	285.0 ± 9.1	140.0 ±36.9
6(e) groupe 1(e) effort avec mixture nutritive	252.0 ±13.4				
6(e) groupe 2(e) effort avec mixture nutritive	542.0 ±59.0	133.8 ±15.5	64.5 ±17.3	250.0 ±15.0	225.0 ±29.3

dans les muscles (B), — par conséquent, une utilisation plus économique des ressources énergétiques.

Nous considérons que l'effet positif du mélange alimentaire appliqué par nous est dû à l'influence globale des constituantes qui y sont incluses. Le mélange d'hydrolysat de caséine et de métabolites du cycle de Crebs exerce un effet prononcé sur les processus de récupération et améliore la capacité d'effort en cas d'un deuxième effort, tout en préservant l'organisme contre un épuisement plus poussé de ses réserves énergétiques. L'utilisation du mélange alimentaire recommandé par nous crée dans l'organisme des conditions propices à l'accomplissement d'un deuxième effort plus intense, sur la base d'une récupération plus complète après le premier effort physique. Ce mélange perfectionne, certes, le mécanisme de la phase

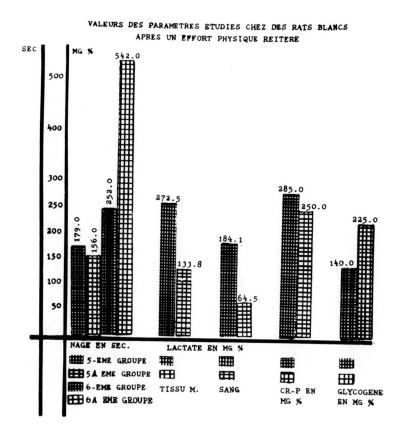

FIGURE 3.

lactique de l'échange d'hydrocarbures, contribuant ainsi indirectement à la meilleure marche des processus d'oxydation dans l'organisme.

Effets trophiques de l'isoprotérénol sur le muscle squelettique du rat

Marie-Christine Thibault et Jacques LeBlanc

Introduction

Parmi les différences observées entre les muscles à contraction lente et les muscles à contraction rapide, il y a celles qui existent au niveau de l'influence du système nerveux sympathique. Ainsi, dans les réponses du muscle aux catécholamines, on observe des effets bêta-adrénergiques différents au niveau de la contraction musculaire provoquée et de la glycogénolyse. Il est par exemple reconnu que le muscle à contraction lente est plus sensible à ce type de stimulation que le muscle à contraction rapide [3]. Certains de ces effets aigus sur les deux types de muscles s'apparentent d'une certaine façon à ceux produits sur le muscle cardiaque. Nous savons également qu'une stimulation répétée des récepteurs bêta-adrénergiques par l'isoprotérénol produit une hypertrophie marquée du muscle cardiaque [1, 28, 30]. Dans ce contexte, l'hypothèse d'un effet trophique de l'isoprotérénol sur le muscle squelettique nous est apparue intéressante. Nous avons donc étudié les effets d'un tel traitement chronique à l'isoprotérénol sur la masse des muscles squelettiques en tenant compte du type de fibres musculaires.

Méthodes

Un groupe de 9 rats Wistar dont le poids moyen initial était d'environ 200 g reçoit, pendant 21 jours, une dose quotidienne d'isoprotérénol de 30 μg/100 g préparée dans le l'huile d'olive. Le groupe contrôle reçoit uniquement la quantité d'huile d'olive correspondante. Le coeur et les muscles *soleus, gastrocnemius* et *tibialis anterior* sont prélevés et pesés chez l'animal décapité 24 heures après la dernière injection. La mesure du diamètre des fibres est effectuée au niveau du *tibialis anterior* dans une région comportant trois types de fibres. Ceux-ci sont distingués histo-

Marie-Christine Thibault et Jacques LeBlanc, Département de physiologie, Faculté de médecine, Université Laval, Québec, Canada.

chimiquement sur des sections transverses par la méthode de Brooke et Kaiser[9] qui consiste à déterminer l'activité de l'adénosine triphosphatase alcaline (pH 9.4) de la myosine après pré-incubation dans un milieu acide (pH 4.3 -4.5). Cette procédure permet de distinguer les fibres de type I à contraction lente et deux types de fibres II (A et B) à contraction rapide. Afin de réduire les erreurs de mesure de diamètre dues à l'obliquité et à la courbure des fibres, toutes les mesures ont été faites selon la méthode de Brooke et Engel [8] qui consiste à mesurer la distance maximale entre les côtés les plus rapprochés d'une fibre.

Résultats

Sous l'influence du traitement à l'isoprotérénol, la masse tissulaire a augmenté significativement pour le coeur (37%, p < .01) et pour les muscles *tibialis anterior* (9%, p < .01) et *gastrocnemius* (8%, p < .05). Nous n'avons observé aucun changement significatif dans la masse du muscle *soleus*.

En ce qui a trait aux diamètres des fibres, nous les avons regroupés par type de façon à comparer la distribution de toutes les valeurs expérimentales à celle des contrôles, comme si les échantillons provenaient d'une même source, tel qu'employé par Brooke et Engel [8]. Des comparaisons furent ensuite effectuées sur la base du nombre de fibres retrouvées dans différentes classes de diamètres, à des intervalles de 5μ tel qu'illustré aux Figures 1, 2 et 3. La concordance des deux distributions fut évaluée par la méthode de Kolmogorov et Smirnov [24]. Nos résultats indiquent que le traitement à l'isoprotérénol augmente le diamètre des fibres de type I, IIA et IIB (p < .001).

Discussion

Il est déjà connu que le coeur et les muscles à contraction rapide augmentent leur tension de secousse maximale et leur vitesse de relaxation sous l'effet d'une seule stimulation à l'isoprotérénol, alors que les muscles à contraction lente comme le *soleus* exhibent les effets complètement opposés [1, 28, 30]. Il a par ailleurs été observé qu'en terme d'influence sur la contraction musculaire provoquée, le *soleus* est plus sensible à une faible dose d'isoprotérénol que le *tibialis anterior* [1, 4, 5]. Ce phénomène est encore plus évident à des fréquences de stimulation électrique physiologiquement significatives pour le *soleus* [5, 10].

En ce qui regarde les effets métaboliques de l'isoprotérénol sur le muscle squelettique, il est généralement reconnu qu'ils consistent

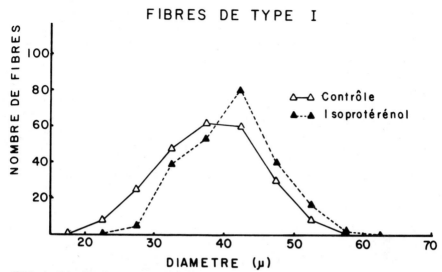

FIG. 1. Distribution des diamètres des fibres de type I dans le *tibialis anterior* des rats contrôles et des rats traités à l'isoprotérénol (30 μg/100 g/jour durant 21 jours)

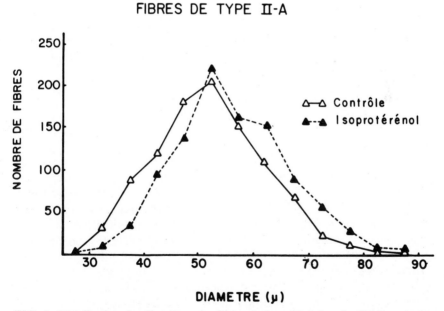

FIG. 2. Distribution des diamètres des fibres de type II-A dans le *tibialis anterior* des rats contrôles et des rats traités à l'isoprotérénol (30 μg/100 g/jour durant 21 jours)

FIBRES DE TYPE II-B

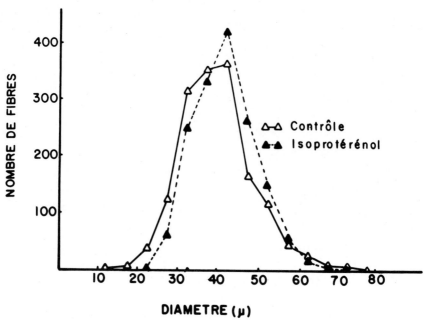

FIG. 3. Distribution des diamètres des fibres de type II-B dans le *tibialis anterior* des rats contrôles et des rats traités à l'isoprotérénol (30 μg/100 g/jour durant 21 jours)

principalement dans la stimulation de la glycogénolyse par l'activation de la phosphorylase. Avec des doses comparables à celles utilisées dans la présente étude, cette stimulation s'accompagne d'une élévation de l'activité de l'adényl cyclase et de la quantité d'AMP cyclique [6, 26, 27]. Mais ici encore, il existe des différences entre les deux types de muscles. En effet, les fibres musculaires à contraction rapide contiennent plus de phosphorylase totale que les autres types de fibres [13, 14]. Nous savons par ailleurs que ces fibres sont caractérisées par un potentiel glycolytique élevé. Une étude a cependant démontré que l'activité de l'adényl cyclase au niveau du sarcolemme est inférieure de 50% dans le muscle à contraction rapide comparativement au muscle à contraction lente [22]. Ces mêmes auteurs ont également rapporté que, sous l'influence d'une seule stimulation à `l'isoprotérénol, le niveau d'activité de l'enzyme augmente de 30% dans les muscles à contraction rapide alors qu'il triple dans le muscle à contraction lente. Il est par ailleurs suggéré que l'activité de base de la phosphodiestérase dans les homogénats de muscles entiers est plus faible dans les muscles à contraction lente que dans les autres muscles [22]. Ces résultats sont contradictoires aux observations faites par Sullivan et Zaimis [27] sur l'effet de l'isoprotérénol sur les concentrations d'AMP cyclique dans le muscle squelettique. Ces auteurs rapportent en effet une augmentation plus marquée de l'AMP cyclique au niveau du *tibialis anterior.*

Des chercheurs ont conclu qu'il n'est pas justifié d'établir une relation entre les effets physiologiques associés à la contraction musculaire et les changements métaboliques causés par une stimulation à l'isoprotérénol sur le muscle squelettique [6, 13, 26]. C'est ainsi que Drummond et al [13] ont démontré que le mécanisme d'activation de la phosphorylase par la contraction musculaire provoquée est fondamentalement différent de celui associé à une stimulation par les amines adrénergiques. De plus, une telle réponse à l'adrénaline est inhibée par la dichloroisoprotérénol, un agent bloquant bêta-adrénergique, alors qu'une activation par stimulation électrique ne l'est pas [26]. Stull et Mayer ont de plus démontré qu'en activant d'une façon maximale la phosphorylase in vivo par l'intermédiaire de l'un ou de l'autre type de stimulation, aucune activation additionnelle n'est décelée lorsque les deux stimuli sont appliqués simultanément.

Quelques études sont maintenant disponibles sur les effets d'un traitement chronique à l'isoprotérénol sur le coeur et les muscles squelettiques. Deshaies et al [11] ont rapporté qu'un traitement de 21 jours à raison de 30µg/100g/jour produit une hypertrophie du muscle cardiaque accompagnée d'une augmentation de la teneur protéique totale. Le taux de dégradation des protéines n'étant apparemment pas affecté par le traitement, les auteurs suggèrent que l'augmentation du taux de synthèse des protéines est le seul facteur responsable de l'accroissement de la teneur en protéines totale du muscle cardiaque.

Récemment, des auteurs finlandais ont par ailleurs étudié certains effets métaboliques d'un tel traitement chronique sur le muscle squelettique [17]. Ils ont observé une augmentation de l'activité des enzymes oxydatives telles la succinate déshydrogénase, la malate déshydrogénase et la citrate synthase au niveau du muscle *gastrocnemius* alors que, parmi l'activité des enzymes hexokinase, phosphofructokinase et lactate déshydrogénase, seule la première a augmenté. Ils n'ont cependant décelé aucun changement dans la concentration en protéines dans l'homogénat de muscle.

Nos résultats confirment ceux de LeBlanc et al [20] et de Deshaies et al [11] qui ont obtenu par un traitement à l'isoprotérénol une augmentation de la masse cardiaque et de celle du *tibialis anterior* de l'ordre de 40% et de 15% respectivement. Dans la présente étude, le *soleus*, un muscle à contraction lente, ne s'est pas hypertrophié sous l'influence du traitement à l'isoprotérénol. Le coeur et les muscles *gastrocnemius* et *tibialis anterior* se sont d'autre part hypertrophiés, indiquant une action préférentielle de l'isoprotérénol sur le muscle du type à contraction rapide. L'augmentation du diamètre des trois types de fibres musculaires dans le *tibialis anterior* indique que le muscle entier est la cible de l'effet trophique de l'isoprotérénol. L'hypertrophie serait la conséquence d'un effet spécifique de la stimulation bêta-adrénergique sur les muscles à contraction rapide.

Les données de la littérature nous indiquent que les muscles à contraction lente et les muscles à contraction rapide réagissent différemment à l'isoprotérénol administrée sous forme d'une seule dose ou sous forme d'un traitement chronique. Certains paradoxes existent cependant au niveau des effets observés. Ainsi, il est étonnant qu'en terme de réponse contractile, le *soleus* soit plus sensible à l'isoprotérénol que le *tibialis anterior* puisque c'est au contraire au niveau de ce dernier que se manifeste la plus grande sensibilité dans les réponses d'hypertrophie du muscle. Ceci s'explique sans doute par le fait que contrairement à ce que l'on observe au niveau du *tibialis anterior* et du muscle cardiaque, les catécholamines agissent sur le *soleus* en diminuant la réponse contractile au lieu de la stimuler. Ainsi, tout comme le muscle cardiaque, le *tibialis anterior* répond au traitment par une hypertrophie qui s'accompagne sans doute également d'une augmentation de la teneur protéique totale. Quoique ces effects, directs ou indirects, soient tous inhibés par un agent bloquant bêta (le propranolol) [2, 25, 27, 30], l'effet inhibiteur de l'isoprotérénol sur le *soleus* n'est pas en relation avec l'effet d'augmentation de la concentration d'AMP cyclique [27] et fait sans doute appel à un type d'effet bêta-adrénergique différent.

Ces effets spécifiques d'un traitement chronique à l'isoprotérénol ressemblent à ceux qu'on observe au niveau du muscle après un entraînement intensif. L'entraînement musculaire intensif de courte durée, produit une hypertrophie du muscle actif [15] et ces effets ne sont pas exclusifs à un type de fibres. Ce sont en effet celles qui sont les plus sollicitées métaboliquement qui s'hypertrophient [23]. Les exercices musculaires intensifs de type levée de poids ont aussi pour effet d'augmenter de façon préférentielle les protéines myofibrillaires responsables de la contraction. L'entraînement en endurance par contre ne modifie pas la masse musculaire et provoque une augmentation prépondérante des protéines sarcoplasmiques [16, 21]. Les effets d'un tel type d'entraînement s'expriment également par une augmentation de la capacité oxydative des fibres.

D'une part, l'hypertrophie produite par l'isoprotérénol s'apparente à un type d'entraînement musculaire intensif. D'autre part, les changements observés au niveau métabolique ressemblent précisément à ceux qui surviennent à la suite d'un entraînement de type d'endurance. L'activité des enzymes impliquées dans le métabolisme oxydatif augmente et de la même façon, l'hexokinase, dont l'activité varie avec la capacité respiratoire dans les différents types de muscles, est la seule enzyme glycolytique qui change sous l'effet du traitement. Un tel effet se situe au niveau des fibres rouges à contraction rapide (i.e. les II-A) après l'entraînement [18].

Ces résultats suggèrent que les changements observés au niveau du muscle squelettique en réponse à l'entraînement puissent dépendre en grande partie de stimulations des récepteurs bêta-adrénergiques au cours du processus de l'adaptation. Ces hypothèses supportent les données de Yakovlev [29]. Selon cet auteur, le système nerveux sympathique influence et stabilise les réponses d'adaptation à un effort accru.

References

1. Bowman, W.C., Goldberg, A.A.J. and Raper, C.: A comparison between the effects of tetanus and the effects of sympathomimetic amines on fast- and slow-contracting mammalian muscles. Br. J. Pharmacol. Chemother. 19:464-484, 1962.
2. Bowman, W.C. and Nott, M.W.: Actions of some sympathomimetic bronchodilator and beta-adrenoceptor blocking drugs on contractions of the cat soleus muscle. Br. J. Pharmacol. 38:37-49, 1970.
3. Bowman, W.W. and Nott, M.W.: Actions of sympathomimetic amines and their antagonists on skeletal muscle. Pharm. Rev. 21:27-72, 1969.
4. Bowman, W.C. and Raper, C.: Adrenotropic receptors in skeletal muscle. Ann. N.Y. Acad. Sci. 139:741-753, 1967.
5. Bowman, W.C. and Zaimis, E.: The effects of adrenaline, noradrenaline and isoprenaline on skeletal muscle contractions in the cat. J. Physiol. (London) 144:92-107, 1958.
6. Brody, T.M. and McNeill, J.H.: Adrenergic receptors for metabolic responses in skeletal and smooth muscles. Fed. Proc. Fed. Am. Soc. Exp. Biol. 29:1375-1378, 1970.
7. Brooke, M.H.: The pathologic interpretation of muscle histochemistry. In Pearson, C.M. and Mostofi, F.K. (eds.): The Striated Muscles, 1973.
8. Brooke, M.H. and Engel, W.K.: The histographic analysis of human muscle biopsies with regard to fiber types. I. Adult male and female. Neurology 19:221-223, 1969.
9. Brooke, M.H. and Kaiser, K.K.: Some comments on the histochemical characterization of muscle adenosine triphosphatase. J. Histochem. 17:431-431, 1969.

10. Denny-Brown, D.E.: On the nature of postural reflexes. Proc. Roy. Soc. Ser. B. Biol. Sci. 104:252-301, 1929.
11. Deshaies, Y., LeBlanc, J. and Willemot, J.: Studies on protein metabolism during isoproterenol-induced cardiac hypertrophy. In Roy, P.-E. and Harris, P. (eds.): Recent Advances in Studies on Cardiac Structure and Metabolism. Vol. 8. The Cardiac Sacroplasm, 1975.
12. Drummond, G.I.: Muscle metabolism. Fortschr. Zool. 18:339, 1969.
13. Drummond, G.I., Harwood, J.P. and Powell, C.A.: Studies on the activation of phosphorylase in skeletal muscle by contraction and by epinephrine. J. Biol. Chem. 244:4235-4240, 1969.
14. Edgerton, V.R. and Simpson, D.R.: The intermediate muscle fiber of rats and guinea pigs. J. Histochem. Cytochem. 17:828-838, 1969.
15. Faulkner, J.A., Maxwell, L.C., Brook, D.A. and Lieberman, D.A.: Adaptation of guinea pig plantaris muscle fibers to endurance training. Am. J. Physiol. 221:291-297, 1971.
16. Gordon, E.E.: Anatomical and biochemical adaptation of muscle to different exercise. JAMA 201:755-758, 1967.
17. Harri, M.N.E. and Valtola, J.: Comparison of the effects of physical exercise, cold acclimation and repeated injections of isoproterenol on rat muscle enzymes. Acta Physiol. Scand. 95:391-399, 1975.
18. Holloszy, J.O. and Booth, F.W.: Biochemical adaptations to endurance exercise in muscle. Ann. Rev. Physiol. 38:273-291, 1976.
19. Kvam, D.C.: Adrenergic receptors for metabolic effects in muscle. Fed. Proc. Fed. Amer. Soc. Exp Biol. 29:1379-1380, 1970.
20. LeBlanc, J., Vallieres, J. and Vachon, C.: Beta-receptor sensitization by repeated injections of isoproterenol and by cold adaptation. Am. J. Physiol. 222:1043-1046, 1972.
21. Mommaerts, W.F.H.M.: Molecular alterations in myofibrillar proteins. In Briskey, E.J. et al (eds.): The Physiology and Biochemistry of Muscle as a Food, 1966.
22. Reddy, N.B., Oliver, K.L., Engel, W.K. and Festoff, B.W.: Neurotrophic control of adenylate cyclase in fast and slow twitch skeletal muscles. Fed. Proc. Fed. Am. Soc. Exp. Biol. 1976.
23. Saltin, B.: Metabolic fundamentals in exercise. Med. Sci. Sports 5:137-146, 1973.
24. Sokal, R.R. and Rohlf, J.: Biometry. San Francisco:Freeman, 1969.
25. Stanton, H.C. and Bowman, Z.: Studies on isoproterenol-induced cardiomegaly in rats. Proc. West. Pharmacol. Soc. 10:87-89, 1967.
26. Stull, J.T. and Mayer, S.E.: Regulation of phosphorylase activation in skeletal muscle in vivo. J. Bio. Chem. 246:5716-5723, 1971.
27. Sullivan, A. and Zaimis: The effect of isoprenaline on cyclic AMP concentrations in skeletal muscle. J. Physiol. 231:102P-103P, 1973.
28. Tashiro, N.: Effects of isoprenaline on contractions of directly stimulated fast and slow skeletal muscles of the guinea-pig. Br. J. Pharmacol. 48:121-131, 1973.
29. Yakovlev, N.M.: The role of sympathetic nervous system in the adaptation of skeletal muscles to increased activity. In Howald, H. and Poortmans, J.R. (eds.): Metabolic adaptation to prolonged physical exercise, 1975.
30. Yamaha, K. and Iizuka, M.: Effect of trimetoquinol on skeletal muscle contraction in rabbits. Comparison with epinephrine and isoproterenol. Jap. J. Vet. Sci. 35:183-191, 1973.

Effects of Overtraining in Two Different Exercise Regimens and Ascorbic Acid Intake Upon Bone Growth in Albino Rats

K. W. Ho, R. R. Roy, W. D. Van Huss,
W. W. Heusner, L. Sive and R. E. Carrow

Introduction

Recent improvements in athletic performance have promoted interest in the implementation of rigorous conditioning programs during the rapid growth period of late childhood and adolescence. The effects of intensive physical training upon the growing child have not been determined. This paper concentrates on one aspect only, bone growth.

Rarick [13] concluded that some unidentified minimum of physical activity is essential for normal bone growth. Increases in bone growth have been reported with low-intensity exercise programs [3, 5, 7]. However, the bones of immobilized limbs have been shown to be longer (although thinner) than those in stressed contralateral limbs [19].

A number of investigators have reported that the linear growth of long bones is retarded as a result of both voluntary and forced exercise [7, 9, 17, 20]. Growth impairment has been observed in junior high school boys competing in athletics [4, 14]. In one study, the growth decrement in height amounted to 0.94 cm over a six-month period [4]. It is conceivable that differences in growth between athletes and nonathletes may be due to a joint dependence of athletic participation and terminal height upon genetic rate of maturation; but a study of Japanese children suggests that maturation cannot be the only factor involved [6]. A group of subjects involved in heavy labor were shorter than otherwise similar subjects. The difference in height was associated primarily with short legs. The

K. W. Ho, R. R. Roy, W. D. Van Huss, W. W. Heusner, L. Sive and R. E. Carrow, Michigan State University, East Lansing, Mich., U.S.A.

epiphyses at the lower end of the femur and at both ends of the tibia showed early closure. Experiments on animals have demonstrated that stressed bones are short and dense [16] and that they can tolerate large lateral forces before breaking [15].

Booth and Gould [2] have taken the position that the adaptation of bone to training is a function of the intensity of the exercise. Their position appears tenable although the precise stimuli and mechanisms are yet to be identified. The alterations observed in bone have been attributed to increased activity of hypertrophied adrenal glands [8] and to epiphyseal pressure [21].

The present study was undertaken to determine the effects of two training programs on long-bone growth in male rats. The two training regimens were more intensive than any heretofore utilized and were designed primarily to overload the aerobic and anaerobic capacities, respectively. Vitamin C supplementation was included for study as a possible preventive of the decrement in bone and overall growth of the exercised animals since vitamin C is closely related to the activity of the pituitary-adrenal axis [21]. The intrinsic supply of vitamin C in the adrenal is depleted as a result of heavy stress and does not appear to be immediately replaced even though the rat is known to synthesize this vitamin [1, 11]. Training has been shown to increase the vitamin C content of the adrenals in rested animals [10, 12]. It was reasoned that supplementation might prevent the vitamin C depletion and thus have a favorable effect upon bone growth.

Methods

Male albino rats (Sprague-Dawley) were assigned randomly to one of the following activity treatment groups: Sedentary Control (CON), Sprint Running (SPT) and Endurance Running (END). In addition, half of the animals in each activity group received vitamin C supplementation (C group) and the remaining animals received a placebo (No C group). Vitamin C supplementation was administered orally by syringe with a dosage of 2.4 mg vitamin C (Merck) in a .1 ml 5% sugar solution per 100 gm of body weight between 19:00 and 21:00 hour daily. The No C groups received only an identical quantity of sugar solution per unit of body weight.

For 12 days prior to the study, the animals were housed in individual spontaneous-activity cages to permit adjustment to laboratory conditions. During the study, all of the animals were housed in individual sedentary cages (24 × 18 × 18 cm). The animals had access to food and water ad libitum. A relatively constant environment was maintained for the animals by daily handling and by automatic control of temperature and lighting.

All treatments were initiated when the animals were 84 days of age and were continued for eight weeks. The CON animals received no exercise and were forced to remain relatively inactive throughout the experiment. The two exercise treatments were conducted once daily, five days per week.

The SPT animals were subjected to an interval training program of high-intensity sprint running. The workload of the SPT program was gradually increased until the 26th day of training. Thereafter, the animals were expected to complete six bouts of exercise with 2.5 minutes of inactivity between bouts. Each bout included five 15-second work periods at a speed of 108 meters/min alternated with four 30-second work periods (Table I).

The END animals were subjected to a demanding program of distance running. The workload was progressively increased so that on the 26th day of training and thereafter, the animals were expected to complete a 60-minute continuous run at a speed of 36 meters/min (Table II).

Both the SPT and END animals were exercised in a battery of individual controlled-running wheels (CRW) previously reported from this laboratory [22]. The animals learn to run in these wheels by avoidance-response operant conditioning. A mild regulated shock current (1.0 or 1.2 ma) provides motivation for animals to run. The apparatus is capable of inducing a group of small laboratory animals to participate in highly specific programs of controlled reproducible exercise and yet allows the animals to respond individually to the exercise program. Following the daily exercise session, the performance of each animal is recorded in terms of total meters run (TMR) and cumulative duration of shock (CDS). The TMR and total expected meters (TEM) are used to calculate the percentage of expected meters: PEM = 100(TMR/TEM). PEM values are used to evaluate and compare training performances. A secondary criterion is provided by the percentage of shock-free time (PSF) which is calculated from the CDS and the total work time (TWT): PSF = 100-100(CDS/TWT).

Ten animals in each subgroup were killed after eight weeks of treatments at 140 days of age. Final body weights were recorded immediately prior to death. Each animal then was anesthetized by an intraperitoneal injection (2 mg/100 gm body weight) of a 6.48% sodium pentobarbital (Halital) solution. The right tibia and fibula complex was removed and trimmed of extraneous tissue. A wet weight was determined immediately using a Mettler Balance. The

Table I. Eight-Week Sprint Running Program and Results for Postpubertal Male Rats in Controlled-Running Wheels

Wk.	Days of Train.	Work Time (min: sec)	Rest Time (sec)	Repetitions per Bout	No. of Bouts	Time Between Bouts (min)	Shock (ma)	Run Speed (m/min)	Total Exp. Meters TEM	Total Work Time (sec) TWT	% of Exp. Meters PEM C	% of Exp. Meters PEM No C	% of Shock Free PSF C	% of Shock Free PSF No C
1	1- 5	00:10	15	10	8	2.5	1.2	54	720	800	79	94	76	83
2	6-10	00:15	30	6	7	2.5	1.2	72	756	630	71	81	70	80
3	11-15	00:15	30	6	6	2.5	1.2	81	729	540	60	68	70	68
4	16-20	00:15	30	5	6	2.5	1.0	90	675	450	56	63	58	65
5	21-25	00:15	30	5	6	2.5	1.0	99	743	450	49	55	54	67
6	26-30	00:15	30	5	6	2.5	1.0	108	810	450	46	54	46	60
7	31-35	00:15	30	5	6	2.5	1.0	108	810	450	44	49	43	50
8	36-40	00:15	30	5	6	2.5	1.0	108	810	450	42	49	39	49

Table II. Eight-Week Endurance Running Program and Results for Postpubertal Male Rats in Controlled-Running Wheels

Wk.	Days of Train.	Work Time (min: sec)	Rest Time (sec)	Repetitions per Bout	No. of Bouts	Time Between Bouts (min)	Shock (ma)	Run Speed (m/min)	Total Exp. Meters TEM	Total Work Time (sec) TWT	% of Exp. Meters PEM C	% of Exp. Meters PEM No C	% of Shock Free PSF C	% of Shock Free PSF No C
1	1- 5	5:00	0	1	3	5.0	1.2	36	540	900	104	90	88	80
2	6-10	15:00	0	1	1	0.0	1.2	36	540	900	82	80	65	66
3	11-15	15:00	0	1	2	1.0	1.0	36	1080	1800	79	80	70	66
4	16-20	15:00	0	1	3	1.0	1.0	36	1620	2700	86	89	75	72
5	21-25	15:00	0	1	4	1.0	1.0	36	2160	3600	76	80	64	65
6	26-30	60:00	0	1	1	0.0	1.0	36	2160	3600	75	75	62	64
7	31-35	60:00	0	1	1	0.0	1.0	36	2160	3600	78	80	70	72
8	36-40	60:00	0	1	1	0.0	1.0	36	2160	3600	75	78	67	73

maximum tibial length was determined to the nearest .1 mm using vernier calipers [9, 21].

The data were analyzed using a two-way (3 × 2) fixed-effects analysis of variance. Newman-Keuls tests (SNK) were used to evaluate differences between pairs of means whenever a significant F-ratio was obtained. The 0.05 level of significance was established for all statistical analyses.

Results

Training Performance

The SPT training program and the relative responses (PEM and PSF) of the C and No C groups are shown in Table I. The program had been planned to be extremely rigorous so as to overload the anaerobic mechanism. The PEM and PSF values attained in the last week of training were only about 45% as contrasted with the usual criteria of 75% for satisfactory completion of an exercise regimen. The animals clearly were unable to meet the training requirements. During the experimental period, it was necessary to destroy three animals due to tibial fractures that occurred during running.

The END program and the relative responses of the C and No C groups are shown in Table II. The PEM results met the standard criterion level of 75%. The PSF results, although lower than the 90% to 95% seen in most CRW training studies, held at about 70% which seems respectable for this intensive program.

No significant differences in training responses were observed between the C and No C groups. No evidence of murine pneumonia was found in either group upon subjective evaluation of the lungs at death [23].

Vitamin C — No Vitamin C Comparisons

The body weight and bone data for both the C and No C groups are shown in Table III. The overall mean value of absolute tibia weight for the three No C groups ($\overline{X}$ = 0.880) was significantly greater (P < .05) than that for the three C groups ($\overline{X}$ = 0.834); however, this was not the case for relative tibia weight. In 13 of 15 comparisons on body weight, bone weight and bone length the values for the C group were less than those for the No C group (P = .008). It is clear that vitamin C did not serve as a preventive for the impairment of growth during training. In fact, these data include greater impairment with the dosage of vitamin C used.

Table III. Effects of Sedentary Control (CON), Sprint Running (SPT) and Endurance Running (END) Activities on Body Weight and Tibia Size in Male Albino Rats (140-Days Old) After Eight Weeks of Treatments*

Treatment Group	Body Weight (g)		Tibia Weight[1] (g)		Relative Tibia Weight ($\times 10^{-3}$)		Tibia Length (mm)		Relative Tibia Length ($\times 10^{-3}$)	
	C[2]	No C[3]	C	No C	C	No C	C	No C	C	No C
CON	512.8 ±12.0	517.3 ±8.7	0.890 ±0.020	1.004 ±0.079	1.91 ±0.03	1.94 ±0.05	4.31 ±0.04	4.32 ±0.02	8.44 ±0.15	8.38 ±0.15
SPT	386.1 ±8.8	408.5 ±8.3	0.592 ±0.021	0.675 ±0.024	1.53 ±0.04	1.65 ±0.06	4.13 ±0.03	4.18 ±0.04	10.73 ±0.16	10.27 ±0.17
END	401.2 ±12.3	415.3 ±8.2	0.934 ±0.018	0.960 ±0.014	2.34 ±0.08	2.32 ±0.04	4.19 ±0.03	4.23 ±0.03	10.51 ±0.33	10.20 ±0.20
	CON>SPT CON>END	CON>SPT CON>END	CON>SPT END>SPT	CON>SPT END>SPT	END>CON> SPT	END>CON> SPT	CON>SPT CON>END	CON>SPT CON>END	SPT>CON END>CON	SPT>CON END>CON

*All values are means ±SE for ten rats. Significant (P <0.05) Newman-Keuls contrasts are shown at the bottom of the columns.
[1] The overall mean of the tibia weight of the No C group is significantly greater than the C group (P < 0.05).
[2] C = vitamin C treatment groups.
[3] No C = placebo groups.

Activity Level Comparisons

All overall comparisons between activity levels were statistically significant. The SNK contrasts shown on the bottom two lines of Table III identify which groups were significantly different (P < .05). The body weights and absolute tibia lengths of the CON animals were greater than those of either the SPT or END animals. It would appear, as in our earlier work [21], that training impaired overall growth. When the relative tibia lengths were compared, however, the mean values for both the SPT and END groups were greater than that for the CON group.

The tibia weight results were very different. Both the absolute and relative tibia weights of the SPT group were significantly less than those of the other groups. The SNK comparisons indicate that the END animals had the heaviest tibias and the SPT animals had the lightest tibias. These results were not anticipated. It had been expected that the greater stress involved in the SPT program would result in heavier bones. The data contradict Wolff's law [18] regarding bone responses to stress.

The tibia of the SPT animals were actually less dense than those of the CON animals. Although breaking force was not measured, it would appear from the three tibial fractures sustained during training that bone strength was altered. The implications of these results to age group athletics are self-evident in that with extremely high-intensity training bone strength may be impaired. Further research is indicated.

References

1. Bacchus, H.: Cytological distribution of cholesterol and ascorbic acid in the adrenal cortex of the rat exposed to cold. Anat. Rec. 110:495, 1951.
2. Booth, F.W. and Gould, E.W.: Effects of training and disuse on connective tissue. *In* Wilmore, J. (ed.): Exercise and Sport Review, Vol. 3, 1975, p. 83.
3. Donaldson, H.H.: Summary of data for the effects of exercise beginning at different ages on the weight or musculature and of several organs of the albino rat. Am. J. Anat. 56:57, 1935.
4. Fait, H.F.: The physiological effects of strenuous activity upon the immature child. FIEP Bull. 26:28, 1956.
5. Heikkinen, E., Suonimen, H., Vihersaari, M. et al: Effect of physical training on enzyme activities of bones, tendons, and skeletal muscles in mice. Proc. Int. Symp. Exercise Biochem. 2nd., 1973, p. 448.
6. Kato, S. and Ishiko, T.: Obstructed growth of long bones due to excessive labor in remote corners. *In* Kato, K. (ed.): Proc. Int. Cong. Sport Sci., Tokyo, 1964, p. 479.
7. Kiiskinen, A. and Heikkinen, E.: Effect of prolonged physical training on the development of connective tissues in growing mice. Proc. Int. Symp. Exercise Biochem. 2nd., 1973, p. 253.

8. King, D.W. and Pengelly, R.G.: Effect of running on the density of rat tibias. Med. Sci. Sports 5:68, 1973.

9. Lamb, D., Van Huss, W.D., Carrow, R.E. et al: Effects of prepubertal physical training on growth, voluntary exercise, cholesterol and basal metabolism in rats. Res. Q. 40:123, 1969.

10. Namyslowski, L.: Effect of training on the adaptation of rat adrenals to efforts. Endokrynol. Pol. 9:223, 1958.

11. Namyslowski, L.: Course of return of ascorbic acid content in rat adrenals following exhaustive exercise. Rocz. Panstw. Zakl. Hig. 8:265, 1957.

12. Namyslowski, L.: Influence of stress on ascorbic acid content of rat adrenals. Rocz. Panstw. Zakl. Hig. 7:425, 1956.

13. Rarick, G.L.: Exercise and growth. In Johnson, W. (ed.): Science and Medicine of Exercise and Sports. New York:Harper and Bros., 1960, p. 440.

14. Rowe, F.A.: Growth comparisons of athletes and non-athletes. Res. Q. 4:108, 1933.

15. Saville, P.D. and Smith, R.: Bone density, breaking force and leg muscle mass as functions of weight in bipedal rats. Am. J. Phys. Anthrop. 25:35, 1966.

16. Saville, P.D. and Whyte, M.P.: Muscle and bone hypertrophy. Clin. Orthop. 65:81, 1969.

17. Slonaker, J.R.: The effect of a strictly vegetable diet on the spontaneous activity, the rate of growth and longevity of the albino rat. Stanford University Publications, April 2, 1912, pp. 1-52.

18. Stedman's Medical Dictionary 22nd Ed., Baltimore:Williams and Wilkins, 1972, p. 687 (Wolff's Law).

19. Steinhaus, A.H.: Chronic effects of exercise. Phys. Rev. 13:103, 1933.

20. Tipton, C.M., Matthes, R.D. and Maynard, J.A.: Influence of chronic exercise on rat bones. Med. Sci. Sports 4:55, 1972.

21. Van Huss, W.D., Heusner, W.W. and Mickelsen, O.: Effect of prepubertal exercise on body composition. In Franks, D. (ed.): Exercise and Fitness, 1969. Chicago:Athletic Institute, 1970, p. 201.

22. Wells, R.L. and Heusner, W.W.: A controlled running wheel for small animals. Lab. Anim. Sci. 21:904, 1971.

23. Yevich, P.P., Van Huss, W.D., Carrow, R.E. et al: Pulmonary pathology to be considered in exercise research in the rat. Res. Q. 40:251, 1969.

Energy Metabolism and Fatigue During Archery Training

K. Tsuji, H. Takeyama, H. Koishi,
Y. Katayama and C. Shimoshima

We carried out the investigation and measurements as described below in order to obtain certain basic data to be used in designing a physical training program for archers. First, energy metabolism during training was measured for six of the subjects to clarify the intensity of archery training. Second, food intake and time study were continuously investigated in seven Olympic candidates for five days during a summer training session. Parallel to these examinations, the level of fatigue was estimated by differences in salivary pH, by the Flicker test, the Donaggio urine reaction, the level of endurance associated with a fully drawn bow position and by the subjective feelings at pre- and posttraining. Furthermore, a physical fitness test was administered to 12 of the subjects on the fourth day of the five-day training period.

Table I shows the results of the physical fitness tests for the Olympic candidates. Their physical constitution was as follows: average body height, about 171 cm; average body weight, about 66 kg; average girth of chest, about 92 cm. These data indicate that the athletes have good constitutions for Japanese.

Energy metabolism associated with target archery was determined from expiratory gases collected in a Douglas bag and analyzed for O_2 and CO_2 contents.

The results of the energy metabolism determination are shown in Table II. The average basal metabolic rate was 1.06 kcal/min, while rest metabolism averaged 1.24 kcal/min. During training, energy consumption increased to a mean of 3.59 kcal/min. As a result of calculations, a relative metabolic rate of 2.3 was obtained. This value corresponds approximately with that obtained for walking at 4

K. Tsuji, Laboratory of Health and Physical Education, Osaka Institute of Technology, Osaka; H. Takeyama, Laboratory of Health and Physical Education, Osaka Prefectural University, Osaka; H. Koishi, Y. Katayama and C. Shimoshima, Department of Food and Nutrition, Faculty of Sci. Living, Osaka City University, Osaka, Japan.

Table I. Physical Fitness Test

Variables	Olympic Candidates N: 12
Body height (cm)	170.9 ± 3.2
Body weight (kg)	66.3 ± 5.8
Girth of chest (cm)	92.3 ± 3.6
Balance (sec)	45.6 ± 6.8
Harvard step test (index)	58.9 ± 4.1
Vertical jump (cm)	51.8 ± 5.4
Vital capacity (cc)	4300.0 ± 386.0
Grip strength (kg) R.	46.8 ± 4.0
Grip strength (kg) L.	43.0 ± 3.1
Back lift strength (kg)	142.0 ± 15.5
Trunk bending (cm)	11.4 ± 2.7
Trunk extension backward (cm)	58.3 ± 4.5
Strength of pull (kg)	48.5 ± 4.2
Strength of push (kg)	50.6 ± 5.4

Confidence limit ($P < 0.05$)

Table II. Energy Metabolism in Target Archery

Subject (age)	Basal Metabolism kcal/min	kcal/m/h	At Rest kcal/min	Exercise kcal/min	Energy Requirement kcal/min	R.M.R.
T.H. (20)	1.07	39.0	1.25	3.38	2.13	2.0
T.N. (21)	1.02	36.7	1.24	3.95	2.71	2.7
M.S. (21)	1.08	38.4	1.30	4.10	2.80	2.6
Y.E. (21)	1.05	37.8	1.23	3.53	2.30	2.2
T.T. (21)	1.09	39.0	1.24	3.40	2.16	2.0
S.K. (21)	1.02	38.9	1.18	3.18	2.00	2.0
M.	1.06	38.3	1.24	3.59	2.35	2.3
C.L.	±0.03	±0.95	±0.04	±0.38	±0.22	±0.35

R.M.R.: $\dfrac{T - R}{B}$

T : total energy consumption (kcal)
R : resting energy consumption (kcal)
B : basal metabolism (kcal)

Values are mean ± half range of confidence interval
(confidence limits at $P < 0.05$).

km/hr, indicating that the intensity of archery training is classified into relatively light exercise groups.

Our candidates recorded the kinds and amount of food consumed during one meal. From these records an analysis of food intake could be performed.

Table III shows the composition of food consumed by the subjects per day. As main foods, 472 gm of cereal, 255 gm of meat, poultry, or fish, 251 gm of milk and 350 gm of vegetables were consumed daily.

As shown in Table IV, the intake of nutrients per day was as follows: protein, 102.2 gm; lipid, 76.2 gm and carbohydrate, 544 gm. From these values, the protein, lipid and carbohydrate contents of the consumed food were calculated to be 12.5%, 21.2% and 66.5%, respectively. This indicates that the intake of nutrients was balanced. On the other hand, the average caloric intake was 3399 kcal/day. This value is 13% higher than the 3000 kcal/day which is required for "relatively heavy work" on the basis of nutrient allowance. Therefore, the level of energy intake during training was appropriate. With respect to vitamins, the intake of vitamins A and B_1 and nicotinic acid may not be sufficient, since these vitamins are destroyed to a certain extent by cooking.

Figure 1 shows the result of the time study investigation. The upper part shows the time distribution and the lower part presents

Table III. Food Composition Analysis

Food Item	8/20	8/21	8/22	8/23	8/24	Average
1. Cereals	483	490	469	477	443	472.3 ± 22.3
2. Potatoes and starches	67	0	59	0	0	25.2 ± 43.0
3. Sugars and sweeteners	142	93	80	64	65	88.8 ± 39.8
4. Confectioneries	0	10	0	0	0	2.1 ± 5.7
5. Oils and fats	16	23	14	20	19	18.6 ± 4.5
6. Seeds and nuts	0	12	0	1	23	7.1 ± 12.5
7. Pulses	266	62	161	73	18	116.0 ±122.5
8. Fish and shellfish	6	86	6	107	0	40.9 ± 63.6
9. Meat, poultry and whales	86	360	286	41	299	214.3 ±175.6
0. Eggs	171	125	57	174	145	134.4 ± 59.2
1. Milk	0	411	238	360	245	250.8 ±196.9
2. Vegetables, leafy green and yellow	55	50	9	1	49	32.9 ± 32.0
3. Other vegetable	200	477	235	241	234	317.4 ±250.1
4. Fruits	3	12	158	169	148	98.0 ±103.0
5. Fungi	0	0	0	0	0	0
6. Seaweeds	3	2	1	1	1	1.7 ± 1.2
7. Beverages	277	994	68	378	614	466.4 ±439.9
8. Seasonings and others	88	91	71	51	70	74.4 ± 19.8
Total	1864	3498	1912	2158	2373	2361.1 ±828.6

Table IV. Nutritional Evaluation

Nutrients		8/20	8/21	8/22	8/23	8/24	Average	Dietary Allowance Individual	A Little Heavier Work
Energy (kcal)		3580	3673	3072	3285	3383	3399 ±296.4	2652	3000
Protein (g)		93.7	108.9	92.5	104.4	111.4	102.2 ± 10.8	81.3	70.0
protein calorie ratio	(%)	10.3	12.7	11.9	13.4	14.1	12.5 ± 1.8		
animal prot./total prot.	(%)	35.8	50.6	45.0	57.7	58.7	49.5 ± 11.8		
protein/B.W.	(%)	1.43	1.66	1.41	1.59	1.70	1.56± 0.2		
Lipid (g)		98.2	71.4	58.1	66.7	86.6	76.2 ± 19.9		
lipid calorie ratio	(%)	25.3	19.2	16.8	19.4	24.6	21.1 ± 4.6		
Carbohydrate (g)		562.7	584.9	540.9	534.9	496.2	544.0 ± 41.2		
carbohydrate calorie ratio	(%)	64.4	68.1	71.3	67.2	61.4	66.5 ± 4.7		
cereal calorie ratio	(%)	46.2	46.1	52.6	49.4	45.2	47.9 ± 3.9		
Calcium (mg)		633	927	569	650	556	667 ±187.0	629	600
Iron (mg)		18.6	21.9	15.3	16.2	14.7	17.3 ± 3.6	10.9	10.0
Vitamin A (I.U.)		1899	2089	945	1764	1907	1721 ±557.0	2000	2000
Vitamin B$_1$ (mg)		1.26	1.54	1.19	1.40	1.23	1.32± 0.2	1.19	1.4
Vitamin B$_2$ (mg)		1.10	2.03	1.36	1.51	1.63	1.53± 0.4	1.33	1.5
Vitamin C (mg)		115	88	58	63	79	81 ± 28.4	67.6	60.0
Nicotinic acid (mg)		16.1	20.9	21.4	19.2	22.4	20.0 ± 3.1	21.2	24.0

Average values are confidence limits (P < 0.05)

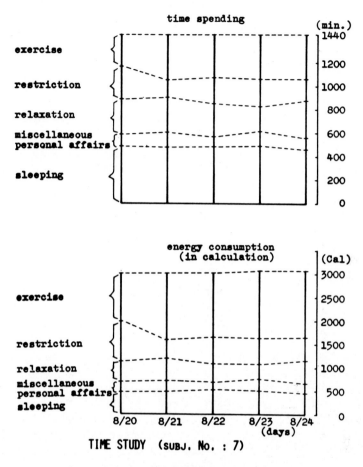

FIGURE 1.

that of the energy consumption. As shown in the upper figure, the exercise time was less on the first day than on the other four because of some preliminary arrangements. However, the respective times for relaxation, miscellaneous personal affairs and sleeping were nearly constant during the five-day period. The energy consumption per day was 3020 kcal. This value agrees well with the energy intake of 3399 kcal/day calculated on the basis of food intake.

Figure 2 presents the results of the determination of the level of fatigue occurring during the training period. The level of fatigue is reflected in the differences between the daily pre- and postpractice values and fatigue becomes marked as the values for the differences descend below the zero line. No significant differences in pre- and

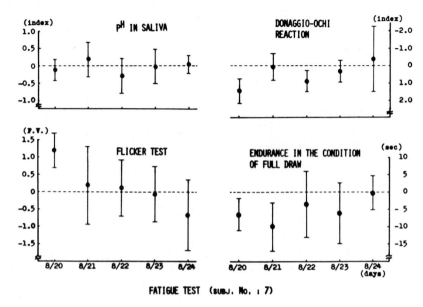

FATIGUE TEST (SUBJ. No. : 7)

FIGURE 2.

postpractice salivary pH were observed. The value of the Flicker test, however, was higher at prepractice on the first day of the training period, but pre- and postpractice differences in the test values became smaller as training progressed. On the last day, however, the difference became negative indicating the development of fatigue. The Flicker test is useful as a measure of the amount of stimulation of the eye and the level of mental fatigue is reflected by the test value. In this case, it seems that mental fatigue developed gradually during training. In the case of the Donaggio urine reaction, the value was relatively high at prepractice on the first day, but differences in the values between pre- and postpractice gradually decreased during the latter half of the training period. Muscle fatigue was estimated by the endurance level associated with a fully drawn bow position. On the first day, the value was higher at prepractice than at postpractice. The differences in these values decreased gradually and no difference was observed on the last day.

Table V shows the average frequency of the subjective feelings of fatigue obtained by the inquiry. No consistent results were obtained when comparing pre- with postpractice data. However, differences for the A group seem to be relatively larger than those for groups B and C.

Table V. Number of Subject Complaints (Average)

	Before Practice			After Practice		
	A	B	C	A	B	C
1st	0.71	0.43	0.00	1.29	0.00	1.00
2nd	1.71	0.14	0.29	2.00	0.14	0.29
3rd	2.29	0.29	0.14	1.71	0.14	0.29
4th	2.00	0.00	0.14	2.14	0.00	0.00
5th	1.57	0.00	0.14	1.29	0.00	0.14

A: physical, B: psychological, C: sensory. Each contains ten questions.

Conclusion

First, energy metabolism was measured and an average R.M.R. of 2.3 was obtained. Second, the energy consumption agreed well with the energy intake calculated on the basis of the food intake. The intake of protein, lipid and carbohydrate was sufficient with respect to the nutrient allowance for "relatively heavy work," but the intake of vitamins A and B_1 and nicotinic acid was not quite sufficient due to some destruction of these vitamins by cooking. Third, slight fatigue was observed in the latter half of the training period only on the basis of the Flicker test. No fatigue was indicated by other tests.

Influence of the Level of Physical Fitness on the Cardiovascular Response to Norepinephrine in Men

M. Jobin, M. Boulay, S. Dulac, A. Labrie,
J. Côté and J. LeBlanc

Introduction

Increased catecholamine (CA) secretion occurs during physical activity, especially with exercises of high intensity and long duration [16]. It is still debated, however, whether repeated exposure to high CA levels, such as might occur during regular training for endurance, leads to a change in the sensitivity to these amines. Increased sensitivity to the metabolic effects of CA probably results from training, as judged from the enhanced lipolytic response to noradrenalin (NA) of incubated fat tissue from trained animals [1, 12].

With regard to the cardiovascular effects of CA, conflicting results have been obtained. Pavlik and Frenkl [13] found a reduced pulse and blood pressure response to NA in trained men, whereas the response to isoproterenol (beta-stimulator) was unaltered, indicating a selective reduction of the alpha-receptors sensitivity in these subjects. On the other hand, experiments based on the effects of beta-receptor blockade [3] suggested that the reduced cardiovascular response to exercise observed after two months of training resulted from a reduced sensitivity of the beta-receptors to CA. In the present study, the influence of the level of fitness on the sensitivity to CA was examined by assessing the cardiovascular effects of NA infused in human volunteers with different levels of physical conditioning.

Methods

Forty male volunteers, age 18 to 30, with no previous history of endocrine or cardiovascular disease were chosen from a university

M. Jobin, M. Boulay, S. Dulac, A. Labrie, J. Côté and J. LeBlanc,
Department of Physiology and Department of Physical Education, Laval
University, Quebec, Canada.

271

student population to cover a wide range of levels of training. Highly trained subjects were competitors in long-distance events: running, cross-country skiing or cycling. The physical characteristics of the subjects were measured a few days prior to the NA test. Maximum oxygen uptake ($\dot{V}O_2$ max) was measured on a bicycle ergometer by stepwise increase of the workload and the oxygen uptake and pulmonary ventilation were measured using a closed-circuit gas analysis system (Dargatz Magna Test). The percentage of total body weight as fat was determined by the hydrostatic weighing technique [11]. The NA test was scheduled at 8:00 in the morning, and the subjects were instructed to fast and to avoid smoking and unnecessary activity before coming to the lab. Before the test, the subjects laid supine for 30 minutes. Subsequently, a vein of the left arm was cannulated and normal saline was perfused at a rate of 1 ml/min by means of a continuous infusion apparatus (B. Braun, Melsingen). After 15 minutes, saline was replaced by a solution of NA in saline (Levophed, Winthrop), which was infused for 30 minutes at a rate of 0.1 μg/kg/min and 1 ml/min. During the whole test, including 15 minutes of recovery, the heart rate was recorded by ECG and blood pressure was measured at one-minute intervals by auscultatory method (right arm). Thirty milliliter blood samples were drawn from the right arm on three occasions: at the end of saline perfusion and after 15 and 30 minutes of NA perfusion. These were used for the determination of various blood constituents in the assessment of the metabolic effects of NA [8].

Statistical Analysis

To better illustrate the effects of training, two groups of ten subjects (trained and nontrained), corresponding to the highest ($\dot{V}O_2$ max larger than 65 ml/kg/min) and the lowest level of fitness ($\dot{V}O_2$ max smaller than 45 ml/kg/min), were picked from our group of 40. Although the data of these two groups were generally used for comparison by the Student's t test, the relationships between the $\dot{V}O_2$ max and the various cardiovascular parameters were also evaluated by correlation tests involving the data of all the subjects.

Results

It is obvious from the $\dot{V}O_2$ max data (Table I) that the "trained" and "nontrained" groups had markedly different levels of fitness. The significantly higher body weight in the nontrained group is entirely accounted for by a higher percentage of body fat, and the lean body mass shows no significant difference. As expected a highly

Table I. Characteristics of Subjects

Group	Age (year)	Height (cm)	Weight (kg)	Body Fat (%)	Lean Body Mass (kg)	Max $\dot{V}O_2$ (ml/kg/min)	Max $\dot{V}O_2$ (l/min)
Nontrained subjects (n=10)	26.9 ± 1.7	1.71 ±7.14	72.95 ± 3.29	21.12 ± 1.29	57.23 ± 1.86	38.76 ± 1.04	2.82 ±0.14
Trained subjects (n = 10)	21.0 ± 1.9	1.71 ±8.21	64.24* ± 2.93	8.37** ±1.21	58.72 ± 2.40	69.61** ± 1.02	4.46 ±0.17
All subjects (n = 40)	24.2 ± 3.3	1.73 ±7.31	70.08 ± 1.45	12.35 ± 0.99	61.17 ± 1.12	54.61 ± 1.85	3.79 ±0.12

* = p < .05   ** = p < .01

significant negative correlation (r = −0.75; p < 0.01) was found
between the $\dot{V}O_2$ max and the percentage of body fat.

The blood pressure data pertaining to these two groups are
summarized in Figure 1. At rest, the trained subjects had
significantly lower blood pressures than the nontrained subjects. The
respective systolic pressures were 107 for trained and 118 mm Hg for

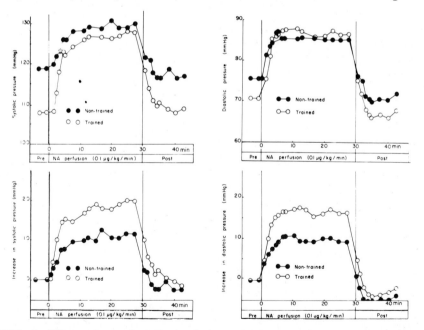

FIG. 1. Effect of noradrenalin perfusion on systolic (*left side*) and diastolic
blood pressures in trained and nontrained subjects. Upper part: absolute values;
lower part: increases.

nontrained groups (p < 0.05) while the corresponding diastolic values were 70 and 75 mm Hg (p < 0.05). When the relationship between the resting systolic or diastolic pressures of our 40 subjects and their $\dot{V}O_2$ max was analyzed, a significant negative correlation was found in both cases.

During NA perfusion, the systolic and diastolic pressures increased in all subjects. However, the pressure rises were significantly larger in the trained group, who had lower resting values, in such a way that the levels during NA perfusion did not differ between the two groups (Fig. 1).

The results obtained on the heart rate are shown in Figure 2. At rest, the trained subjects had a much slower heart rate, which reflects their higher level of training. Indeed, a highly significant negative correlation was found between the resting heart rate of our 40 subjects and their $\dot{V}O_2$ max. NA perfusion caused bradycardia in all subjects. The absolute and relative decrease was significantly smaller in the trained than in the nontrained group.

Discussion

Our results show that the trained subjects have significantly lower diastolic and systolic blood pressures at rest. This inverse

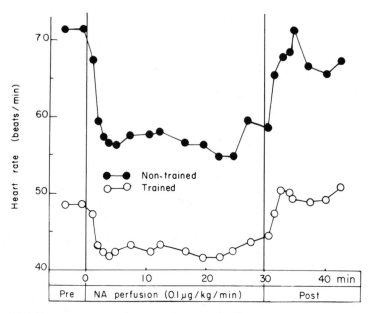

FIG. 2. Effect of noradrenalin perfusion on the heart rate of trained and nontrained subjects.

relationship between the blood pressure values and the $\dot{V}O_2$ max, which may be a very important beneficial effect of training, has already been reported by some authors [6, 7, 9, 17], but denied by others [4, 5]. Lower blood pressure values at rest in trained subjects may indicate a decreased sympathetic tone and are compatible with the findings of lower urinary excretion of NA at rest in trained rats [2, 10].

With regard to the sensitivity to NA, the results obtained in this experiment are difficult to interpret. An increased sensitivity to NA could be suggested by the larger pressure increase recorded in the trained group under NA. However, the absolute blood pressure values recorded during NA were the same in trained and nontrained subjects, despite presumedly identical levels of circulating NA in both groups during perfusion. Therefore, this would suggest that the sensitivity of the cardiovascular system to NA was the same in trained and nontrained subjects.

The blood pressure response to NA results mainly from the vasoconstrictive effect of this amine, an effect mediated by the alpha-receptors. On the other hand, indirect evidence from this experiment [8] and from others indicates that training produces an increased sensitivity to the metabolic effects of NA, which are beta-receptor mediated. The evidence suggests that physical training produces an increased sensitivity to NA with regard to the actions mediated by the beta-receptors, but no change in the response to alpha-receptor stimulation.

Another possibility could be suggested. The blood pressure recorded during NA infusion might be seen as the result of two opposing effects, the alpha effects, characterized by vasoconstriction and increased peripheral resistance, and the beta effects characterized by vasodilatation of certain areas. If the sensitivity of both types of receptors was altered in the same direction by training, it is conceivable that the pressure response to NA be unaltered.

Our results confirm the well-documented association between a slow resting heart rate and a high level of training (Fig. 2). Infusion of NA produced in all subjects a bradycardia which was doubtless due to a reflex vagal action produced by the elevation of blood pressure. Since the blood pressure rise during NA was larger in the trained group, one could expect a more marked bradycardia in this group, and even more so if, as suggested by Tipton [14, 15], the bradycardia of trained subjects is larger for a given vagal stimulus. In our study, however, the NA-induced bradycardia was smaller in the trained than in the nontrained group, whether expressed in absolute or in relative change. It is quite possible that the marked resting bradycardia of our trained subjects (48/min) imposed a limit to the NA action. The results obtained in the present study, therefore, do not show any clearcut effect of training on the sensitivity of the cardiovascular system to NA.

References

1. Askew, E.W., Dohm, G.L., Huston, R.L. et al: Response of rat tissue lipases to physical training and exercise. Proc. Soc. Exp. Biol. Med. 141:123-127, 1972.
2. Bernet, F. and Denimad, J.: Evolution of the sympathico-adrenal response to exercise during physical training in the rat. In Howald and Poortmans (eds.): Metabolic Adaptation to Prolonged Physical Exercise. Birkhauser Verlag, Bâle 1975, pp. 326-332.
3. Brundin, T. and Cernigliaro, C.: The effect of physical exercise on the sympatho-adrenal response to exercise. Scand. J. Clin. Lab. Invest. 35:525-530, 1975.
4. Ekblom, B., Astrand, P.O., Saltin, B. et al: Effect of training on circulatory response to exercise. J. Appl. Physiol. 24:518-529, 1968.
5. Häggendal, J., Hartley, L.H. and Saltin, B.: Arterial noradrenaline concentration during exercise in relation to the relative work loads. Scand. J. Clin. Lab. Invest. 26:337-342, 1970.
6. Hollmann, W.: Der arbeit-und trainingseinfluss auf kreislauf und atmung. Darmstadt 1957.
7. Jokl, E.: Obesity. In Larson, L. (ed.): Encyclopedia of Sport Sciences and Medicine. N.Y., 1971, pp. 1173-1180.
8. LeBlanc, J., Dulac, S., Boulay, M. et al: The influence of the level of physical fitness on the metabolic response to norepinephrine in men. This Congress.
9. Mellerowick, H.: Effects of training on the heart and circulation. In Grupe, D., Kurz, D. and Tepel, J.M. (eds.): The Scientific View of Sport: Perspectives, Aspects, Issues. Berlin, 1972.
10. Ostman, I. and Sjöstrand, N.O.: Reduced urinary noradrenaline excretion during rest, exercise and cold stress in trained rats: A comparison between physically trained rats, cold acclimated rats and warm acclimated rats. Acta Physiol. Scand. 95:209-218, 1975.
11. Parizkova, J.: Impact of age, diet, and exercise on man's body composition. Ann. N.Y. Acad. Sci. 110:661-675, 1963.
12. Parizkova, J. and Stankova, L.: Influence of physical activity on a treadmill on the metabolism of adipose tissue in rats. Br. J. Nutr. 18:325-331, 1964.
13. Pavlik, G. and Frenkl, R.: Sensitivity to catecholamines and histamine in the trained and untrained human organism. Eur. J. Appl. Physiol. 34:199-204, 1975.
14. Tipton, C.M., Barnard, R.J. and Tharp, G.D.: Cholinesterase activity in trained and non-trained rats. Int. Z. Angew. Physiol. 23:34-39, 1966.
15. Tipton, C.M., Barnard, R.J. and Tharp, G.D.: Training and its cholinergic consequences. J. Sport Med. Phys. Fitness 6:63-69, 1966.
16. von Euler, U.S.: Sympatho-adrenal activity in physical exercise. Med. Sci. Sports 6:165-173, 1974.
17. Wilmore, J.H., Royce, J., Girandola, R.N. et al: Physiological alterations resulting from a 10-week program of jogging. Med. Sci. Sports 2:7-11, 1970.

Physiological and Biochemical Correlates of Fitness

J. A. White and A. H. Ismail

Introduction

The purpose of this investigation was (1) to determine the relationships between selected physiological and biochemical variables before, during and after exercise and (2) to determine the value of biochemical variables alone in physical fitness.

Subjects

Twenty-two male subjects, aged 27 to 57, were used in this investigation. Two groups were established, one sedentary and one active (both N = 11), based upon the physical fitness criterion of Ismail et al [5]. The physical characteristics and physiological changes of the subjects are given in Table I. All gave their informed consent and had undergone medical examinations before participating in the investigation.

The Program

The physical fitness program was conducted three days per week during the lunch period between 12.00 and 13.30 hr, and was of four-month duration. Each session consisted of a warm-up, calisthenics and progressive running followed by recreational activities. The intensity of subject participation in the program was carefully matched with each individual's capabilities and rate of progression made during the course of the program.

General Testing Procedure

On reporting to the laboratory the subject was allowed to rest in the supine position for ten minutes before performing graded

J. A. White, Department of Physical Education, Liverpool Institute of Higher Education, Notre Dame College, Mount Pleasant, Liverpool, England and A. H. Ismail, Department of Physical Education (Men), Purdue University, West Lafayette, Indiana, U.S.A.

Table I. Physical Characteristics and Physiological Changes of Two Groups of Subjects Participating in Study

Age ($\bar{X}$ ± S.E. yr) Active Group 44.6 ± 2.5 (range = 27-54) Sedentary Group 43.7 ± 2.5 (range = 28-57)
Height ($\bar{X}$ ± S.E. cm) 181.3 ± 1.6 182.9 ± 2.2

		Active Group			Sedentary Group		
		Pretest ($\bar{X}$ ± S.E.)	(P)	*Posttest* ($\bar{X}$ ± S.E.)	*Pretest* ($\bar{X}$ ± S.E.)	(P)	*Posttest* ($\bar{X}$ ± S.E.)
Weight (kg)		82.9 ± 3.4	N.S.	81.6 ± 3.2	102.3 ± 7.8	N.S.	96.7 ± 6.1
% Lean		84.2 ± 1.6	N.S.	85.4 ± 1.7	77.1 ± 1.2	N.S.	77.8 ± 1.3
Blood pressure mm Hg	Syst.	126.4 ± 4.3	N.S.	124.8 ± 4.1	133.1 ± 3.6	<0.01	125.3 ± 2.8
	Diast.	77.8 ± 1.7	N.S.	79.0 ± 2.0	88.7 ± 3.5	N.S.	83.7 ± 3.0
	Pulse	47.7 ± 2.9	N.S.	46.3 ± 3.8	44.4 ± 2.2	<0.05	41.6 ± 1.6
Heart rate	Rest	58.7 ± 2.4	N.S.	54.0 ± 2.2	66.7 ± 2.8	<0.01	57.6 ± 1.7
	Low	110.0 ± 4.1	N.S.	102.6 ± 3.8	124.4 ± 5.4	<0.01	106.7 ± 6.2
	High	157.3 ± 3.8	<0.05	145.8 ± 3.8	154.6 ± 2.4	<0.01	136.2 ± 3.8
				166.6 ± 3.0			159.5 ± 3.6
Oxygen intake $\dot{V}O_2$ ml kg^{-1} min^{-1}	Low	22.6 ± 1.2	N.S.	21.4 ± 1.7	24.8 ± 2.0	N.S.	23.4 ± 1.6
	High	45.4 ± 1.6	N.S.	43.8 ± 2.2	36.4 ± 2.0	N.S.	37.8 ± 1.8
				54.2 ± 2.2			45.9 ± 2.2
Respiratory quotient	Low	0.82 ± 0.02	N.S.	0.79 ± 0.02	0.85 ± 0.02	N.S.	0.82 ± 0.01
	High	0.92 ± 0.02	<0.05	0.89 ± 0.03	0.94 ± 0.02	<0.05	0.88 ± 0.02
				0.96 ± 0.02			0.92 ± 0.02
% Predicted $\dot{V}O_2$ max	Low	45%		39%	59%		47%
	High	92%		78%	88%		76%
				98%			94%

Low/High = intensity of exercise

exercise seated on a bicycle ergometer (Monark, Sweden). This was followed by a 15-minute recovery period in the supine position. Venous blood samples were taken from the antecubital vein at rest, during low and high intensity exercise and after recovery and later analyzed for serum hormone and substrate concentrations. The subject's respiratory and cardiac responses were monitored at each stage of exercise and $\dot{V}O_2$, RQ and HR were determined.

Each subject was studied in the postabsorptive state between 08.00 and 12.00 hr at the same time of day initially (pre test) and at the conclusion of the fitness program (post test) in an attempt to minimize the effects of diurnal and intra-individual variation in the biochemical variables under investigation. All subjects were familiarized with the bicycle ergometer test before the investigation.

Two exercise levels were selected to produce relatively low ($\sim$ 50% predicted $\dot{V}O_2$ max) and relatively high ($\sim$ 90% predicted $\dot{V}O_2$ max) work intensities in each group of subjects. Maximal oxygen uptake capacity ($\dot{V}O_2$ max) was predicted using the procedure of Åstrand and Ryhming [1], with a correction factor for age.

The Ergometer Test

In the pretest, exercise consisted of low intensity exercise of ten-minute duration at 600 kpm min^{-1} and a pedaling frequency of 50 rpm. This involved work at 59% and 45% of predicted $\dot{V}O_2$ max for the sedentary and active groups, respectively. Following the low intensity exercise bout the subjects immediately performed a bout of high intensity exercise which involved an increase in the workload of 150 kpm min^{-1}, until the relative work output demanded 88% and 92% of predicted $\dot{V}O_2$ max for the sedentary groups and the active groups, respectively.

The same procedures were utilized in the posttest, whereby all subjects performed their identical pretest workloads. As a result low intensity exercise now involved 47% and 39% of predicted $\dot{V}O_2$ max and high intensity exercise 76% and 78% of predicted $\dot{V}O_2$ max for the sedentary and active groups, respectively. Consequently, the reduction in the relative intensity of work performed at each level of exercise in the posttest was attributed to the training effects of the fitness program which are outlined in Table I. Furthermore, in order to accommodate for the increased work capacity of the subjects resulting from participation in the program, an additional high intensity level was introduced in the posttest, which demanded a relative work output of 94% and 98% of predicted $\dot{V}O_2$ max for the sedentary and active groups, respectively.

Data

Standardized procedures were utilized for the collection of physiological data which included age, height, weight, blood pressure, $\dot{V}O_2$, HR and RQ. Percent lean body weight was estimated using the Wilmore and Behnke procedure [11] and physical fitness score using the Ismail criterion [5]. Standard clinical methods were used for the determination of glucose [4] and free fatty acids [2, 10]; a modified competitive protein binding technique for corticosteroids [3, 8]; and radioimmunoassay procedures for growth hormone [7, 9] and insulin [12].

Statistical Analysis

The intercorrelation matrices determined by the Pearson product moment procedure were factor analyzed using the principal axis components method with orthogonal factor rotation according to Kaiser's criterion [6]. Discriminant function analysis was applied to determine the ability of specific biochemical variables to differentiate between fitness groups. (Detailed correlation matrices, factor analytic solutions and discriminant function analyses are available upon request.)

Results

The changes in factor structure of physiological variables from pre- to posttests are shown in Table II and may be summarized as follows:

Rest

Latent hormone-substrate interactions were related to blood pressure and enhanced fitness status, while the influence of the corticosteroid variable was reduced possibly due to lowered anticipatory stress levels. Age and anaerobic performance continued to be important especially related to submaximal performance, whereas growth hormone and free fatty acids were depressed. Finally, the relationship between weight and fitness status was accentuated at the expense of the height variable.

Low Intensity Exercise

A stability in factor structure existed in terms of physique, fitness correlates and corticosteroids which may indicate a unique factor unaffected by the program. On the other hand, the impor-

Table II. General Factor Structure Identified at Each Stage of Exercise in the Pre- and Postprogram Tests

	Pretest Factors	% Variance	Posttest Factors	% Variance
Rest	1. Blood pressure, fitness status, insulin and glucose	19.9	4. Hormone-substrates and blood pressure	15.1
	2. Fitness correlates, corticosteroids and free fatty acids	18.7 ⎤	1. Physique, blood pressure, submaximal performance and free fatty acids	18.6 ⎤
	3. Age, anaerobic performance, growth hormone and free fatty acids	15.5 ⎥ 67.9	3. Age, anaerobic capacity and submaximal performance	16.0 ⎥ 66.4
	4. Height, fitness status and submaximal performance	13.8 ⎦	2. Weight and fitness correlates	16.7 ⎦
Low Intensity Exercise	1. Physique, fitness correlates and corticosteroids	18.7 ⎤	2. Physique, fitness correlates and corticosteroids	18.2 ⎤
	2. Physique, fitness status, submaximal performance and substrate levels	17.6 ⎥ 65.8	1. Physique, blood pressure, submaximal performance and free fatty acids	19.5 ⎥ 65.0
	3. Blood pressure, fitness status and insulin	15.9 ⎥	4. Submaximal performance, growth hormone and glucose	12.4 ⎥
	4. Age, anaerobic performance and substrate behavior	13.6 ⎦	3. Age, anaerobic and submaximal performance	14.9 ⎦

Table II. General Factor Structure Identified at Each Stage of Exercise in the Pre- and Postprogram Tests (Continued)

	Pretest Factors	% Variance	Posttest Factors	% Variance
High Intensity Exercise	1. Stature, fitness status, growth hormone, corticosteroids and glucose	19.9	1. Stature, fitness status, growth hormone and glucose	21.7
	2. Blood pressure, insulin and glucose	18.4	4. Blood pressure and corticosteroids	12.5
	3. Physique, fitness correlates and maximal performance	18.0	2. Physique, fitness correlates and work performance	19.4
	4. Age, anaerobic performance and free fatty acids	12.6	3. Age, work performance, conditioned substrate behavior	15.3
		68.9		68.9
			1. Fitness status, growth hormone and energy substrate behavior	22.2
			2. Physique, submaximal and maximal performance, ergometry	18.0
			3. Age, anaerobic capacity, submaximal performance and growth hormone	16.8
			4. Blood pressure and hormone levels	14.5
				71.5

Recovery

1. Physique, fitness correlates and corticosteroids	20.2	
2. Blood pressure, fitness status, growth hormone and insulin	18.5	
3. Body size, fitness status and glucose	16.7	66.8
4. Age and anaerobic performance	11.4	

4. Growth hormone, insulin and free fatty acid interactions	11.9	
2. Physique, blood pressure, submaximal performance and glucose	19.7	
1. Weight, fitness status and substrate behavior	21.1	70.4
3. Age, submaximal performance and free fatty acids	17.7	

tance of lipid substrates for energy after the program probably indicated enhanced oxidative capacity. Furthermore, submaximal performance appeared to be less dependent upon glucose availability following conditioning, which accompanied the disappearance of the factor relating blood pressure, fitness status and insulin level. Finally, the stable age and anaerobic performance factor became allied to submaximal work performance.

High Intensity Exercise

The influence of the corticosteroid variable was reduced probably as a result of the training effects of the program. Nevertheless, corticosteroid level was still related to blood pressure level after conditioning. The stability of physique, fitness correlates and work performance factor possibly indicated a unique relationship unaffected by the program. However, the degree of anaerobic state was reduced at this level of exercise with work performance becoming related to augmented free fatty acid importance, with the age variable maintaining its presence.

The factor structure which emerged at the new high intensity level of exercise in the posttest reflected the demands of the work performed. Fitness status became critically related to substrate availability, with corticosteroids absent in view of the uniform stress of a "near maximal" response. Physique and work performance appeared to be related to the use of the ergometer test instrument. Age and anaerobic capacity reflected the submaximal performance response, and the interrelationship between blood pressure and serum hormone levels probably reflected the metabolic stress incurred at this stage.

Recovery

A purely biochemical factor emerged which replaced the physiological components physique and fitness status relating to recovery from stress as identified by the corticosteroid component. The interaction of blood pressure and hormone levels diminished with glucose availability assuming importance. Furthermore, fitness status was allied to general substrate availability during recovery. Finally, the age component became unrelated to anaerobic performance and was allied to submaximal performance and lipid substrate availability in recovery.

The ability of biochemical variables to classify subjects into the correct fitness category was determined by performing a discriminant function analysis using the most powerful discriminator variables identified at each stage of exercise in the pre- and posttests as shown in Table III. The pretest data resulted in only one misclassification per group and the magnitude of coefficients indicated that corticosteroid level at high intensity exercise represented the most important discriminator variable between active and sedentary subjects. The posttest data resulted in no misclassifications in either group and the magnitude of coefficients indicated that corticosteroid level at low intensity exercise was the best overall discriminator item. It was concluded therefore that corticosteroid level in response to exercise stress was the most important biochemical variable in distinguishing between active and sedentary subjects who had been initially classified according to physiological criteria alone.

Table III. Discriminant Function Analyses Utilizing Most Powerful Biochemical Variables at Each Phase of Activity to Classify Subjects in Pre- and Postprogram Tests

Variable	Phase of Activity	Coefficients[+] (Active v. Sedentary)
Pretest		
1. Growth hormone	Rest	1.984
2. Corticosteroids	Low ⎱ Intensity	0.098
3. Corticosteroids	High ⎰ Exercise	3.118
4. Corticosteroids	Recovery	2.928
Number of Incorrect Classifications per Group		1
Mahalanobis D^2		4.841
Corresponding F Ratio		5.66*
Posttest		
1. Corticosteroids	Rest	4.766
2. Corticosteroids	Low ⎱	6.992
3. Corticosteroids	High ⎰ Intensity Exercise	6.745
4. Growth Hormone	High	2.014
5. Corticosteroids	Recovery	1.289
Number of Incorrect Classifications per Group		0
Mahalanobis D^2		5.961
Corresponding F Ratio		5.01*

[+]All coefficients multiplied by 100.
*Significant at the 0.01 level.

References

1. Astrand, P.-O. and Ryhming, I.: A nomogram for calculation of aerobic capacity (physical fitness) from pulse rates during submaximal work. J. Appl. Physiol. 7:218-221, 1954.

2. Dole, V.P.: A relationship between non-esterified and fatty acids in plasma and the metabolism of glucose. J. Clin. Invest. 35:150-154, 1956.

3. Few, J.D. and Cashmore, G.C.: The determination of plasma cortisol by competitive protein binding. Ann. Clin. Biochem. 8:205-209, 1971.

4. Hoffman, W.S.: A rapid photoelectric method for the determination of glucose in blood and urine. J. Biol. Chem. 120:51-61, 1937.

5. Ismail, A.H., Falls, H.B. and MacLeod, D.F.: Development of a criterion for physical fitness tests. J. Appl. Physiol. 20:991-999, 1965.

6. Kaiser, H.F.: The varimax criterion for analytic rotation in factor analysis. Psychometrika 23:187-200, 1963.

7. Molinatti, G.M., Massara, F., Strumia, E. et al: Radioimmunoassay of human growth hormone. J. Nucl. Biol. Med. 13:26, 1969.

8. Murphy, B.E.P.: Protein binding and the assay of nonantigenic hormones. Rec. Prog. Horm. Res. 25:565-610, 1969.

9. Pennisi, F.: A fast procedure for radioimmunoassay of human growth hormone. J. Nucl. Biol. Med. 12:137, 1968.

10. Trout, D.L., Estes, E.H. Jr. and Friedberg, S.J.: Titration of free fatty acids of plasma: A study of current methods and a new modification. J. Lipid Res. 1:199-202, 1962.

11. Wilmore, J.H. and Behnke, A.R.: An anthropometric estimation of body density and lean body weight in young men. J. Appl. Physiol. 27:25-31, 1969.

12. Yalow, R.S. and Berson, S.: Immunoassay of endogenous plasma insulin in man. J. Clin. Invest. 39:1157-1159, 1960.

Characteristics of Well-Trained Long-Distance Runners From the Biochemical Viewpoint

Tatsuya Tsutsumi

It seems that well-trained long-distance running champions of the first class must generally have efficient mechanism of energy supply during physical exercise, and it is said that the rate of decrease in muscle glycogen as an energy source is almost equal in trained and untrained men, if the intensity of exercise is regulated properly according to their physical fitness.

The present experiment was made for the purpose of elucidating the characteristic aspects of physical functions of well-trained champions of long-distance running from the biochemical viewpoint. Comparative observations were made on the heart rate, oxygen uptake and changes in physiological substances in the blood, imposing controlled physical exercise upon well-trained and untrained men according to their physical capacity.

The subjects of the experiment were three university distance running champions of the first class (22 years of age, 164.2 cm and 55.3 kg on the average) and three physically untrained laboratory workers (33.7 years, 164.5 cm and 57.0 kg on the average). The exercise consisted of 70 minutes of running on a treadmill of 3° inclination. The running speed was regulated in each subject so that they became almost exhausted in about 70 minutes. As the result, the speed and the duration of running were on the average 213 meters/min × 71 minutes in the champions and 143 meters/ min × 65 minutes in the laboratory workers, respectively. In other words, the intensity of the exercise was 1.5 times as strong in the former as in the latter. However, the average heart rate during the exercise was rather similar to each other, viz., 163 beats/min in the champions and 167 beats/min in the laboratory workers. This fact seems to suggest that the relative intensity ($\%\dot{V}O_2$ max) was almost equal in the two groups.

Tatsuya Tsutsumi, Department of Biochemistry, Physical Fitness Research Institute, Meiji Life Foundation of Health and Welfare, Tokyo, Japan.

Regarding the oxygen intake, it became steady after 20 minutes of running in both groups, as shown in Figure 1, but the average level was a little higher in the champions (2.7 l/min) than in the laboratory workers (2.3 l/min). The difference, of course, seemed to be related to the absolute intensity of the exercise. The fact also suggests that the average maximum oxygen intake was different in the two groups, because the relative intensity of the exercise was similar in both groups as far as the heart rate was concerned.

Figure 2 shows the changes in serum GOT and GPT, and Figure 3 shows those in serum LDH during and after the above-mentioned

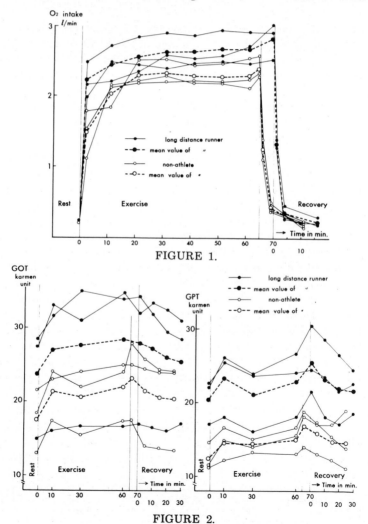

FIGURE 1.

FIGURE 2.

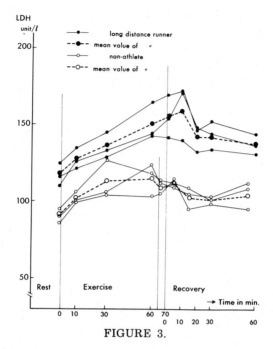

FIGURE 3.

exercise. It is noted that the activity of these enzymes was obviously augmented at the beginning of exercise to reach a plateau or to turn to a slower increase thereafter. After the cessation of exercise, the activity levels became slowly lower, but did not reach the initial resting level even after 60 minutes. There was no difference between the trained and the untrained in the pattern of changes in these enzymes. Since the increase in these enzymes in the blood is caused by insufficient supply of oxygen to the tissue cells, the similarity of the above-mentioned pattern in two groups seems to be related to the similarity in relative exercise intensity and in oxygen deficit in the two groups. Otherwise, the fact might suggest that the oxygen debt was not sufficiently large to cause significant increase in these enzymes in the blood so that no appreciable difference between two groups could be found.

Figure 4 shows the changes in serum triglycerides (TG) and cholesterol (Ch) during and after the exercise. Just as in the case of the enzymes in the blood, triglycerides and cholesterol showed a rapid increase at the beginning of exercise and maintained thereafter rather constant levels during the exercise. No significant differences between the two groups in the levels at the end of the exercise could be found. The increase in serum triglycerides can be caused by venous infusion of catecholamine and the catecholamine secretion is

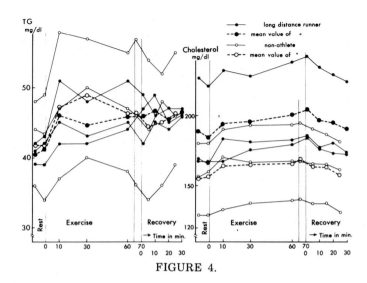

FIGURE 4.

said to increase exponentially as the intensity of exercise (%V̇O₂ max) increases. Therefore, the above-mentioned similarity of the increase in serum triglycerides in two groups seems to be related to the similarity in the exercise intensity and also in the catecholamine secretion in both groups. Regarding the increase in serum cholesterol, it seems to keep pace with serum triglycerides.

However, it is highly noteworthy that the serum free fatty acids (FFA), which seem to be an important energy source of physical exercise and can be augmented by catecholamine secretion, presented patterns of changes different from serum triglycerides, as shown in Figure 5. It is evident that the serum FFA show in both groups a decrease in the early stage of exercise, followed by a gradual increase during exercise and a marked increase in the recovery stage reaching a peak value about ten minutes after the cessation of exercise. The increase after the exercise, especially the peak value ten minutes after the exercise, is obviously smaller in the champion group than in the untrained group. It seems to me that the peak value ten minutes after the exercise is a good indicator of mobilization of FFA into the blood from the fat deposit and also an indicator of FFA combustion in the muscles. Accordingly, Figure 5 seems to suggest that the combustion of deposited fat through FFA mobilization was less in the champion group than in the untrained group.

Figure 6 shows the changes in the blood sugar during and after the exercise. In the case of the untrained group, the blood sugar level became lower in the early stage of exercise and then recovered the

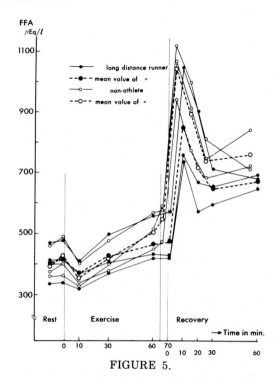

FIGURE 5.

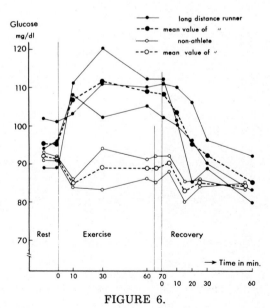

FIGURE 6.

initial level to maintain it thereafter. On the other hand, in the champion group, the blood sugar level rose in the early stage of exercise to a level higher than the resting level, maintained it until the end of the exercise and decreased after the cessation of exercise to recover the resting level in 60 minutes. Since the sugar uptake of the muscles is said to increase along with the rise of the blood sugar level during the exercise, the sugar supply to the muscles from the storage in the liver seems to be more abundant in the champion group than in the untrained group. As aforementioned, the increase in serum FFA, mostly caused by the catecholamine secretion, was a little less in the champion group, although the degree of augmentation of catecholamine secretion was considered to be similar in the two groups. This fact must be related to a greater increase in blood sugar during the exercise in the champion group.

Figure 7 shows the changes in blood lactate. The blood lactate increased in the early stage of the exercise to reach a plateau which maintained its level until the end of the exercise. It is noteworthy that the increase in blood lactate in the untrained group was three times as much as in the champion group. This fact seems to be

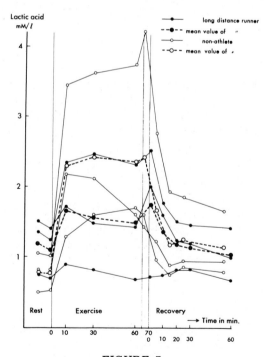

FIGURE 7.

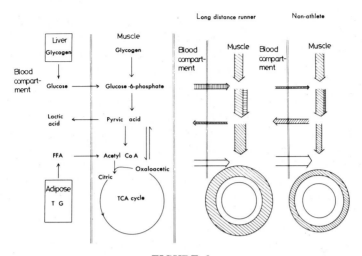

FIGURE 8.

related either to less lactate production or to more uptake and oxidation of lactate in the champion group.

The abovementioned findings led the author to the concept that the biochemical characteristics of the trained long-distance runners consist in the changes of blood substrates as energy source somewhat different from those in the untrained men. The characteristics are schematically illustrated in Figure 8. The trained runners have a large capacity of oxygen uptake and oxidation. However, the fat used through FFA in combustion as the fuel seems to be rather small in quantity, while the carbohydrate used through pyruvic acid is abundantly oxidized in the champion group. On the other hand, it is said that the rate of loss in muscle glycogen is similar in the trained and the untrained. Accordingly, the glycogen supply from the liver seems to be abundant in the trained and they have a large capacity of oxidizing the pyruvic acid. It is presumed that the trained distance runners can maintain their high speed for a long time by abundant oxidation of carbohydrate, but in economizing the use of muscle glycogen. This point seems to be an aspect of the characteristics of excellent long-distance runners from the biochemical viewpoint.

Influence of Adrenergic Stimulation on the Sinoatrial Node

R. L. Hughson, J. D. Fitzgerald,
J. R. Sutton and N. L. Jones

Introduction

Resting cardiac frequency decreases following a period of aerobic training. We have observed both in humans [3] and in animals [2] a reduction of intrinsic sinoatrial frequency (ISF) with training. The present study investigated the effect of increased sympathetic activity on the sinoatrial node in eliciting changes in the properties of the ISF. In addition, the chronotropic responses to noradrenalin and to exercise were studied.

Methods

Male Sprague-Dawley rats were assigned to four groups of ten animals. Two groups acted as controls, an active group, and a group which exercised on a treadmill for 45 minutes at 19 m/min, five days/week for ten weeks. The other two groups received subcutaneous injections of noradrenalin suspended in oil five days/week; one group was inactive, the other exercised on the treadmill. Measurements were made of resting cardiac frequency and ISF before and at the completion of the ten-week exercise period. The ISF was taken as the cardiac frequency 20 minutes following the IP injection of atropine sulphate (3 mg/kg) and propranolol (8 mg/kg). The measurements at ten weeks were made 48 hours after the last exercise or drug administration. At the completion of the ten-week study, the hearts of these animals were removed and the right atrium of each was placed in an isolated organ bath. Dose-response curves to the chronotropic effects of noradrenalin were obtained. Measurements of sodium and potassium contents were made on the plasma and the ventricular homogenate.

R. L. Hughson, J. D. Fitzgerald, J. R. Sutton and N. L. Jones, Department of Medicine, McMaster University Medical Centre, Hamilton, Ontario, Canada.

Results

Effects on ISF

Ten weeks of treadmill training produced a significant reduction in resting cardiac frequency in the exercised control animals (Fig. 1). Neither of the noradrenalin-pretreated groups had a resting cardiac frequency different from control. The decrease in ISF of the exercised control group was significantly greater than that of the inactive control animals. In contrast, the inactive noradrenalin-pretreated group demonstrated a reduction in ISF, while the exercised noradrenalin-pretreated animals showed no greater reduction in ISF than the inactive control.

Changes in ISF may result from alterations in the electrophysiological properties of the sinoatrial nodal cells. The slope of the prepotential, the threshold potential and the maximum diastolic repolarization can influence intrinsic discharge frequency of the sinoatrial node. From the measurements of sodium and potassium contents of the myocardium and plasma, we have information concerning the latter factor influencing ISF, the maximum diastolic repolarization. While the Ko^+/Ki^+ ratio of the exercised animals was reduced from the inactive control, the ratio in the noradrenalin-pretreated inactive animals was greater, and the ratio in noradrenalin-pretreated exercised animals was similar to inactive controls (Fig. 2). On the basis of the Nernst equation, this would imply a more negative maximum diastolic repolarization in the exercised control

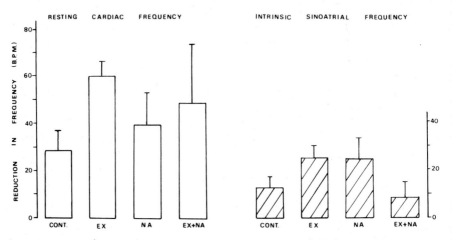

FIG. 1. *Left*, the reduction in resting cardiac frequency. *Right*, the reduction in ISF over the ten-week study.

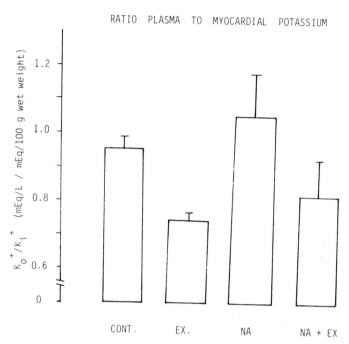

FIG. 2. Ratio of plasma to myocardial potassium (K_o^+/K_i^+).

animals and a more positive maximum diastolic repolarization in the noradrenalin-pretreated inactive animals. Thus, factors other than changes in maximum diastolic repolarization appear to be affecting the ISF.

Noradrenalin Responses

The chronotropic dose-response curves (Fig. 3) show that in comparison with inactive control, there is a small reduction in maximum response of the exercised control animals. The two noradrenalin-pretreated groups are more sensitive to noradrenalin in vitro, as shown by the significant left shift in the dose-response curves. We do not have any information to indicate whether the increased sensitivity is related to the neuronal uptake mechanisms or to the receptor itself. This increased sensitivity in the noradrenalin-pretreated groups with no change in sensitivity of the exercised control animals does not support the recent reports by Ekblom et al [1] and others that the chronotropic sensitivity to catecholamines is reduced following training.

The reduction in maximum chronotropic response in the isolated atrial preparation was related to the reduction in the in vitro ISF

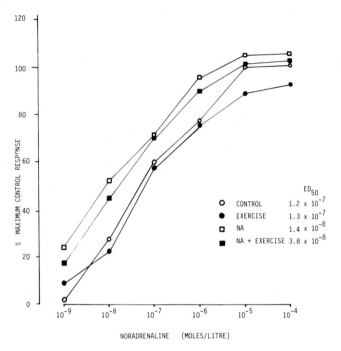

NORADRENALINE   (MOLES/LITRE)

FIG. 3. Noradrenalin chronotropic dose-response curves.

(Fig. 4). The linear relationship between maximum sinoatrial response to noradrenalin (Y) and the in vitro ISF (X) is expressed by the equation $Y = 0.62 X + 172$, $r = 0.60$. This indicates that electrophysiological factors which establish the ISF also impose limitations on the maximum in vitro response to noradrenalin. To determine whether this in vitro observation has any application to the limitation of maximum cardiac frequency in vivo, we studied the cardiac frequency response of a further group of animals during maximal treadmill exercise and under anesthesia for the maximum noradrenalin response.

Maximum in Vivo Cardiac Frequency

Untrained female Sprague-Dawley rats were exercised on one occasion on the treadmill to exhaustion at 30 m/min, with the grade of the treadmill increased by 3% every two minutes. Cardiac frequency was monitored during exercise with limb lead electrodes on a standard electrocardiograph. ISF was determined previously in these same animals by the IP injection of atropine and propranolol. Following these experiments, the same animals were anesthetized

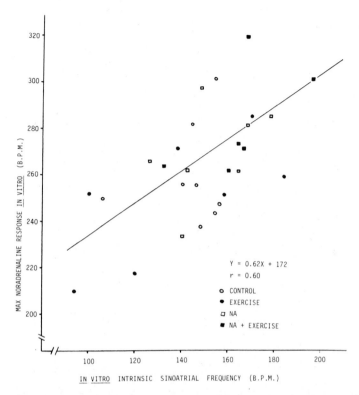

FIG. 4. Maximum noradrenalin response in vitro vs. the in vitro ISF, and the ED_{50} for each group.

and ganglionic blockade was achieved with 6 mg/kg hexamathonium to prevent a reflex bradycardia from noradrenalin-induced hypertension. Noradrenalin was injected IV in increasing doses until a maximum cardiac frequency response was observed. Figure 5 shows on the left the positive relationship between maximum exercise cardiac frequency and the ISF, and on the right the positive relationship between maximum noradrenalin-stimulated cardiac frequency and the ISF. This in vivo evidence gives further support to our hypothesis derived previously from in vitro studies that the maximum sinoatrial frequency is limited by electrophysiological factors which establish the ISF. Thus, the frequent observations of reduced maximum cardiac frequency with physical training may be explained by the accompanying reduction of ISF.

The results of the present study suggest that changes in the intrinsic properties of the sinoatrial node with physical training are not due to increased sympathetic activity. Rather, the ISF, the

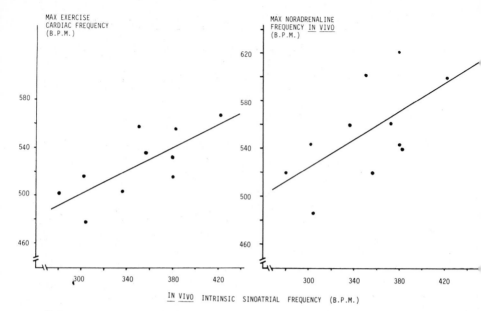

FIG. 5. *Left*, the maximum exercise cardiac frequency (Y) vs. the in vivo ISF
(X) Y = 0.49 X + 355, r = 0.76. *Right*, the maximum noradrenalin-stimulated
cardiac frequency (Y) measured in vivo vs. the in vivo ISF (X),
Y = 0.58 X + 350, r = 0.61.

Ko^+/Ki^+ ratio and the chronotropic sensitivity to noradrenalin
following exercise were not related to increased catecholamine
activity, but to some other aspect of the physical training itself.

References

1. Ekblom, B., Kilbom, A. and Soltysiak, J.: Physical training, bradycardia and
   autonomic nervous system. Scand. J. Clin. Lab. Invest. 32:251-256, 1973.
2. Hughson, R.L., Sutton, J.R., Fitzgerald, J.D. and Jones, N.L.: Intrinsic
   sinoatrial frequency and norepinephrine response of the exercised rat.
   Unpublished 1976.
3. Sutton, J.R., Cole, A., Gunning, J. et al: Control of heart rate in healthy
   young men. Lancet 2:1398-1400, 1967.

Effect of Submaximal Exercise on Canine Ventricular Fibrillation Threshold

Albert K. Dawson

Introduction

The American College of Sports Medicine has set down some strict guidelines for graded exercise stress testing and exercise prescription writing for persons with possibly latent or overt ischemic heart disease [1]. The work of Bruce and Kluge [4] and of Friedman et al [6] indicates that such precautions are probably well justified. However, controlled animal experiments studying the risk of sudden death due to the earliest phase of acute myocardial ischemia, in conjunction with moderate rhythmic exercise, are still lacking. The electrical determination of ventricular fibrillation thresholds (VFT) is a well-established technique for reproducibly quantitating and comparing ventricular electrical stability. Numerous investigators have utilized VFT experiments to study the effects of coronary ligation, drug administration, autonomic nervous system stimulation, hypothermia and various other interventions related to ventricular electrical stability [8]. In the present study a chronic dog preparation was used to examine the effect of submaximal treadmill exercise on VFT. In addition, the risk of suffering spontaneous ventricular fibrillation during the earliest phase of acute myocardial ischemia was compared during conditions of rest and moderate exercise.

Methods

Twenty-five adult mongrel dogs of either sex weighing 17 to 30 kg were studied. On the day of surgery each dog was anesthetized with 25 to 30 mg/kg sodium pentobarbital (IV) and administered

Albert K. Dawson, Laboratory of Physiological Hygiene, School of Public Health, University of Minnesota, Minneapolis, Minn., U.S.A. Present address: Medtronic, Inc., Minneapolis, Minn.
Supported in part by A.H.A. Grant-in-Aid # 73 829.

600,000 units of penicillin (IM). Under aseptic conditions and positive pressure ventilation, a left thoracotomy was performed at the fifth intercostal space. The anterior descending coronary artery was isolated 1.0 to 1.5 cm distal to its origin and a snare made of surgical monofilament nylon (size 2), enclosed in a polyethylene sleeve (tubing size P.E. 320), was placed around it and anchored with two small sutures to the epicardium. Next, two platinum-iridium electrodes of a "corkscrew" tipped configuration (Medtronic Model 6917) were screwed into the left ventricular myocardium 1 to 3 cm apart and within the region of projected ischemia. Following this, the animal's chest was closed and the distal ends of the electrodes and snare were buried in a subcutaneous pocket just caudal to the left scapular region. Following three to four weeks of recovery, the subcutaneous pocket was opened, aseptically, under a local anesthetic and the distal ends of the electrodes and snare were exposed. Baseline VFT were determined by the method of Bacaner [3] with the following modifications. The single, constant current rectilinear pulse used to scan the vulnerable period of the cardiac cycle had a width of 2 ms and, for the normal or nonischemic thresholds, was initiated every 10th to 15th sinus beat. The R-wave from a modified lead III ECG was used to synchronize each stimulus pulse delivered to the vulnerable period. Both nonischemic and ischemic VFT were recorded in milliamps of current required to produce fibrillation. Three nonischemic and one ischemic VFT were measured in each dog at baseline. To obtain the ischemic VFT the snare around the anterior descending coronary artery was rapidly tightened by an amount predetermined during surgery to produce complete occlusion. A stopwatch was then started, and the ischemic changes in the myocardial electrogram were monitored continuously from one of the myocardial electrodes for the first seven to eight minutes of the occlusion. After this initial phase, scanning of the vulnerable period was begun with the 2 ms pulse being delivered very sixth sinus beat. The total duration of ischemia from occlusion to fibrillation was recorded along with the VFT. In all cases, defibrillation was accomplished by D.C. transthoracic countershock delivered following 15 to 30 seconds of fibrillation. For the ischemic VFT determination, the snare was released following resuscitation and the myocardial electrogram was monitored for signs of return to normal. Coronary artery occlusion was never maintained longer than 20 minutes. Following baseline VFT determinations each animal was randomly assigned to either an exercise or a control group. One or two days later treatment VFT were determined in all dogs in a manner consistent with baseline determinations. For the control group treatment VFT were measured while the dogs were, again, standing quietly at rest. For the exercise group treatment VFT were measured while each dog ran on a motor driven treadmill at 3.0 to 3.5 mph and 30% grade. For the ischemic run, coronary occlusion, starting the stopwatch and starting the treadmill was carried out in that order in as rapid a sequence as was possible.

Results

Nonischemic and ischemic VFT data were collected on 13 exercise and 12 control dogs. Tables I and II present these data together with the differences between baseline and treatment VFT for the exercise and control groups. The means of the nonischemic differences for exercise and control dogs were −1.47 ± 4.84 and 2.09 ± 5.10 mA, respectively. These means were not significantly different from one another. The means of the ischemic differences for exercise and control dogs were 4.38 ± 2.88 and −0.25 ± 3.52 mA, respectively. These means were significantly different from one another (0.001 < p < 0.01). Five of the 13 exercise dogs fibrillated

Table I. VFT (mA) for Exercise Dogs

Dog	Nonischemic			Ischemic		
	Baseline	Treatment	Difference	Baseline	Treatment	Difference
E1	41.0	42.5	−1.5	35	30	5
E2	18.7	19.5	−0.8	16	13	3
E3	20.0	18.5	1.5	18	8	10
E4	43.5	45.0	−1.5	16	13	3
E5	21.7	28.0	−6.3	22	18	4
E6	50.0	50.0	0.0	3	3	0
E7	31.7	35.0	−3.3	10	6	4
E8	25.3	40.0	−14.7	22	16	6
Mean	31.49	34.81	−3.32	17.75	13.38	4.38
± S.D.	±11.99	±11.76	±5.15	±9.39	±8.42	±2.88
E9	30.5	30.0	0.5	10	S*	
E10	22.5	20.0	2.5	19	S	
E11	32.0	27.5	4.5	22	S	
E12	25.5	23.5	2.0	17	S	
E13	29.0	31.0	−2.0	14	S	
Mean	30.11	31.58	−1.47	17.23		
± S.D.	±9.60	±10.29	±4.84	±7.68		

*"S" denotes the occurrence of spontaneous ventricular fibrillation before vulnerable period scanning with the 2 ms pulse began.

Table II. VFT (mA) for Control Dogs

	Nonischemic			Ischemic		
Dog	Baseline	Treatment	Difference	Baseline	Treatment	Difference
C1	32.3	34.0	-1.7	25	31	-6
C2	41.3	33.6	7.7	20	27	-7
C3	50.0	53.5	-3.5	20	18	2
C4	22.6	23.6	-1.0	20	20	0
C5	23.6	19.3	4.3	6	5	1
C6	32.3	29.0	3.3	12	14	-2
C7	50.3	44.7	5.6	44	43	1
C8	36.0	33.5	2.5	13	7	6
C9	29.0	32.3	-3.3	26	24	2
C10	39.5	42.3	-2.8	25	24	1
C11	26.7	26.0	0.7	10	10	0
C12	60.0	46.7	13.3	21	22	-1
Mean	36.97	34.88	2.09	20.17	20.42	-0.25
± S.D.	±11.68	±10.15	±5.10	±9.87	±10.73	±3.52

spontaneously early in the ischemic treadmill run (all within the first eight minutes of coronary ischemia). Hence, the statistical analysis of ischemic VFT was limited to only 8 exercise and 12 control animals.

Table III presents the drop in VFT during coronary occlusion for the exercise group. Table IV shows these data for the control group. As shown in these tables, the means of the differences (baseline — treatment) for exercise and control dogs were -7.70 ± 6.13 and 2.34 ± 6.88 mA or -23.32 ± 17.99 and 2.71 ± 13.59 percent,* respectively. Within both pairs these means were significantly different from one another $(0.001 < p < 0.01)$. Paired T-tests were also applied directly to the groups of data. From this a significant difference was found at the 1% level when baseline and treatment data for ischemic exercise dogs were compared (Table I). Again, significance at the 1% level was found when the baseline drop in VFT during coronary occlusion was paired with the corresponding treatment data for the exercise group (Table III). However, a comparison of nonischemic data for the exercise group showed no significant change from baseline to treatment. No significant differences whatsoever were seen within the control group when baseline and treatment data were compared.

---

*The unit "percent" refers to the measurement of the drop in VFT during coronary occlusion as follows:

$$\frac{(\text{nonischemic VFT}) - \text{ischemic VFT}}{\text{nonischemic VFT}} \times 100$$

Table III. Drop in VFT During Coronary Occlusion for Exercise Dogs

Dog	Milliamps			% of Nonischemic Value*		
	Baseline	Treatment	Difference	Baseline	Treatment	Difference
E1	6.0	12.5	-6.5	14.6	29.4	-14.8
E2	2.7	6.5	-3.8	14.4	33.3	-18.9
E3	2.0	10.5	-8.5	10.0	56.8	-46.8
E4	27.5	32.0	-4.5	63.5	71.1	- 7.6
E5	-0.3	10.0	-10.3	-1.4	35.7	-37.1
E6	47.0	47.0	0.0	94.0	94.0	0.0
E7	21.7	29.0	-7.3	68.4	82.8	-14.4
E8	3.3	24.0	-20.7	13.0	60.0	-47.0
Mean	13.74	21.44	-7.70	34.56	57.89	-23.32
± S.D.	±16.84	±14.05	±6.13	±35.22	±23.94	±17.99

*Same footnote as on page 304.

Table IV. Drop in VFT During Coronary Occlusion for Control Dogs

Dog	Milliamps			% of Nonischemic Value*		
	Baseline	Treatment	Difference	Baseline	Treatment	Difference
C1	7.3	3.0	4.3	22.6	8.8	13.8
C2	21.3	6.6	14.7	51.6	19.6	32.0
C3	30.0	35.5	-5.5	60.6	66.4	-5.8
C4	2.6	3.6	-1.0	11.5	15.2	-3.7
C5	17.6	14.3	3.3	74.6	74.1	0.5
C6	20.3	15.0	5.3	62.8	51.7	11.1
C7	6.3	1.7	4.6	12.5	3.8	8.7
C8	23.0	26.5	-3.5	63.9	79.1	-15.2
C9	3.0	8.3	-5.3	10.3	25.7	-15.4
C10	14.5	18.3	-3.8	36.7	43.3	-6.6
C11	16.7	16.0	0.7	62.5	61.5	1.0
C12	39.0	24.7	14.3	65.0	52.9	12.1
Mean	16.80	14.46	2.34	44.55	41.84	2.71
± S.D.	±10.55	±10.54	±6.88	±24.30	±26.36	±13.59

*Same footnote as on page 304.

Discussion

This study presents experimental evidence to support the hypothesis that moderate rhythmic exercise may increase the risk of sudden death due to ventricular fibrillation during an acute myocardial ischemic event. Not only was the measured VFT (mA) consistently at its lowest during the ischemic exercise, but the fact that five out of 13 dogs fibrillated spontaneously early in the course of this run points dramatically to the seriousness of this increased ischemic risk. It should be emphasized that this enhanced risk of sudden death was found only during acute ischemia. There was no hint of increased risk during exercise for the nonischemic heart.

All coronary occlusions were limited to less than 20 minutes. Burgess and her co-workers [5] have shown that the maximum vulnerability to ventricular fibrillation in the dog usually occurs within the first 30 minutes following coronary occlusion. Jennings et al [7] have shown that focal myocardial necrosis can occur in the dog after as little as 22 minutes of transient ischemia. Hence, by limiting each occlusion to less than 20 minutes it was felt that each dog would be studied during or very near to its peak vulnerability without any substantial risk of creating an infarct. The avoidance of infarct production in this study was very important, since each dog served as its own control. Data gathered both on dogs [9] and on humans [2] indicate that an infarct may have a stabilizing effect on the ventricle. Apparently, the highest risk of sudden death in ischemic heart disease is associated with the earliest phase of acute myocardial ischemia and not with the later infarct formation phase.

References

1. ACSM Guidelines For Graded Exercise Testing and Exercise Prescription. Philadelphia:Lea & Febiger, 1975.
2. Baum, R.S., Alvarez, H., III and Cobb, L.A.: Survival after resuscitation from out-of-hospital ventricular fibrillation. Circulation 50:1231-1235, 1974.
3. Bacaner, M.B.: Quantitative comparison of bretylium with other antifibrillatory drugs. Am. J. Cardiol. 21:504-512, 1968.
4. Bruce, R.A. and Kluge, W.: Defibrillatory treatment of exertional cardiac arrest in coronary disease. JAMA 216:653-658, 1971.
5. Burgess, M.J., Abildskov, J.A., Millar, K. et al: Time course of vulnerability to fibrillation after experimental coronary occlusion. Am. J. Cardiol. 27:617-621, 1971.
6. Friedman, M., Manwaring, J.H., Roseman, R.H. et al: Instantaneous and sudden deaths: Clinical and pathological differentiation in coronary artery disease. JAMA 225:1319-1328, 1973.
7. Jennings, R.B., Sommers, H.M., Smyth, G.A. et al: Myocardial necrosis induced by temporary occlusion of a coronary artery in the dog. Arch. Pathol. 70:68-78, 1960.
8. Surawicz, B.: Ventricular fibrillation. Am. J. Cardiol. 28:268-287, 1971.
9. Thompson, P.L., Lohrbauer, L.A. and Lown, B.: Strenuous exercise during acute stages of myocardial infarction in dogs. (Abst.) Circulation 44 (Suppl. II):60, 1971.

Prepubertal Exercise and Myocardial Collateral Circulation

R. L. Rasmussen, R. D. Bell and G. D. Spencer

Introduction

A renewed interest in the effects of physical activity programs on the health of specific populations has led to many diverse studies involving the use of various types and intensities of exercise. However, few of these studies have been concerned with the prepubertal age group even though it is a time when the organism is undergoing significant cellular changes.

Recent investigations [1-3, 5-7] concerned with myocardial capillary development agree that capillarization can be augmented to a certain degree, dependent upon the age of the organism and the specific stimulus to such development. The experiments of Tomanek [7], Bell and Rasmussen [1], Poupa and Rakusan [3] and others agree that physical exercise is one such appropriate stimulus for additional capillary development beyond that occurring due to the aging process in the hearts of young animals. However, few, if any, experiments have investigated the effects of different exercise programs on the exact degree of myocardial capillary development. The present experiments represent an attempt to describe the effect of different exercise programs on the capillary-fiber (C-F) ratio in prepubertal animals.

Methods and Materials

Initial Experiment

Forty prepubescent male albino rats, 4 weeks of age (Wistar), were randomly divided into exercise (n = 20) and control (n = 20) groups as follows: (1) *exercise group* — animals exercised for six weeks before the onset of puberty and (2) *control group* — animals in a sedentary state for the six weeks before puberty.

R. L. Rasmussen, Department of Physical Education, St. Francis Xavier University, Antigonish, Nova Scotia; R. D. Bell and G. D. Spencer, College of Physical Education, University of Saskatchewan, Saskatoon, Saskatchewan, Canada.

The exercise group was subjected to an exercise program which consisted of a 30-minute swim daily, five days a week for six weeks. A weight equal to 4% body weight was attached to the tip of the tail of each animal during each exercise period.

All animals received standard laboratory chow and water ad libitum throughout the duration of the experiment.

Following the training program all animals were individually anesthetized with an overdose of ether. After anesthesia the animals were fastened to a dissection board and the abdominal and chest cavities were opened via a midline incision. The inferior vena cava was clamped with a hemostat to reduce venous return to the heart and the aorta was exposed, isolated and cannulated with an 18-gauge needle retrograde to the normal flow of blood. When the aorta was cannulated successfully, the needle was connected to the perfusing apparatus and the heart was perfused at a pressure of approximately 65 mm Hg for several moments, until it was uniformly dark on the surface or judged to be as completely perfused as possible. The perfusate was a solution of 2.0% carbochrome ink, 0.2% heparin and 97.8% Locke's solution. The perfusate was maintained at a temperature of 30 C. The heart was then tied off around the base, removed from the animal and fixed in a 10% formalin solution for 24 hours. Next a mid-ventricular section approximately 1 cm thick was obtained by a transverse ablation of the ventricles, midway between the apex and the base of the heart. After being embedded in paraffin, ventricular tissue sections, each approximately 15μ thick, were cut on a Leitz microtome and subsequently stained simultaneously with a standard hematoxylin and eosin stain (Fig. 1).

Myocardial C-F ratios were determined for all animals in accordance with previously discussed procedures [1]. This initial experiment involving rats and using swimming as the exercise regime indicated that prepubescent exercise can have a positive effect on the myocardial C-F ratio. In fact, at death, the exercised animals showed an increase in their C-F ratio of approximately 31% above that of the nonexercised control animals.

The next logical step, it seemed, was to see if these results could be replicated using a different species of animal and a different exercise protocol. Also, in order to investigate the influence of aging, as well as the exercise, an initial sacrifice group was to be included.

Experiment 2

Forty prepubescent male guinea pigs, 3 weeks of age (colored English short haired), were randomly divided into exercise (n = 15)

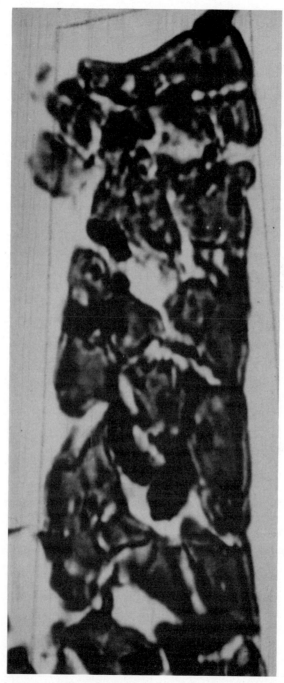

FIG. 1. Cross-section of the endocardium showing myocardial muscle fibers and capillaries.

and control (n = 15) groups. In addition ten animals served as the initial sacrifice group: (1) *exercise group* — animals exercised for five weeks before the onset of puberty; (2) *control group* — animals in a sedentary state throughout the experiment; and (3) *initial sacrifice group* — those killed at the onset of the experiment in order to establish a base value for the C-F ratio.

The exercise group was subjected to daily 30-minute training sessions, six days a week for five weeks. In this experiment the exercise consisted of running on a motor-driven treadmill.

An increasing intensity exercise program was maintained throughout the schedule by increasing the speed of the treadmill (5 m/min every week from an initial speed of 10 m/min to a maximum of 30 m/min). At the beginning of the third week of the training period the treadmill grade was also increased (5% each week to a maximum of 10% during the final week of training).

Feeding and care of the animals was similar to the initial experimeñt.

Sacrifice and perfusing techniques were also similar with the following exceptions: (1) the anesthetic was sodium pentobarbital, (2) the anticoagulant and vasodilator was papaverine and (3) the perfusing pressure was approximately 120 mm Hg.

Myocardial C-F ratios were determined as in the initial experiment.

A two-tailed "t" test was used in both experiments to determine the significance of difference between the mean C-F ratio values of the exercise and control groups (P < .05).

Results

As stated earlier, in the study using rats and swimming as the exercise, it was found that the exercise had a favorable influence on capillary development.

The mean C-F ratio for the exercise group was 0.894, which was significantly greater than the control group mean value of 0.620 (Fig. 2).

In the guinea pig experiment and using treadmill running as the exercise, similar results were also obtained.

The mean C-F ratio of the exercise group (0.941) was significantly greater than that of the control group (0.740). This reflects a 21% increase in capillary development. As might be expected, both groups had significantly greater mean values than the initial sacrifice group mean value of 0.539. (Fig. 3).

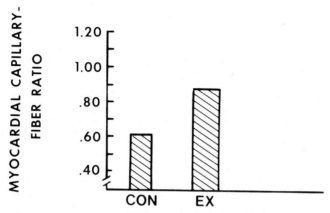

FIG. 2. Mean myocardial C-F ratio for prepubescent white rats.

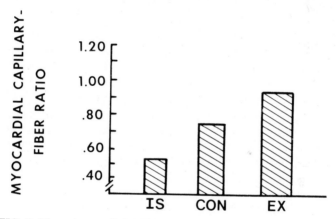

FIG. 3. Mean myocardial C-F ratio for prepubescent guinea pigs.

Discussion

During the developing years of life the internal structure of the heart is in a state of constant change [4] and the myocardial C-F ratio reflects this changing status as it develops from a ratio of approximately 1:6 (six fibers supplied by one capillary) at birth to an approximate 1:1 ratio at adulthood, if the stress of exercise is not an added factor.

The results of the Saskatchewan studies suggest that exercise can further effect this ratio in the hearts of animals, especially when the stress is imposed during the prepubertal stage of life, while the heart is in its developmental stage.

From the studies reported here, the question remains open as to whether these effects persist into adulthood. However, in a rat study previously reported [1], groups of both control and exercise animals were taken through to maturity. Again, the mean C-F ratio of the postpubescent exercise group remained significantly higher than that of the postpubescent control group.

Further experiments are now warranted to investigate the effects of various intensities of prepubertal exercises on adult animal myocardial C-F ratios.

References

1. Bell, R.D. and Rasmussen, R.L.: Exercise and the myocardial capillary-fiber ratio during growth. Growth 38:237-244, 1974.
2. Burt, J.J. and Jackson, R.: The effects of physical exercise on the coronary collateral circulation of dogs. J. Sports Med. Phys. Fitness 5:203-206, 1965.
3. Poupa, O. and Rakusan, K.: The terminal microcirculatory bed in the heart of athletic and non-athletic animals. In Physical Activity in Health and Disease. Baltimore:The Williams and Wilkins Co., 1966, pp. 18-29.
4. Roberts, J.T. and Wearn, J.T.: Quantitative changes in the capillary-muscle relationship in human hearts during growth and hypertrophy. Am. Heart J. 21:217-233, 1941.
5. Rakusan, K. and Poupa, O.: Capillaries and muscle fibers in the heart of old rats. Gerontologia 9:107-112, 1964.
6. Stevenson, J.A.F., Feleki, V., Rchnitzer, R. and Beaton, J.R.: Effect of exercise on coronary tree size in the rat. Circ. Res. 15:265-269, 1964.
7. Tomanek, R.J.: Effects of age and exercise on the extent of the myocardial capillary bed. Anat. Record 167:55-62, 1970.

Etude noninvasive de la fonction myocardique chez les athlètes entraînés

J. Turcot, J. L. Laurenceau, J. G. Dumesnil,
M. C. Malergue et M. Boulay

Introduction

Les effets de l'entraînement sur le coeur de l'athlète ont fait l'objet de nombreuses études depuis quelques années. Les recherches se sont surtout orientées vers les variations de volume cardiaque utilisant pour cela la radiographie [1, 6, 8, 12, 14] et vers la détection de l'hypertrophie myocardique par l'électrocardiographie. Le but de cette recherche est d'étudier la fonction ventriculaire gauche de l'athlète et également la fonction intrinsèque du myocarde par une méthode noninvasive. Nous avons donc utilisé l'échocardiographie, technique basée sur la réflexion des ultrasons permettant d'évaluer les différentes structures cardiaques ainsi que les dimensions des cavités et l'épaisseur des parois cardiaques de façon dynamique.

Méthode

Cette étude porte sur 47 sujets âgés de 20 à 29 ans (moyenne 24 ans) répartis en trois groupes. Le groupe I comprend 30 sujets normaux et sédentaires, ce sont en majeure partie des étudiants gradués de la faculté de médecine de l'université Laval, âgés de 24 ans en moyenne (19 à 29 ans); il ne suivent aucun programme d'entraînement régulier et sont en bonne santé physique. Le groupe II est constitué de 11 athlètes de fond (6 marathoniens et 5 skieurs nordiques). Les coureurs de fond parcourent en moyenne 73 miles par semaine et les skieurs nordiques pratiquent leur sport à raison de 12 heures par semaine. Le groupe III est formé de 6 gymnastes s'entraînant également 12 heures par semaine. La moyenne d'âge des athlètes est de 24 ans (écart 23 à 27 ans); ils font partie d'équipes

J. Turcot, Boursier de la Fondation Canadienne des Maladies du Coeur et J. L. Laurenceau, J. G. Dumesnil, M. C. Malergue et M. Boulay, Institut de Cardiologie de Québec et Université Laval, Québec, Canada.

inter-universitaires de l'Université Laval et sont considérés comme des athlètes de haute compétition. Ils s'entrainent depuis bientôt 5 ans et ce, durant la presque totalité de l'année. Les échocardio-grammes sont faits au repos en décubitus dorsal. Nous utilisons une sonde de 2.25 MHz avec un foyer acoustique de 10 cm relié à un échographe commercial (SKF: Ekoline 20A); l'électrocardiogramme en dérivation D2 est enregistré simultanément. A partir des enregis-trements, les mesures suivantes sont effectuées: diamètres diastol-iques (Dd) ventriculaires gauche et droit, diamètre systolique (Ds) ventriculaire gauche, épaisseur diastolique (E.D.) et épaisseur systol-ique (E.S.) du septum et de la paroi postérieure ainsi que leur temps de contraction (Tc). Les volumes ventriculaires gauches télé-diastoliques (V.T.D.) et télé-systoliques (V.T.S.) ainsi que la fraction d'éjection (E.F.) sont calculés selon la méthode décrite par Feigen-baum [4]: V.T.D. = Dd^3, V.T.S. = Ds^3, E.F. = V.T.D. − V.T.S./V.T.D. La vitesse de raccourcissement d'une fibre circon-férentielle (Vcf) est calculée selon la méthode de Cooper et coll [2]. Les indices d'épaississement du septum et de la paroi postérieure sont calculés selon la méthode de Dumesnil et coll [3]: pourcentage d'épaississement (%E) = E.D. − E.S./ED × 100, vitesse d'épaississe-ment corrigée (V.E.C.) = E.D. − E.S./Tc × 1/Ed. La masse ventricu-laire a été calculée d'après la méthode de Troye et coll [13]. L'analyse statistique de nos résultats a été faite à l'aide des tests de "t" de Student sur système APL 360.

Résultats

Les résultats de l'étude sont réunis dans les tableaux I et II. Plusieurs données sont corrigées pour la surface corporelle étant donné la plus petite taille des athlètes de fond et des gymnastes comparativement aux sujets sédentaires. La fréquence cardiaque est abaissée chez les deux groupes d'athlètes et de façon significative (p < .05) chez les athlètes de fond. La vitesse de raccourcissement d'une fibre circonférentielle (V.C.F.) est également abaissée de façon significative chez les athlètes. Chez les athlètes de fond, les diamètres et les volumes ventriculaires gauches ainsi que le volume d'éjection systolique sont plus élevés comparativement aux sédentaires (Fig. 1). Pour les mêmes données, les gymnastes ont des valeurs comparables aux sédentaires. Les épaisseurs diastoliques des parois ventriculaires ainsi que leurs indices d'épaississement ne diffèrent pas de façon significative chez les trois groupes de sujets. Bien que le %E et la V.E.C. puissent apparaître diminués chez les gymnastes, il n'y a toutefois pas de différence statistique significative. D'une part, il

Tableau I. Etude de la fonction ventriculaire gauche, indices globaux

	Sédentaires N = 30	Athlètes de fond N = 11	Gymnastes N = 6
Age	24.8 ± .8 (o)	24 ± .7	23 ± .6
Surface corporelle (m²)	1.86 ± .02	1.74 ± .03 (*)	1.73 ± .02 (*)
F.C.	72 ± 2.4	55 ± 4.8 (*)	63.8 ± 2.3
V.C.F. (circ/sec)	1.36 ± .05	1.073 ± .05 (**)	1.11 ± .094 (*)
Dd (mm)	48.7 ± .85	54.4 ± 1.06 (*)	48 ± 2.53
Dd (mm)/s.c.	26.25 ± .47	30.4 ± .91 (**)	27.67 ± 1.17
Ds (mm)/s.c.	16.32 ± .41	19.52 ± .92 (**)	18.22 ± .52
D.V.D. (mm)	9.37 ± 2.79	9.45 ± 7.04	8.62 ± .585
F.E. (%)	74.8 ± 1.36	71.1 ± 1.74	70.3 ± 3.23
V.T.D. (ml)/s.c.	63.6 ± 3.07	83.5 ± 7.3 (**)	66.2 ± 9.6
V.T.S. (ml)/s.c.	15.7 ± 1.15	23.6 ± 3.26 (**)	18.7 ± 2.3
V.E. (ml)/s.c.	46.9 ± 2.49	60.1 ± 4.2 (**)	47.3 ± 7.6
M.V. (g)/s.c.	106 ± 4.2	115.3 ± 8.7	108 ± 7.9

N = Nombre de sujets; (o) = Moyenne ± écart type; F.C. = Fréquence cardiaque; S.C. = Surface corporelle (m²); Dd = Diamètre diastolique; Dd/s.c. = Diamètre diastolique corrigé; Ds/s.c. = Diamètre systolique corrigé; D.V.D./s.c. = Diamètre du ventricule droit/corrigé; F.E. (%) = Fraction éjection; V.T.D. = Volume télé-diastolique corrigé (ml); V.T.S. = Volume télé-systolique corrigé (ml); V.E. = Volume d'éjection systolique corrigé (ml); V.C.F. = Vitesse de raccourcissement des fibres circonférentielles; M.V. = Masse ventriculaire gauche corrigée (g); (*) P ≤ .05 comparé aux sédentaires; (**) P ≤ .01 comparé aux sédentaires.

s'agit d'un petit nombre de sujets et d'autre part, toutes les valeurs sont comprises dans l'écart observé chez les sédentaires.

Discussion

Il est bien connu que les athlètes entraînés peuvent présenter des modifications radiologiques et électrocardiographiques suggestives d'hypertrophie cardiaque. Grâce à l'échocardiographie, des études plus détaillées des structures cardiaques ont pu être effectuées chez ces individus. Dans une étude récente, Morganroth et coll [10] ont observé une augmentation du volume ventriculaire avec épaisseur normale des parois chez des athlètes soumis à un exercice isotonique (athlètes de fond) tandis qu'une groupe de lutteurs et de lanceurs de poids (exercice isométrique) ont un volume ventriculaire gauche normal mais une épaisseur de paroi et une masse ventriculaire augmentées. Roeske et coll [11] ont étudié un groupe de joueurs de basketball; certains présentaient une augmentation des dimensions ventriculaires gauches et d'autres une augmentation de l'épaisseur de

Tableau II. Etude de la contractilité par échocardiographie sur le ventricule gauche

Groupes	E.D. (mm)	E.S. (mm)	T.C. (s)	ΔE (mm)	%E	V.E.S. (mm/s)	V.E.C.
Sédentaires							
P. post.	7.33 ± .22 (o)	12.7 ± .24	.34 ± .006	4.96 ± .26	67.6 ± 5.5	14.78 ± .83	2.02 ± .16
Septum	10.5 ± .23	15.1 ± .29	.29 ± .007	4.56 ± .26	43.8 ± 3.13	15.6 ± .93	1.51 ± .10
Athlètes de fond							
P. post.	7.18 ± .26	12.5 ± .36	.38 ± .007 (**)	5.36 ± .33	75.9 ± 6.07	13.94 ± 1.05	1.98 ± .17
Septum	9.81 ± .44	13.8 ± .51 (*)	.32 ± .01 (*)	4 ± .02	43 ± 3.77	12.6 ± .13	1.31 ± .13
Gymnastes							
P. post	8.1 ± .16	12.1 ± .3	.35 ± .01	4 ± .36	49 ± 4.92	11.4 ± 1.29	1.41 ± .17
Septum	9.8 ± .16	13.3 ± .55 (*)	.25 ± .01 (*)	3.5 ± .67	36 ± 7.48	14 ± 3.01	1.44 ± .32

(o) = Moyenne et écart type; P. post = Paroi postérieure; E.D. = Epaisseur diastolique; E.S. = Epaisseur systolique; T.C. = Temps de contraction; ΔE = Gain d'épaisseur; %E = Pourcentage d'épaississement; V.E.S. = Vitesse d'épaississement systolique; V.E.C. = Vitesse d'épaississement corrigée; μE/s = Unités d'épaississement par seconde; (*) P ⩽ .05 comparé aux sédentaires; (**) P ⩽ .01 comparé aux sédentaires.

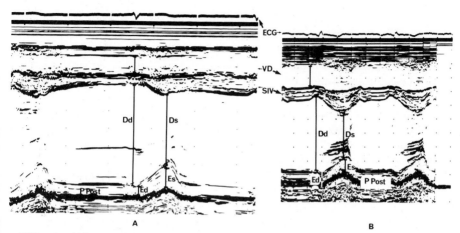

FIG. 1. (A) Echocardiogramme d'un athlète de fond, avec un diamètre télé-diastolique augmenté (5.9 cm). L'épaisseur des parois et les indices d'épaississement sont normaux. (B) Echocardiogramme d'un sujet sédentaire. Diamètre télé-diastolique = 5.2 cm. Echelle de l'échocardiogramme (distance entre deux points): 1 cm verticale, 0.2 sec. horizontale. V.D. = Ventricule droit; S.I.V. = Septum inter-ventriculaire; Dd = Diamètre diastolique; Ds = Diamètre systolique; Ed = Epaisseur diastolique; Es = Epaisseur systolique; P. post. = Paroi postérieure; ECG = Electrocardiogramme.

la paroi. La dimension ventriculaire droite était également augmentée chez certains sujets tandis que la fraction d'éjection (E.F.) et la V.C.F. pouvaient être considérées comme normales.

Notre étude démontre bien que les athlètes soumis à un exercice isotonique peuvent présenter une dilatation ventriculaire gauche et un volume d'éjection systolique augmenté. Ces modifications sont associées à une diminution de la fréquence cardiaque; tel que suggéré par Frick et coll [5], il s'agit vraisemblablement d'un mécanisme d'adaptation normal permettant d'assurer un plus grand débit cardiaque à l'effort maximal. Contrairement à Roeske et coll [11], nous n'avons pas retrouvé de dilatation ventriculaire droite. Les sujets exécutant des exercices isométriques (gymnastes) ont des volumes ventriculaires et une masse ventriculaire à peu près comparables aux sujets sédentaires. La différence entre nos résultats et ceux de Morganroth et coll pourrait suggérer qu'il y a une différence dans le stress imposé (gymnastique vs lutte et lancer du poids) ou que nos athlètes étaient moins entraînés. Etant donné le petit nombre de sujets, d'autres études seront nécessaires afin de déterminer si un entraînement physique intensif peut effectivement entraîner une hypertrophie des parois cardiaques. La diminution de la V.C.F. chez les deux groupes d'athlètes doit être interprétée avec une certaine prudence. Notre expérience personnelle démontre que cet indice peut être fortement influencé par les changements de fréquence cardiaque, une fréquence cardiaque plus basse se traduisant par une V.C.F. diminuée. De plus, les valeurs de V.C.F. chez les sédentaires sont légèrement supérieures à celles retrouvées habituellement dans la littérature ainsi qu'à celles obtenues chez un autre groupe de sujets normaux étudiés dans notre laboratoire [3].

Plusieurs études chez l'animal [9] et certaines chez l'homme [7] ont suggéré que l'hypertrophie cardiaque pouvait s'accompagner d'une diminution de la fonction myocardique intrisèque. Il semblerait que les indices d'épaississement soient plus sensibles aux atteintes de la fonction contractile [3, 7]; ceux-ci furent donc utilisés pour étudier de façon plus précise la fonction myocardique des athlètes. Ces indices sont normaux chez tous les sujets étudiés; ces résultats suggèrent encore davantage que les modifications cardiaques rencontrées chez l'athlète représentent probablement des mécanismes d'adaptation physiologiques n'entraînant pas d'altérations pathologiques. Les mêmes études devront être répétées à long terme afin de savoir si l'entraînement prolongé a les mêmes effets.

En conclusion, cette étude démontre qu'il est désormais possible d'étudier de façon non-invasive tant la physiologie cardiaque que la fonction myocardique intrinsèque de l'athlète; elle permet d'envisager une évaluation plus précise des effets à court et à long terme de l'exercice. Les résultats suggèrent en outre que les modifications cardiaques rencontrées chez l'athlète sont un phénomène physiologique d'adaptation.

Références

1. Arstila, M. and Koirikko, A.: Electrocardiographic and vectocardiographic signs of left and right ventricular hypertrophy in endurance athletes. J. Sports Med. Phys. Fitness 14:166, 1964.
2. Cooper, R., O'Rourke, R.A., Karliner, J.S. et al: Comparison of ultrasound and cineangiographic measurements of the mean rate of circumferential fiber shortening in man. Circulation 46:914, 1972.
3. Dumesnil, J.G., Laurenceau, J.L. and Labatut, A.: L'épaississement myocardique, un critère valable pour apprécier la fonction ventriculaire gauche régionale. Ann. Cardiol. Angeiol. 24(6):491, 1975.
4. Feigenbaum, H.: Echocardiography. Lea and Febiger, 1972.
5. Frick, M.H.: Coronary implications of hemodynamics changes caused by physical training. Am. J. Cardiol. 22:417, 1968.
6. Keys, A. and Friedell, H.L.: Size and stroke of the heart in young men in relation to athletic activity. Science 88:456, 1958.
7. Laurenceau, J.L. and Dumesnil, J.G.: Relation entre épaississement ventriculaire régional et fonction myocardique dans les hypertrophies cardiaques concentriques. Nouv. Presse Méd. 33:4, 1975.

8. Lichtman, J., O'Rourke, R.A., Klein, A. and Karliner, J.S.: Electrocardiogram of the athletes. Arch. Intern. Med. 132:763, 1973.
9. Meerson, F.Z. and Kapelka, V.I.: One contractile function of the myocardium in two types of cardiac adaptation to a chronic load. Cardiology 57:183, 1972.
10. Morganroth, J., Maron, B.J., Henry, W.L. et al: Comparative left ventricular dimensions in trained athletes. Ann. Intern. Med. 82:521, 1975.
11. Roeske, W.R., O'Rourke, R.A., Klein, A. et al: Non-invasive evaluation of ventricular hypertrophy in professional athletes. Circulation 53:286, 1976.
12. Roskamm, H.: Optimum patterns of exercise for healthy adults. Can. Med. Assoc. J. 22:895, 1967.
13. Troy, B.L., Pombo, J. and Rackley, C.E.: Measurement of left ventricular wall thickness and mass by echocardiography. Circulation 45:603, 1972.
14. Van Ganse, W., Versee, L., Eyelenbasch, W. and Vuylstrek, K.: The electrocardiogram of athletes: Comparison with untrained subjects. Br. Heart J. 32, 160: 1970.

Relationship Between Blood Pressure and Workload During a Stress Test on Young Men and Women

J. L. Bonnardeaux and J. Bonneau

Introduction

System analysis theory of the cardiovascular system shows that two components are involved: (1) the controlled system which is composed of a mechanical section and an exchanger section and (2) the controlling system, which comprises neuronal and humoral sections [10] (Fig. 1).

In order to evaluate cardiovascular reserves for training or prevention of disease, the most common measurement is the tissular maximum oxygen consumption in one minute ($\dot{V}O_2$max) calculated by extrapolation of the heart rate at a given workload. Electrocardiographic changes are also used [3]. Anyone concerned with cardiovascular systems can estimate $\dot{V}O_2$max, but the data are mostly related to the exchanger section of the cardiovascular system rather than to the mechanical section. In order to study the cardiovascular response to physical workloads, it is possible to use a factor which reflects the properties of this mechanical section. In the design of a cardiovascular index, we have to take into account the heart rate and blood pressure values and relate these to muscular and heart work. A good index would enable an accurate analysis for the response of the cardiovascular system at a defined workload to be established, in order to analyze the mechanical efficiency and to facilitate the prescription of safety training programs, or the prediction of cardiovascular degeneracy diseases [5, 7, 14].

Methods

Three hundred subjects, 143 males and 157 females, aged 19 to 30, were evaluated. After a stabilizing period of 45 minutes, the

J. L. Bonnardeaux and J. Bonneau, Département de kinanthropologie, Université du Québec à Montréal, Montréal, Québec, Canada.

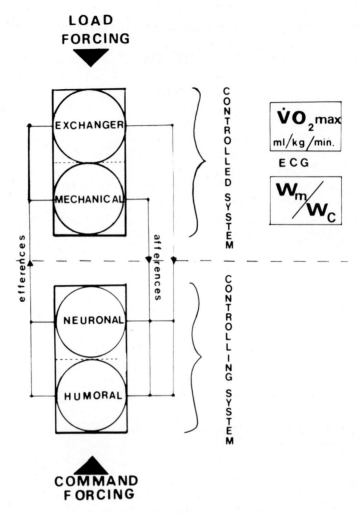

FIGURE 1.

following measurements were taken: body height (cm) and weight (kg), four skinfolds (mm): brachial, subscapular, supra-iliac, ombilical. Lung functions were examined by measuring the forced vital capacity (CV) and the forced expiratory volume in half a second and one second (FEV$_{.5}$; FEV$_1$) with a spirometer "Pulmonar 705." Cardiovascular functions were evaluated at rest, taking blood pressures, heart sound and heart rate with a 12-lead ECG. During physical work a two-state stress test was designed using an ergometric bicycle Monark 805 previously calibrated. In the first stage, the subjects were required to ride three minutes at 360 kgm/min (women) and 540 kgm/min (men) at a constant rhythm of 1 Hz and followed by three minutes of rest. This stage served to warm up the subject and eliminate any psychological factors. A second workload level was then determined in order to obtain 80% of the maximal heart rate in five minutes. This second workload was calculated by taking into account the heart rate response at the previous workload and the age of the subject. The subjects then receive five further minutes of recuperation. Throughout the test the following parameters were taken at one-minute intervals: ECG in CM5, heart rate, systemic arterial pressure. A computer program gave a physiological evaluation report of each subject and all the data were compiled in a file for statistical analysis by the SPSS library programs. The calculations performed for the report were height, weight, percentage of fat and body density. The two last parameters were obtained using the Brozek [2] formula. For the pulmonary functions, the ratio between observed and predicted forced vital capacity, and the $FEV_{.5}/CV$, was carried out using the Miller et al [12] classification. In the cardiovascular functions heart rate, diastolic and systolic pressures were entered and differential and mean pressures were calculated, thence the blood flow, vascular resistances and cardiac work were estimated. Subjects showing anomalous pressure responses in the stress test, i.e., systolic blood pressure of over 120 plus 1/10 kpm [11], were classified as high pressure response. Cardiac work was estimated in two ways: the Hellerstein et al [6] index $W_h = P_s \times F_h/1000$ and our own equation derived from $W_h = P$ mean $\times$ cardiac output, and applied in the form: $W_h = P$ mean $\times 0.0136 \times (F_h \times V P_s \times F_h/2)/1000$. At 80% of the maximal cardiac frequency the percentage of deviation between the two formulae was 5%. The descriptive statistical analysis of alpha-numeric parameters was carried out by the SPSS library program of the UQAM computer and is reported below.

Results

Figure 2 shows a display of six parameters measured in the population and represented in six histograms. The first shows the relative frequency of males and females in the population and the second that of normal and overweight persons. Overweight was distinguished from a normal subject by levels of body fat over 19% for men and 20% for women. The forced vital capacity observed was compared to that predicted. If the ratio between CV observed/CV

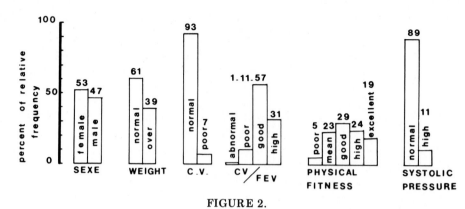

FIGURE 2.

predicted was under 65% the subject was classified as poor. The fourth histogram refers to the Miller et al classification of pulmonary function, and it shows that the population was rather normal. The physical fitness classification of the population was made by comparison of the indirect $\dot{V}O_2$ max measurement computed with the Von Dobëln et al [15] formula with that given in the tables of physical fitness of the American Heart Association (1971) for this purpose. The distribution presented a skewness to the right, brought about by a mean of $\dot{V}O_2$ max higher than the American value, as we have demonstrated elsewhere [1]. Finally, the last two columns identified as systolic pressure show the detection of anomalous pressure responses during physical work, as defined by John Merriman [11]. All systolic pressures measured which were over the prediction were classified as "High" and 11% of the population exhibited this type of response.

In Table I, one can see the mean and standard deviations of cardiovascular values obtained during the examination at rest and during physical work. Comparing the values between males and females, there is no significant difference (t-test). Cardiac output and peripheral vascular resistance were estimated and they are compatible with known data [4, 13].

The relationship between the cardiovascular parameters was established using the correlation coefficient (Pearson). Our results show that workload is well correlated with systolic pressure (r = 0.89) also with the peripheral vascular resistance (r = 0.82); and cardiac work (r = 0.75). Nevertheless there is also an important correlation between systolic pressure and heart rate (r = 0.95).

In the scattergram of these parameters, one can see two patterns of response during physical work. In Figure 3 we have reported the

Table I. Cardiovascular Parameters

	Males (N = 137)		Females (N = 153)	
	At Rest	During Work	At Rest	During Work
Systolic blood pressure mm Hg	125 ± 8.5	188 ± 21	118 ± 9.3	163 ± 17
Diastolic blood pressure mm Hg	73 ± 9.2	81 ± 18	70.5 ± 9.8	75.8 ± 17
Heart rate bts/min	73 ± 16	156 ± 17	76 ± 11	163 ± 15
Predicted cardiac output L/min	4.8 ± 1.2	18.9 ± 4.5	4.6 ± 0.9	18.8 ± 2.7
Predicted peripheral vascular resistance Arbitrary units	2.5 ± 0.8	0.06 ± 0.02	2.5 ± 0.7	0.08 ± 0.03

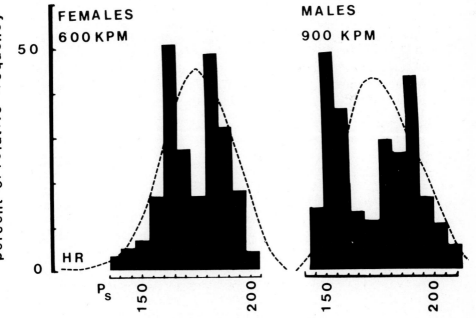

FIGURE 3.

histogram of heart rate (HR) in dotted lines and systolic pressure (P_s) in black columns during a given workload for males and females. It is interesting to see a higher increase in cardiac frequency than in arterial tension and contrarily a higher increase in systolic pressure than in heart rate. We have therefore computed the various factors as follows:

— W_m/W_c, which is the ratio between muscular work and estimated cardiac work;

— A_1, the coefficient of linear regression between the systolic pressure at work as a function of the workloads plus the systolic pressure at rest ($P_{s\,W-} = P_{s,r} + A_1 \times$ kpm)

— A_2 the slope of the linear curve between systolic pressure as a function of heart rate: ($P_s = A_2 \times HR_W + HR_r$)

   — KPM = workload
   — P_s = systolic pressure
   — HR = heart rate
   — (W = work, r = rest)

   Table II shows the results obtained from the statistical computation. The values of the three factors are reported and as there were no significant differences between males and females, we have presented in a third row the mean of paired values. One can see in Table II that numerical values of the various factors are different and that the first factor is more easily handled than the others. The histograms in Figure 4 have been drawn on the assumption that W_m/W_c reflects the type of response in blood pressure or cardiac frequency during work since Wc contains these two parameters. Relative frequency for the physical fitness indices as shown in Figure

Table II. Cardiovascular Factors

	Males (N = 137)	Females (N = 153)	Both (Males Females) (N = 300)
Estimated Cardiac work (kgm/min)	29.2 ± 4.7	26.6 ± 5.5	27.2 ± 4.8
Muscular work (kgm/min)	922 ± 251	606 ± 172	749 ± 270
W_m/W_c	32.4 ± 6.6	22.8 ± 5.7	28.2 ± 5.6
A_1	0.068 ± 0.03	0.074 ± 0.03	0.070 ± 0.03
A_2	0.76 ± 0.02	0.52 ± 0.02	0.59 ± 0.02

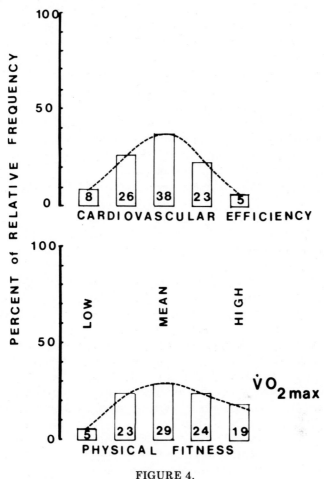

FIGURE 4.

2 and the cardiovascular efficiency indices which are classified poor, 21; low, 21-27; mean, 28-34; good, 35-41; high, 42-   for both sexes are shown in Figure 4. As we can see in the figure the distribution of the cardiovascular efficiency is normal and exhibits some differences compared with the physical fitness curve. These differences are brought about by the systolic pressure parameter which is not included in the $\dot{V}O_2$max computation.

Conclusions

From this research, it appears that when an evaluation of the cardiovascular system is carried out, not only the heart rate but also the behavior of blood pressure throughout the whole system should be observed during an increase of physical work of the body. First, it seems that the patterns of blood pressure response triggered by physical work are not homogeneous. The two patterns described here could result from the action of the controlling system as we stated previously. On the other hand, the efficiency of the cardiovascular system must be related with heart rate and blood pressure. Hence the use of the slope of the curve derived from the relationship between blood pressure and cardiac frequency is probably useful for the analysis of responses triggered by the nervous section and/or the humoral section of the controlling system. Since we do not know more about the type of responses, it is difficult at this time to interpret the values of the slope. The second factor derived from the John Merriman [11] formula allows us to establish the critical values of systolic pressure during physical work. The equation is easy to handle and very useful for the determination of anomalous pressure responses, and also probably in screening for the detection of labile hypertension. Moreover, the coefficient of linear regression derived from the Merriman equation (A_1) for the prediction of labile hypertension could also be useful. In any event the cardiovascular efficiency during work established by the ratio between muscular and cardiac power has many advantages. First, it has a large range of values which reflect the low and high efficiencies. Second, it is accurate and repeatable. Third, in low values one can predict cardiovascular problems, and/or cardiovascular degeneracy, and in high values it is possible to prescribe training programs to develop endurance or resistance of the heart in conjunction with $\dot{V}O_2$ max data. It is also possible to reevaluate the efficiency of training programs since the cardiovascular factor has good accuracy, and it is easy to calculate with the simplest formula. Finally, it is possible to reproduce the same values of the cardiovascular factor within short periods of time and with different types of stress tests [9]. Therefore, it would appear that these results suggest that for general use, the W_m/W_c ratio, called the cardiovascular index, will be at the present time most indicative of the performance of the mechanical section.

References

1. Bonnardeaux, J.L., Bonneau, J. and Johnson, F.: 44 Congres A.C.F.A.S., 1976, p. 10.
2. Brozek, J.: Ann N.Y. Acad. su 110:131-167, 1963.
3. Bruce, A.R. and McDonough, J.R.: N.Y. Acad. Med. Bull. S2, 45:1288-1305, 1969.

4. Ferguson, R.J., Faulkner, J.A., Julius S. and Conway, J.: J. Appl. Physiol. 25:450-454, 1968.
5. Folle, L.E., Gighiero, J., Sadi, I. et al: Cardiology 55:105-113, 1970.
6. Hellerstein, H.K., Hornsten, T.R., Goldbarg, A. et al: Can. Med. Ass. 96:758-765, 1967.
7. Julius, S., Pascual, A.V. and Sannerstedt, R.: Circulation 43:382-390, 1971.
8. Kattus, A.A.: Am. Heart. Assoc. N.Y., 1972, p. 15.
9. Lange Andersen, K., Shephard, R.J., Denolin, H. et al: Fundamentals of Exercise Testing. Geneva:W.H.O., 1971.
10. McAdam, W.E.J.: An Analog Simulation of the Mammalian Cardiovascular System. M.S. Thesis. Northwestern University, 1961.
11. Merriman, J.: Conference Nationale sur la Santé et l'excellence physique. Appendice C, 1972, pp. 151-155.
12. Miller, W.F., Wu, N. and Johnson, R.L.: Anesthesiology 17:480-493, 1956.
13. Rowell, B.L.: Circulation. Med. Sci. Sports 1:15-22, 1969.
14. Sannerstedt, R.: Am. J. Med. Sci. 258:70-79, 1969.
15. Von Döbeln, W., Åstrand, I. and Bergstrom, A.: J. Appl. Physiol. 22:934-938, 1967.

Use of Transitory Electrode Device for Electrocardiography to Measure Heart Rate in Men and Women Immediately Following Judo Pressure Training

P. W. R. Elliott

Introduction

Judo, as a sport involving considerable physical contact, presents problems to anyone trying to determine the maximal heart rates achieved during practice. Radio telemetric techniques are not only expensive, and usually available for only one subject in any session, but they involve wearing a transmitter plus electrodes which constitutes a hazard to both the subject and his opponent. Padding the transmitter sufficiently to prevent a fall on it from causing either damage to the transmitter or injury to the subject converts it to a very bulky object. This can be used to record from a subject during fairly light practice (Fig. 1), but would be quite unacceptable in hard training or in contest.

The next best thing to recording during practice is to record the heart rate as soon as possible after practice. There is minimum time loss (and therefore minimum reduction in heart rate from the level achieved during judo) when the pulse is taken manually with a stop-watch, but it is very difficult to count accurately at such high rates, even more so if there is any irregularity of rhythm. To attach standard ECG electrodes involves a considerable time lag between cessation of activity and beginning of a recording from which heart rate can be measured. In some sports, this delay can be minimized by previously attaching disposable adhesive electrodes to the subject, but in judo, these are seldom still satisfactorily attached at the end of a few minutes of hard training.

When Brooke and Knowles [1] described a simple transitory electrode device for rapid electrocardiography during exercise, this

P. W. R. Elliott, Department of Physiology, Sheffield University, England.

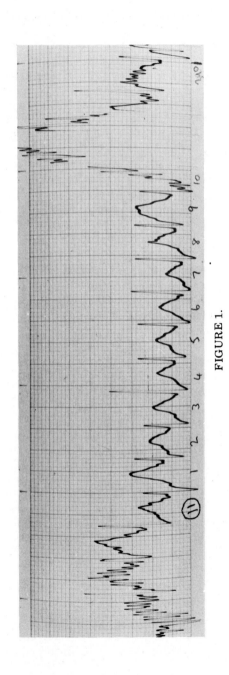

FIGURE 1.

appeared to be the answer to most of these problems, and this paper discusses the results obtained using this device.

Method

The device consists of two standard ECG electrode plates attached to the ends of a piece of pliable tubing (Fig. 2). The recordings were made on a Cambridge VS 4 portable electrocardiograph. Most recordings were made at judo squad training sessions on weekends, when I did not have any skilled assistants; therefore, one of the coaches held the electrodes in place while I operated the recorder.

For men (Fig. 3), one electrode was placed on the sternal angle and attached to the right arm lead, and the other was placed over the apex beat and attached to the left leg lead. The recording was made on lead II (Fig. 4).

For women, the use of leotards made the precordial region rather inaccessible and therefore the electrodes were placed on the wrists and attached to the right arm and left arm leads, respectively. The recording was made on lead I. Each subject was encouraged to adopt

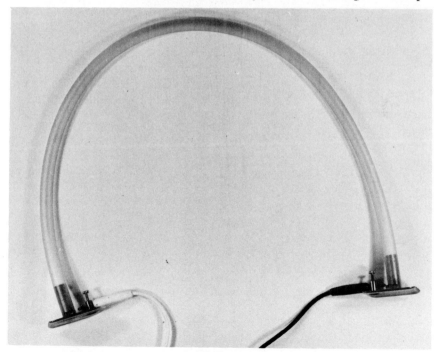

FIGURE 2.

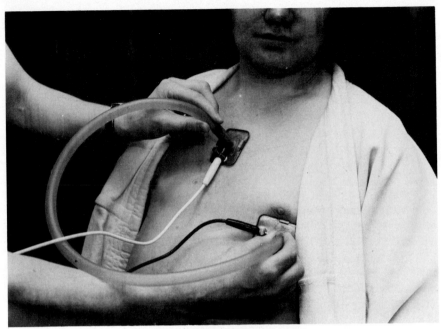

FIGURE 3.

the position she found most comfortable in her exhausted state, and recordings were therefore usually taken from the dorsal aspect of the wrists (Fig. 5). The traces obtained were of lower voltage than those from the precordial region in men, but were quite adequate both for calculation of heart rate and for observing any arrhythmia (Fig. 6). If electrical interference was troublesome, efficient earthing was rapidly achieved by asking the subject to grip the earth lead between the teeth; this was found to be well tolerated by the subject.

Recordings were made after pressure training in judo and in the same individuals after other forms of vigorous activity. In judo pressure training, the subject was fighting continuously for six to ten minutes during which, as soon as his opponent began to tire, he was replaced by a fresh opponent. A high pressure of activity was therefore maintained. The coach in charge of training decided when the subject was nearing exhaustion. As soon as the coach told the subject to come over to the electrocardiograph, the event-marker button was depressed, so that the time elapsing between cessation of judo and the first heart beat recorded could be measured. For safety considerations, the ECG equipment had to be situated well clear of the judo mat area. Despite this, satisfactory recordings were achieved

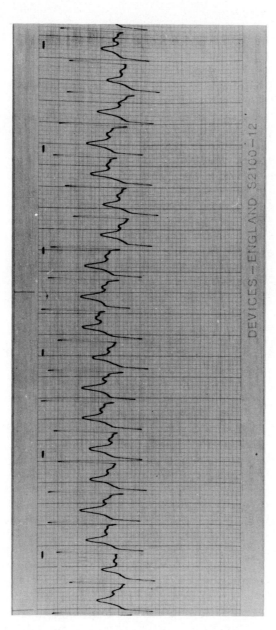

FIGURE 4.

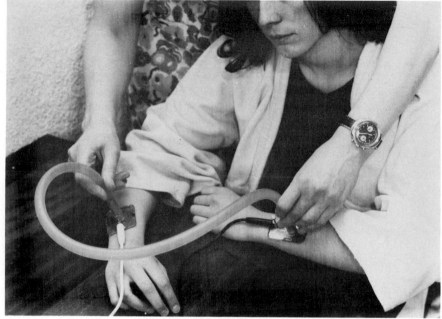

FIGURE 5.

within as little as 4.8 seconds of the subject releasing his last
opponent.

Results

By measuring the time taken for each cardiac cycle, as
represented by the R-R interval on the ECG trace, using callipers and
metal-backed paper, it was found that the length of the cardiac cycle
began to increase within as little as 0.6 second of beginning
recording, and some increase had always occurred within 20 seconds
of cessation of judo.

A typical trace gave the results shown in Table I. Thus the first
recorded increase in cardiac cycle duration occurred 19.7 seconds
after cessation of exercise, and the second recorded increase in
duration occurred 36.0 seconds after cessation of exercise. Since four
or five of the 6.64 seconds which elapsed before the first recorded
beat would have been occupied by the subject running from the judo
mat to the ECG equipment, this means that some decrease in heart
rate will inevitably have occurred before a recording could be
obtained by attaching standard ECG electrodes.

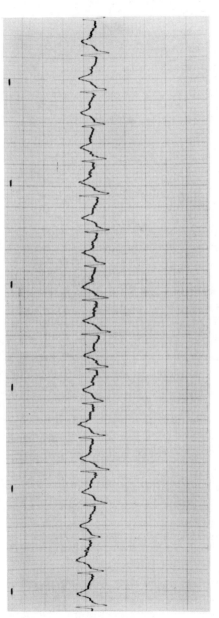

FIGURE 6.

Table I. Beat-by-Beat Measurement of Cardiac Cycle Duration
in Male Subject (AG)

Time After Cessation of Exercise (sec)	Number of Measured Cardiac Cycle	Duration of Each Cardiac Cycle	Equivalent Heart Rate
6.64	1-43 inclusive	304 msec	197/min
19.70	44-94 inclusive	320 msec	188/min
36.00	95-132 inclusive	336 msec	179/min

Traces were obtained from several members of an area squad of men attending monthly training sessions and from several members of the British Judo Association National Young Women's Squad attending a full week's training course. On these traces, measurements were made of the first measurable cardiac cycle recorded (together with the time at which it was obtained after cessation of judo pressure training), plus the cardiac cycle duration at 10 seconds, 20 seconds and 30 seconds after cessation of exercise. Some of the results obtained are shown in Table II (men) and Table III (women), the cardiac cycle duration being expressed in milliseconds and also converted to the equivalent heart rate in each case.

The reason for the longer time lag in the case of the women's squad was simply due to the layout of the training area. The ECG equipment was on a stage overlooking the judo mat, and the subjects therefore had a greater distance to travel than in the case of the men's squad. For this reason, the first cardiac cycle recorded was

Table II. Cardiac Cycle Duration Following
Judo Pressure Training in Male Subjects

	Time Lag Before 1st C.C. Measured	First C.C.	C.C. at 10 sec	C.C. at 20 sec	C.C. at 30 sec
RR	5.60 sec	288 msec 208/min	288 msec 208/min	296 msec 203/min	296 msec 203/min
DW	4.80 sec	320 msec 188/min	328 msec 183/min	352 msec 170/min	376 msec 160/min
TC	4.80 sec	304 msec 197/min	328 msec 183/min	344 msec 174/min	360 msec 167/min

Table III. Cardiac Cycle Duration Following
Judo Pressure Training in Female Subjects

	Time Lag Before 1st C.C. Measured	First C.C.	C.C. at 10 sec	C.C. at 20 sec	C.C. at 30 sec
JW	11.36 sec	312 msec 192/min	–	328 msec 183/min	336 msec 179/min
CA	9.40 sec	280 msec 214/min	288 msec 208/min	296 msec 203/min	312 msec 192/min
JS	12.00 sec	280 msec 214/min	–	296 msec 203/min	328 msec 183/min
NC	13.20 sec	304 msec 197/min	–	320 msec 188/min	336 msec 179/min
CB	14.72 sec	288 msec 208/min	–	304 msec 197/min	320 msec 188/min
VT	8.12 sec	272 msec 221/min	296 msec 203/min	296 msec 203/min	312 msec 192/min
EW	13.28 sec	312 msec 192/min	–	320 msec 188/min	334 msec 174/min
JM	16.00 sec	304 msec 197/min	–	320 msec 188/min	336 msec 179/min

sometimes more than 10 seconds after the subject had relinquished hold of her opponent, but was always less than 20 seconds after.

Having established that a recording could always be obtained within 20 seconds, I then began to compare the heart rate achieved by judo pressure training with the heart rate achieved in the same individuals by some other form of vigorous activity, such as shuttle running or circuit training. The cardiac cycles were measured in the same way, and a comparison made of the rates at 20 seconds after cessation of the two different activities. Table IV shows the results from four of the women's squad recorded after circuit training in one session and after judo pressure training in another session.

Results so far seem to concur with what many judo coaches believe — that none of the noncompetitive forms of training (such as shuttle running and circuit training) are as effective as judo itself in increasing cardiac activity. This device is therefore seen to provide a satisfactory means of recording the heart rate as soon as possible after judo. I hope in the future to obtain recordings in the actual contest situation at championships, when mental as well as physical stress plays a large part.

Table IV. Comparison of Effects on Heart Rate of Circuit Training
With Effects of Judo Pressure Training in Female Subjects

	C.C. Duration and Heart Rate 20 sec After Judo	C.C. Duration and Heart Rate 20 sec After Circuit
JW	328 msec 183/min	352 msec 170/min
CA	296 msec 203/min	304 msec 197/min
CB	304 msec 197/min	336 msec 179/min
JS	296 msec 203/min	352 msec 170/min

Conclusion

It has been found possible, using the transitory electrode device described by Brooke and Knowles, to obtain accurate measurement of cardiac cycle duration, and hence heart rate, within a few seconds of judo pressure training, to make these recordings without skilled assistance on a large number of subjects within a short period of time and to compare the heart rates so achieved with those achieved by other forms of strenuous activity in the same individuals.

Acknowledgments

I thank the members and coaches of the British Judo Association National Young Women's Squad and of the B.J.A. Yorkshire and Humberside Men's Squad for their cooperation, and Mrs. L. Griffiths and Mr. P. Ayton for their assistance in preparation of slides.

Reference

1. Brooke, J.D. and Knowles, J.E.: A simple transitory electrode device for rapid electrocardiography during exercise. Br. J. Sports Med. 6:13-14, 1971.

Blood Flow in the Extremities
of Athletes

It is well known that certain characteristics of all organs of the body develop in the course of systematic sport training, especially those of the cardiovascular system. Besides the well-known changes of structure and functions of the heart of athletes some modifications of the blood vessel functions are developed too. The main function of the vessels is the distribution of blood in the organism.

With respect to the peculiarities of this function in well-trained athletes the investigations in our laboratory show the following. In a group of men, consisting of 550 persons both athletes and nontrained men of the same age, we registered the blood flow in the forearm and calf at rest, during exercise in the resting extremities and also after exercise.

We found that the adaptative changes of the functions of peripheral circulation are dependent upon the mode of training. As a result of endurance training the blood flow in extremities at rest decreases. The trained arm of tennis players had a statistically significant smaller blood flow than the opposite arm. In both arms of tennis players the blood flow was smaller than in the arms of nontrained men.

In basketball players the blood flow at rest was decreased in comparison with that of nontrained men not only in the forearm but also in the calf.

On the other hand, intensive training of strength (weightlifting) leads to a certain increase in the blood flow in the extremities. For instance, a group of students revealed blood flow in the calf at rest of 2.8 ml/100 ml tissue/min. Six months of regular training in weightlifting increased the resting blood flow to 4.8 ml, but three weeks after the interruption of the training it returned to the former level.

During exercise there appears a pronounced vasoconstriction in the resting extremities with a following postexercise hyperemia

P. Ozolin, Latvian Research Institute of Experimental and Clinical Medicine, Riga, U.S.S.R.

341

which in some conditions, that is, in nontrained men after moderate exercise (800 kpm/min for five min) is even larger than that in working limbs.

The reduction of blood flow in resting limbs during exercise is more pronounced in nontrained men (blood flow reduced by 33%) than in well-trained athletes (by 17%).

Hyperemia in extremities after moderate exercise (75 to 150 w) has an approximately similar volume in athletes and nontrained men. After maximal exercise the volume of hyperemia is considerably larger in nontrained men. This indicates that the peripheral circulation at exercise is more affected in nontrained men than in athletes.

We registered separately the blood flow in muscles and in skin. In one forearm the skin blood flow was arrested by iontophoresis of adrenalin. It was observed that the reduction of blood flow of the resting arm developed in a parallel manner in muscles and skin. From this it may be concluded that the characteristic qualities of peripheral blood flow depend upon the vasomotor reflex mechanism.

A decrease of supply of blood causes the activation of the tissue receptors. The increase of afferent impulses impeded the working capacity of muscles in a reflexive way. In experiments on cats it was found that the deafferentiation of the extremities by means of cutting of the hind roots of the spinal cord causes an increase of the working capacity of the calf muscles of 20.5%. The same effect is obtained from the exclusion of receptors of the bone marrow by means of extirpation of marrow from tibia. The occlusion of arteries of one arm of man causes a definite decrease of the working capacity of the opposite arm. Thus, the reduction of the blood flow in the resting extremities has a negative effect on the working capacity of men.

From the foregoing it may be concluded that along with the increase of the vagus effect on the heart of athletes the activity of sympathetic vasoconstrictive fibers at rest increases as well. During exercise the vasoconstrictor mechanisms in the athletes activates in a smaller degree than in nontrained men, which leads to a better blood supply not only of the active muscles but also of the other organs. This is one of the main conditions accounting for the enhanced working capacity of athletes.

Anatomical Shunt and the Alveolar to Arterial Oxygen Difference at Rest and During Exercise

N. Gledhill, A. B. Froese and J. Dempsey

It is well known that normal subjects at rest have an alveolar to arterial oxygen difference of 7 to 10 mm Hg [2, 7]. During exercise, due to the disproportionate increase in ventilation relative to cardiac output, an increase is commonly observed in alveolar PO_2. At the same time, the arterial PO_2 remains constant or perhaps increases slightly. With increasing intensity of exercise, the alveolar to arterial oxygen difference (A-a DO_2) increases progressively, reaching 25 to 30 mm Hg in heavy exercise [1, 13, 22]. Some investigators have reported an initial drop prior to the subsequent rise, but these studies differed in methodology from the current investigation [12, 24].

Widening of the A-a DO_2 could result from the combined effects of anatomical venous-to-arterial shunt, nonuniformity in the matching of ventilation to perfusion (i.e., an uneven distribution of $\dot{V}_A/\dot{Q}$ ratios) and diffusion impairment [8, 14, 18]. Previous investigators have calculated that for normal subjects, both at rest and during exercise, there is no limitation in diffusion [1, 19, 20]. Therefore, the increased A-a DO_2 during exercise must result from an increased nonuniformity in the distribution of $\dot{V}_A/\dot{Q}$ ratios or an increase in the volume and/or desaturation of anatomically shunted blood.

Recently, a new technique has been developed by Wagner et al which permits a detailed evaluation of these options [21]. By infusing intravenously a solution of inert gases with varying solubilities, sampling arterial blood and expired gas, and measuring cardiac output and minute ventilation, it is possible to derive the distribution of $\dot{V}_A/\dot{Q}$ ratios in the lung. This technique yields no information concerning topographical location, but determines the amount of blood and gas equilibrating at given $\dot{V}_A/\dot{Q}$ ratios. It is

N. Gledhill, York University, Toronto; A. B. Froese, Hospital for Sick Children, Toronto, Canada; and J. Dempsey, University of Wisconsin, U.S.A.
Supported by NRC Grant MA-5363 and York University, Faculty of Arts.

possible from this information to evaluate gas exchange throughout the lung.

We employed the inert gas technique to determine the distribution of $\dot{V}_A/\dot{Q}$ ratios of five healthy male subjects, age 23-31, at rest and during graded exercise on a bicycle ergometer. With increasing intensity of exercise, gas was exchanged at progressively higher ratios of ventilation to perfusion and, contrary to the increasing topographical uniformity in the matching of ventilation to perfusion reported in radioactive tracer studies [5, 6], we observed an increasing nonuniformity in the distribution of $\dot{V}_A/\dot{Q}$ ratios [11]. The recovered distributions, together with concurrently measured traditional indices of gas exchange, were then used to calculate anatomical shunt and to partition the A-a DO_2.

The distributions recovered in the current study were based on 50 discrete gas exchange compartments, but in order to simplify the explanation, the present discussion will deal with a theoretical four-compartment model as seen in Table I. The amount of alveolar ventilation ($\dot{V}_A$) and blood flow ($\dot{Q}$) going to each of the four gas exchange units is shown together with the associated $\dot{V}_A/\dot{Q}$ ratio. Summation of the compartmental $\dot{V}_A$ and $\dot{Q}$ values yields the total alveolar ventilation (5.0 liters/min) and perfusion (5.2 liters/min), hence the overall $\dot{V}_A/\dot{Q}$ ratio of .96. The majority of blood and gas in this theoretical lung is matched at a $\dot{V}_A/\dot{Q}$ ratio of 1.0, and there is an intrapulmonary (i.e. nonanatomical) shunt fraction of .1 liters/min ($\dot{V}_A/\dot{Q} = 0.0$). In addition the amount of dead space ventilation is also determined from the inert gas data.

In the investigations conducted at rest and during exercise, the composition of inspired gas was known, and the composition of mixed venous blood was calculated from the measured $\dot{V}O_2$ and $\dot{V}CO_2$. Therefore, using the equation below, it was possible to calculate compartmental gas exchange for the recovered distribu-

Table I. Alveolar Ventilation and Perfusion
Going to Gas Exchange Compartments of a
Given $\dot{V}_A/\dot{Q}$ in a Theoretical Lung

$\dot{V}_A$ l/min	$\dot{Q}$ l/min	$\dot{V}_A/\dot{Q}$
0.0	0.1	0.0
0.5	1.0	0.5
4.0	4.0	1.0
0.5	0.1	5.0
5.0	5.2	0.96

tions. Corresponding values calculated for the theoretical four-compartment lung appear in Table II.

$$\frac{\dot{V}_A}{\dot{Q}} = K \frac{C_{\acute{c}}O_2 - C_{\bar{v}}O_2}{P_IO_2 - P_AO_2}$$ (a similar relationship exists for CO_2)

Blood which perfuses unventilated alveoli ($\dot{V}_A/\dot{Q} = 0.0$) is not involved in gas exchange while traversing the lung; therefore, the end-capillary partial pressures are unchanged from mixed venous levels. In the theoretical lung seen in Table II, the majority of gas and blood is ⸤quilibrated at an alveolar and end-capillary PO_2 of 105 mm Hg and PCO_2 of 40 mm Hg. It is evident that the high $\dot{V}_A/\dot{Q}$ ratio depicted here has its most marked effect on CO_2 removal.

The amount of blood and gas going to each compartment in the resting and exercise distributions was known (as illustrated for the theoretical lung in Table I). Also, the compartmental gas tensions at which equilibrium was attained was known. Therefore, the weighted contributions from all compartments were summed to give overall gas exchange values for the lung. This computation is illustrated schematically for the four-compartment lung in Figure 1.

Mixed alveolar air is a summation of the ventilation weighted partial pressures, and mixed end-capillary blood is a summation of the perfusion weighted partial pressures. Even though equilibrium is achieved in all compartments, an alveolar to end-capillary O_2 difference develops. This is due to the fact that compartments with high $\dot{V}_A/\dot{Q}$ ratios, by virtue of this high ratio of alveolar ventilation to blood flow, affect gas tensions more than blood. That is, arterial blood is weighted more by the lower O_2 tensions, and alveolar gas is weighted by the higher O_2 tensions. Thus, nonuniformity of $\dot{V}_A/\dot{Q}$ ratios in the lung results in an alveolar to mixed end-capillary O_2 difference and the increasing nonuniformity in the distribution of

Table II. Compartmental Gas Exchange Values Corresponding to Each $\dot{V}_A/\dot{Q}$ Ratio in a Theoretical Four-Compartment Lung

$\dot{V}_A/\dot{Q}$	$P_{\acute{c}}O_2, P_AO_2$ mm Hg	$P_{\acute{c}}CO_2, P_ACO_2$ mm Hg
0.0	40	45
0.5	70	43
1.0	105	40
5.0	130	25

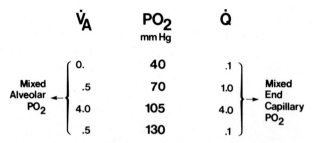

FIG. 1. Calculation of overall gas exchange for the lung from compartmental values. Arterial blood is weighted by the lower $\dot{V}_A/\dot{Q}$ compartments with lower O_2 tensions and alveolar air is weighted by the higher $\dot{V}_A/\dot{Q}$ compartments with higher O_2 tensions.

$\dot{V}_A/\dot{Q}$ ratios observed during exercise must therefore account for at least a portion of the increased A-a DO_2.

However, it is important to note that although the inert gas technique is a very sensitive procedure for detecting intrapulmonary shunt, it does not detect true anatomical shunt from bronchial and thebesian admixture. Therefore, gas tensions calculated for the distributions recovered via this technique are actually mixed end-capillary values prior to the admixture of anatomical shunt. In the current study, no intrapulmonary shunt was detected either at rest or during exercise. The measured arterial and calculated end-capillary oxygen tensions for the recovered distributions appear in Table III together with the alveolar to mixed end-capillary (A-ċ) and alveolar oxygen differences.

It can be assumed that both at rest and during exercise there is no impairment of diffusion [1, 19, 20]. The difference between the mixed end-capillary O_2 tension ($P_{\dot{c}}O_2$) and the measured arterial O_2 tension (P_aO_2) seen in Table III is due to anatomically shunted blood. Therefore, of the A-a DO_2 at rest ($\sim$ 10 mm Hg), approximately 4 mm Hg is due to anatomically shunted blood, and of the A-a DO_2 during exercise ($\sim$ 17 mm Hg), approximately 8 mm Hg is

Table III. Calculated Mixed End-Capillary and Measured
Arterial Oxygen Tensions for the Distributions Recovered
at Rest and During Exercise

	n	$P_{\dot{c}}O_2$ mm Hg	P_aO_2 mm Hg	A-ċ DO_2 mm Hg	A-a DO_2 mm Hg
Rest	5	93.0	88.7	6.7	10.4
Exercise	4	98.9	91.4	9.3	17.1

due to anatomically shunted blood. The remaining portion of the A-a O$_2$ difference in both cases must be due to nonuniformity in the distribution of $\dot{V}_A/\dot{Q}$ ratios. This latter effect was also confirmed by the recovered A-ć DO$_2$ (Table III) which resulted from the nonuniformity.

Since the difference between the measured P$_a$O$_2$ and predicted P$_ć$O$_2$ is a result of anatomically shunted blood, it is possible to use this information to calculate the anatomical shunt fraction from the formula:

$$\frac{\dot{Q}_S}{\dot{Q}_T} = \frac{C_aO_2 - C_ćO_2}{C_{\bar{v}}O_2 - C_ćO_2} \qquad [23].$$

Such calculations show that both at rest and during exercise, an anatomical shunt of less than 1% of the cardiac output can account for the entire difference between the predicted P$_ć$O$_2$ and the measured P$_a$O$_2$. This estimate is quite compatible with values reported by several authors, who have calculated flow through the thebesian veins to be between 0.25% and 0.4% of the total cardiac output [4, 15-17] and bronchial venous flow to be less than 1% of the cardiac output [3, 9, 10].

In order to schematically illustrate the partitioning of the A-a DO$_2$, a simplified representation of the lung and the factors which contribute to the A-a DO$_2$ is shown in Figure 2.

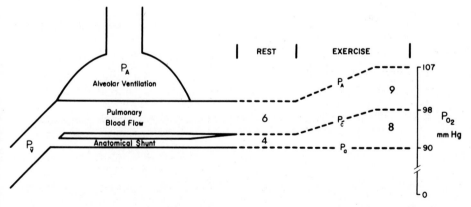

FIG. 2. Schematic representation of the partitioning of the A-a DO$_2$ at rest and during exercise. Anatomical shunt accounts for 4 mm Hg of the A-a DO$_2$ at rest and 8 mm Hg of the difference during exercise. Nonuniformity of $\dot{V}_A/\dot{Q}$ ratios accounts for 6 mm Hg of the A-a DO$_2$ at rest and 9 mm Hg of the difference during exercise.

The alveolar partial pressure at equilibration is determined by the F_IO_2, the mixed venous gas tension, and the ratio of ventilation to perfusion. As pointed out in the analysis of the theoretical lung, a variation of $\dot{V}_A/\dot{Q}$ ratios will create a gradient between the alveolar and mixed end-capillary O_2 tensions. When the partially desaturated anatomical shunt component is added, there is a further reduction in the calculated mixed end-capillary PO_2 to the measured arterial value.

During exercise, since gas is exchanged at higher $\dot{V}_A/\dot{Q}$ ratios, the alveolar oxygen tension increases, and the mixed end-capillary oxygen tension also increases, but because of the increased dispersion during exercise, it does not increase by an equal amount, so that the alveolar to mixed end-capillary oxygen difference widens. Also, due to the increased desaturation of mixed venous blood during exercise, anatomically shunted blood produces a much greater difference in the end-capillary to arterial O_2 tensions, so that the alveolar to arterial O_2 difference increases substantially from rest to exercise.

Thus, of the measured A-a O_2 difference at rest, approximately 4 mm Hg was due to anatomically shunted blood, and the remaining 6 mm Hg was due to nonuniformity of $\dot{V}_A/\dot{Q}$ ratios throughout the lung. Of the measured A-a O_2 difference during exercise, approximately 8 mm Hg was due to anatomically shunted blood, with the remaining 9 mm Hg being due to nonuniformity of $\dot{V}_A/\dot{Q}$ ratios.

References

1. Asmussen, E. and Nielson, M.: Alveolo-arterial gas exchange at rest and during work at different O_2 tensions. Acta Physiol. Scand. 50:153-166, 1960.
2. Asmussen, E. and Nielson, M.: Studies on the regulation of respiration in heavy work. Acta Physiol. Scand. 12:171-188, 1946.
3. Aviado, D.M., de Burgh Daly, M., Lee, C.Y. and Schmidt, C.F.: The contribution of the bronchial circulation to the venous admixture in pulmonary venous blood. J. Physiol. 155:606-622, 1961.
4. Bachofen, H., Hobi, H.J. and Scherrer, M.: Alveolar arterial N_2 gradients at rest and during exercise in healthy men of different ages. J. Appl. Physiol. 34:137-142, 1973.
5. Bake, B., Bjure, J. and Widimsky, J.: The effect of sitting and graded exercise on the distribution of pulmonary blood flow in healthy subjects studied with the ^{133}Xenon Technique. Scand. J. Clin. Lab. Invest. 22:99-106, 1968.
6. Bryan, A.C., Bentivoglio, L.G., Beerel, F. et al: Factors affecting regional distribution of ventilation and perfusion in the lung. J. Appl. Physiol. 19:395-402, 1964.
7. Dempsey, J.A., Reddan, W.G., Birnbaum, M.L. et al: Effects of acute through life-long hypoxic exposure on exercise pulmonary gas exchange. Resp. Physiol. 13:62-89, 1971.

8. Farhi, L.E. and Rahn, H.: A theoretical analysis of the alveolar-arterial O_2 difference with special reference to the distribution effect. J. Appl. Physiol. 7:699-703, 1955.

9. Fritts, H.W., Hardewig, A., Rochester, D.E. et al: Estimation of pulmonary arteriovenous shunt-flow using intravenous injections of T-1824 dye and KR^{85}. Circulation 23:390-398, 1961.

10. Fritts, H.W., Harris, P., Chidsey, C.A. et al: Estimation of flow through bronchial-pulmonary vascular anastomoses with use of T-1824 dye. J. Clin. Invest. 39:1841-1850, 1960.

11. Gledhill, N., Froese, A.B., Harwood, R.A.R. and Dempsey, J.A.: Distributions of ventilation-perfusion ratios in man during hypoxia and exercise. Fed. Proc. 35:478, 1976.

12. Hesser, C.M. and Matell, G.: Effect of light and moderate exercise on alveolar-arterial O_2 tension differences in man. Acta Physiol. Scand. 63:247-256, 1965.

13. Jones, N.L., McHardy, G.J.R., Naimark, A. and Campbell, E.J.M.: Physiological dead space and alveolar-arterial gas pressure differences during exercise. Clin. Sci. 31:19-29, 1966.

14. Kreuzer, F., Tenny, S.M., Mithoefer, J.C. and Remmers, J.E.: Alveolar-arterial oxygen gradient in the dog at altitude. J. Appl. Physiol. 15:796-800, 1960.

15. Lenfant, C.: Management of factors impairing gas exchange in man with hyperbaric pressure. J. Appl. Physiol. 19 (2):189-194, 1964.

16. Mellemgaard, K., Lassen, N.A. and Georg, J.: Right-to-left shunt in normal man determined by the use of tritium and krypton 85. J. Appl. Physiol. 17:778-782, 1962.

17. Ravin, M.B., Epstein, R.M. and Malm, J.R.: Contribution of thebesian veins to the physiologic shunt in anaesthetized man. J. Appl. Physiol. 20 (6):1148-1152, 1965.

18. Riley, R.L., Cournand, A. and Donald, K.W.: Analysis of factors affecting partial pressures of oxygen and carbon dioxide in gas and blood of lungs: Methods. J. Appl. Physiol. 4:102-120, 1951.

19. Staub, N.C.: Alveolar-arterial oxygen tension gradient due to diffusion. J. Appl. Physiol. 18:673-680, 1963.

20. Turino, G.M., Bergofsky, E.H., Goldring, R.M. and Fishman, A.P.: Effect of exercise on pulmonary diffusing capacity. J. Appl. Physiol. 18:447-456, 1963.

21. Wagner, P.D., Saltzman, H.A. and West, J.B.: Measurement of continuous distributions of ventilation-perfusion ratios: Theory. J. Appl. Physiol. 36 (5):588-599, 1974.

22. Wasserman, K., Van Kessel, A.L. and Burton, G.G.: Interaction of physiological mechanisms during exercise. J. Appl. Physiol. 22:71-85, 1967.

23. West, J.B.: Diffusing capacity of the lung for carbon monoxide at high altitude. J. Appl. Physiol. 17:421-426, 1962.

24. Whipp, B.J. and Wasserman, K.: Alveolar-arterial gas tension differences during graded exercise. J. Appl. Physiol. 27:361-365, 1969.

Effects of Pre and Post O_2-Breathing on Performance Times and Ventilatory Response to Repeated 100-Yard Freestyle Swims

Brian A. Wilson, Ray T. Hermiston,
R. K. Stallman and Harold Burton

Introduction

Although there are several studies indicating that O_2-breathing does not improve performance [11, 14] the bulk of the recent literature indicates that O_2-breathing during a two to eight minute exhaustive work bout prolongs the performance time to exhaustion [3, 7, 17]. It is important to note here that hyperbaric studies due to their effects on gas density must be considered separate from O_2-breathing studies at 1 ATA [6]. Miller [14] has shown that prebreathing of oxygen had no effect on treadmill performance or recovery parameters. This study also demonstrated that O_2-breathing in recovery did not hasten the recovery process.

The direction of O_2-breathing studies to date has been to examine the effects of oxygen on endurance time to exhaustion. The possibility that prebreathing of oxygen may increase the maximal work rate of subjects has been given little attention. Karpovich [12] attempted this type of analysis in short sprint swims and found significant improvement in performance times; however, several important control factors regarding administration of oxygen were lacking in this study [15, 17].

The purpose of the present study was to examine the effects of both pre and recovery O_2-breathing on performance times for repeated 100-yard freestyle swims. The design was double-blind with no subjects aware of the mixtures being inspired.

Brian A. Wilson and R. K. Stallman, Department of Human Kinetics, College of Biological Science, University of Guelph, Guelph, Ontario, Canada and Ray T. Hermiston and Harold Burton, Faculty of Human Kinetics, University of Windsor, Windsor, Ontario, Canada.

Supported in part by University of Guelph Research Advisory Board Grant #80818.

352 B. A. WILSON ET AL

Methods

Thirteen competitive swimmers, five from an age group program (ages 12 to 14) and eight from a university team (ages 18 to 22), volunteered as subjects for the study. The group was composed of nine girls and four boys. The subjects all performed three maximal effort 100-yard freestyle swims separated by five-minute recovery periods on four separate occasions. During two of these trials the subjects inspired 100% O_2 for 15 minutes before the first swim and during the five-minute recovery periods after each swim. For the other two trials the subjects inspired 21% O_2 during the identical time periods. The sequence of gas mixtures was randomized.

The inspired mixtures were delivered to the subjects from concealed compressed gas tanks into a Tissot spirometer, via larger bore tubing (34 mm I.D.) through a low resistance triple-J valve to the subjects. The expired air passed via large bore tubing through a dry test gas meter (Parkinson-Cowan CD-4) fitted with a rotary potentiometer and recorded on a 12-inch strip recorder. The system provided an unlimited supply of humid room air temperature gas for inspiration and continuous monitoring of expired volumes during the nonswimming phases.

Subjects started their swims in less than ten seconds after removing the mouthpiece and took no breaths after finishing each swim until fitted with a mouthpiece for recovery breathing. With the mouthpiece held at water level there was no breathhold required at the end of each swim. Times for the 50 split and 100-yard distance were recorded with electronic timing devices. The subjects were not made aware of their times until the complete series was over. During each swim both breathing and stroke frequency were recorded for each lap.

Test retest data were analyzed with paired t-tests and Pearson correlation coefficients were calculated. A treatments-by-treatments by subjects three way ANOVA was used to examine for possible differences in the parameters between gas mixtures [13].

Results

There were no significant effects ($p > .10$) of O_2-breathing on the performance times for the 100-yard swims or the 50-yard split times. Figure 1 shows the clustering of the air vs. O_2-breathing times about the line of identity. The performance times were further analyzed by rank order analysis and again no significant effects of the breathing mixtures were identified. Stroke frequencies during

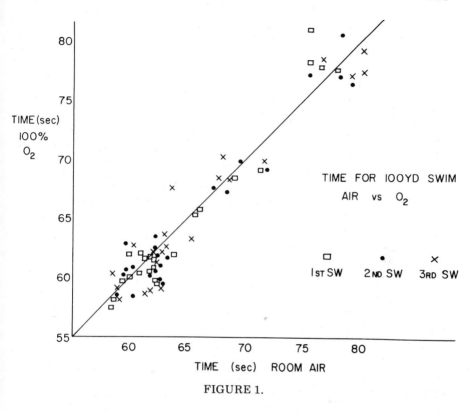

FIGURE 1.

O_2-breathing trials were also not significantly different from the air inspiration trials.

There was a significant decrease in breathing frequencies (p < .05) for the second and third hundreds during O_2-breathing trials. Ventilation was significantly elevated during the prebreathing phase on oxygen but significantly (p < .05) decreased during recovery both after one minute (Fig. 2) and during the total five-minute recovery period (Fig. 3).

The swimmers' subjective feelings regarding the ease and speed of their swims were examined and showed no correlation with the inspired mixture changes.

Discussion

Our data support that of Miller [14] in that there were no significant effects of pre or recovery O_2-breathing on performance times. It has been suggested that the improvement in performance recorded when subjects breathe oxygen during a work bout is related

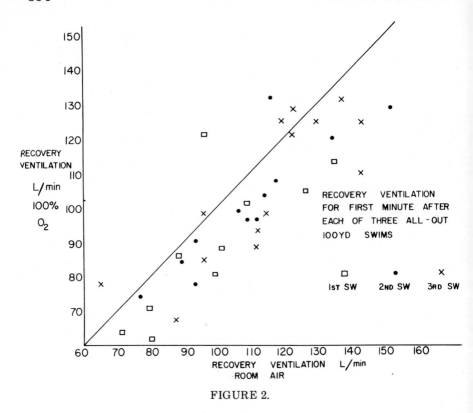

FIGURE 2.

to the effects of oxygen on ventilation during work [17]. If swimmers are aware of the mixtures being inspired, then the increased breath hold time and therefore variations in movement pattern during O_2-breathing may affect performance [12]. Since our subjects inspired room air during all work phases, it is probable that their ventilatory values were similar on air and oxygen trials. Although breathing frequency was significantly reduced during swims two and three on O_2-breathing trials, without tidal volume measurements we are unable to establish the actual inspired volumes during the swims.

Oxygen breathing at rest has been shown to increase ventilation [8, 10]. During light work ventilatory effects of oxygen are minimized, while in heavy work ventilation is significantly reduced by oxygen [1-4, 9, 15-17]. Our data support the resting values reported [8, 10] and extend these findings to show that recovery ventilations after maximal short-term swimming work bouts are decreased for up to five minutes during recovery O_2-breathing. This

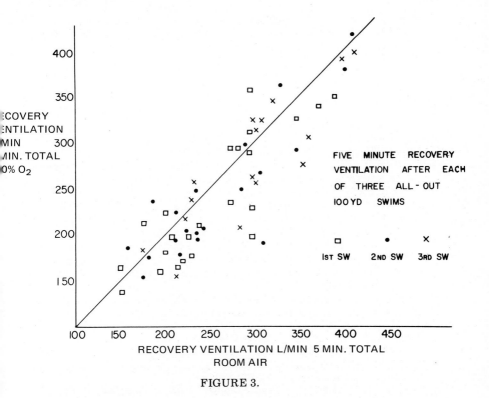

FIGURE 3.

apparent hastening of ventilatory recovery, however, has no measurable effects on the performance times of subsequent swims.

If the decrease in ventilation and subsequent acid-base shifts are the mechanisms by which hyperoxic breathing during a work bout prolongs maximal performance time, then care must be taken in applying our data to other movement situations. In swimming unlike the nonaquatic sports breathing pattern is an inherent part of the skill itself. The strong matching of ventilatory frequency and stroke rate therefore may mask possible O_2-breathing effects. These considerations provide many interesting questions for future research.

References

1. Asmussen, E. and Nielsen, M.: Pulmonary ventilation and effect of oxygen breathing in heavy exercise. Acta Physiol. Scand. 43:365-378, 1958.
2. Asmussen, E. and Nielsen, M.: Studies on the regulation of respiration in heavy work. Acta Physiol. Scand. 12:171-188, 1946.

3. Banister, R.G. and Cunningham, D.J.C.: The effects on the respiration and performance during exercise of adding oxygen to the inspired air. J. Physiol. 125:118-137, 1954.
4. Banister, E.W., Taunton, J.E., Patrick, T. et al: Effect of oxygen at high pressure at rest and during severe exercise. Resp. Physiol. 10:74- 2, 1970.
5. Briggs, H.: Physical exertion, fitness, and breathing. J. Physiol. 54:292-318, 1920.
6. Cook, J.: Work capacity in hyperbaric environments without hyperoxia. Aerospace Med. 41:1133-1135, 1970.
7. Cunningham, D.A.: Effects of breathing high concentrations of oxygen on treadmill performance. Res. Q. 37:491-494, 1966.
8. Dejours, P., Girard, F., Labrousse, Y. and Raynaud, J.: Stimulus oxygène chémoréflexe de la ventilation à basse altitude chez l'homme. I. au repos. J. Physiol. (Paris) 49:115-119, 1957a.
9. Dejours, P., Girard, F., Labrousse, Y. and Raynaud, J.: Stimulus oxygène chémoréflexe de la ventilation à basse altitude chez l'homme. II. au cours de l'exercise musculaire. J. Physiol. (Paris) 49:120-124, 1957b.
10. Dripps, R.D. and Comroe, J. H. Jr.: The effect of inhalation of high and low oxygen concentrations on respiration, pulse rate, ballisto-cardiogram and arterial oxygen saturation of normal individuals. Am. J. Physiol. 149:277-291, 1947.
11. Kaijser, L.: Limiting factors for aerobic muscle performance. The influence of varying oxygen pressure and temperature. Acta Physiol. Scand. Suppl. 346, 1970.
12. Karpovich, P.V.: Effect of oxygen inhalation on swimming performance. Res. Q. Am. Assoc. Health Phys. Educ. 5:24-26, 1934.
13. Lindquist, E.F.: Design and Analysis of Experiments in Psychology and Education. Boston:Houghton-Mifflin, 1953.
14. Miller, A.T.: Influence of oxygen administration on cardiovascular function during exercise and recovery. J. Appl. Physiol. 5:165-168, 1952.
15. Welch, H.G., Mullin, J.P., Wilson, G.D. and Lewis, J.: Effects of breathing O_2-enriched gas mixtures on metabolic rate during exercise. Med. Sci. Sports 6:26-32, 1974.
16. Wilson, B.A., Welch, H.G. and Liles, J.N.: Effects of hyperoxic gas mixtures on energy metabolism during prolonged work. J. Appl. Physiol. 39:267-271, 1975.
17. Wilson, G.D. and Welch, H.G.: Effects of hyperoxic gas mixtures on exercise tolerance in man. Med. Sci. Sports 7:48-52, 1975.

Effects of O_3 on Exercising Humans: Changes in Pulmonary Function and Ventilatory Patterns During Exercise

Anthony J. DeLucia and William C. Adams

Introduction

The inhalation of noxious oxidant gases is known to be highly damaging to the delicate tissues of the respiratory tract of humans. In certain heavily populated areas people are exposed almost daily to elevated concentrations of O_3, the predominant oxidant in photochemical smog and one of the most powerful oxidants known. Much of our knowledge concerning the effects of O_3 on humans has been gained from exposures of resting subjects to relatively high concentrations of the gas, encountered infrequently, if at all, in the atmosphere. Mild exercise has been previously shown to dramatically increase the toxicity of O_3, as gauged by subjective symptoms or quantifiable decrements in pulmonary function.

The objective of our study was to utilize greater exercise demands but lower pollutant concentrations compared to previous O_3 intoxication experiments. We believe this study provides relevant information regarding exercise or work in O_3-containing environments, describing (1) the levels of exercise at which given O_3 concentrations begin to effect normal subjects and (2) the effects on aerobic exercise performance mediated by O_3 inhalation.

Methods

Six nonsmoking male volunteers, aged 21 to 42 years, were subjects for the study (Table I). All were in good health and when tested for aerobic fitness were found to be average or above. Each subject underwent 12 separate one-hour exposures to filtered air or filtered air containing 0.15 ppm O_3 or 0.30 ppm O_3. Resting conditions, as well as separate one-hour exposures while exercising on a bicycle ergometer at workloads requiring 25%, 45%, or 65% of

Anthony J. DeLucia and William C. Adams, Human Performance Laboratory, University of California, Davis, Calif., U.S.A.

Table I. Subject Description

Subject	Age	Height (cm)	Weight (kg)	Max $\dot{V}O_2$ ml/kg/min	Maximum Ventilation lit/min (BTPS)	Ride Time on Max Test
1	42	180	74.1	56.1	157	13 min
2	23	175	64.9	62.4	145	11 min
3	22	180	69.8	44.3	135	9 min
4	27	178	74.5	58.5	155	14 min
5	36	175	73.5	44.1	100	9 min
6	27	189	74.0	40.7	125	9 min

$\dot{V}O_2$ max, were studied for each level of O_3. Subjects were required to inspire the O_3-containing air through the mouth while obtaining their required ventilation volume from the flow through a mixing tube to which the O_3 was added. Expired gas volume was measured using a Parkinson-Cowan dry gas meter, and the expired air was measured for O_2 and CO_2 to allow calculation of $\dot{V}O_2$. Respiratory rate was calculated from a recording of gas temperature during breathing, determined by inserting a subcutaneous temperature probe into the lumen of the rubber mouthpiece of the respiratory valve.

To assess the effects of O_3 on pulmonary function, a short battery of standard pulmonary function tests consisting of residual volume (RV), passive vital capacity (VC), forced expired volume -1 second ($FEV_{1.0}$) and midmaximal flow rate (MMFR) were administered before and after exposure. Recovery measurements of pulmonary function were made 4 and 24 hours postexposure.

Results

The order of occurrence of the 12 protocols was randomized for each subject. By having the nose clipped shut, preventing O_3 odor detection, most subjects were not sure if they had inspired O_3 unless the onset of distinct symptoms allowed them to deduce that they had, in fact, inhaled O_3. The symptoms reported by our subjects are shown in Table II and correspond to those commonly attributed to inhalation of oxidant gases.

$\dot{V}O_2$ and $\dot{V}_E$ were unaltered by O_3 exposure when differences between exposures and filtered air controls were assessed. Respiratory rate (f_R) was also unaffected by O_3 except for progressive increases in f_R observed with the 0.15 ppm and 0.30 ppm experiments combined with exercise at 65% of $\dot{V}O_2$ max. Since $\dot{V}_E$ was held relatively constant, mean tidal volume decreased.

Table II. Subjective Signs Reported Following O_3 Inhalation for One Hour

Workload (% max $\dot{V}O_2$)	O_3 Level	Chest Tightness						Cough						Throat Tickle						Pain on Deep Inspiration						Congestion						Wheezing						Headache					
		1*	2	3	4	5	6	1	2	3	4	5	6	1	2	3	4	5	6	1	2	3	4	5	6	1	2	3	4	5	6	1	2	3	4	5	6	1	2	3	4	5	6
Rest	Filtered Air	–	–	–	–	–	–	–	–	–	–	–	–	–	–	–	–	–	–	–	–	–	–	–	–	–	–	–	–	–	–	–	–	–	–	–	–	–	–	–	–	–	–
25		–	–	–	–	–	–	–	–	–	–	–	–	–	–	–	–	–	–	–	–	–	–	–	–	–	–	–	–	–	–	–	–	–	–	–	–	–	–	–	–	–	–
45		–	–	–	–	–	–	–	–	–	–	–	–	–	–	–	–	–	–	–	–	–	–	–	–	+	–	–	–	–	–	+	–	–	–	–	–	+	–	–	+	–	–
65		–	–	–	–	–	–	+	–	–	–	–	–	–	–	–	–	–	+	–	–	–	–	–	–	–	–	–	–	–	+	–	–	–	–	–	–	–	–	–	–	–	–
Rest	0.15 ppm Ozone	–	+	–	–	–	–	–	–	–	–	–	–	–	–	–	–	–	–	–	–	–	–	–	–	–	–	–	–	–	–	–	–	–	–	–	–	–	–	–	–	–	–
25		–	+	+	–	–	+	–	–	–	–	–	–	–	–	–	–	–	–	–	–	–	–	–	–	–	–	–	–	–	–	–	+	–	–	–	–	–	–	–	–	–	–
45		–	+	+	–	–	–	–	+	–	+	–	–	–	+	+	+	+	–	–	+	+	+	–	+	–	+	–	–	–	–	–	–	–	–	–	–	–	–	–	–	–	–
65		–	+	+	–	–	+	–	+	–	+	–	+	–	+	+	+	+	–	–	+	–	–	+	+	–	–	–	–	–	+	–	–	–	–	–	–	–	–	–	–	–	–
Rest	0.30 ppm Ozone	–	+	–	–	–	–	–	–	–	–	–	–	–	–	–	–	–	–	–	–	–	–	–	–	–	–	–	–	–	+	+	–	–	–	–	–	+	–	–	–	–	+
25		–	+	+	–	–	–	–	–	–	–	+	+	+	+	–	–	+	+	–	–	+	+	+	–	–	–	–	–	+	+	+	–	–	–	–	–	–	–	–	–	–	–
45		+	+	+	–	–	+	+	+	+	+	+	+	+	+	+	+	+	+	+	+	+	+	–	+	+	+	+	+	–	–	+	+	+	+	–	–	–	–	–	–	–	–
65		–	+	–	–	–	+	+	+	+	+	+	+	+	+	+	+	+	+	+	+	+	–	–	+	+	+	+	+	+	+	+	+	–	–	–	–	–	–	–	–	–	–

*Subject number

Residual volume was not significantly affected by O_3 inhalation; however, all three other lung function tests were significantly altered after the most severe protocols. VC, $FEV_{1.0}$ and MMFR were found to decrease 9%, 14% and 21%, respectively (P < .05 to P < .001), following exposure and had returned to normal by four hours postexposure, except in the case of MMFR, which was still 9% lower than pre-exposure control.

Distinct differences in individual susceptibility to O_3 were noticed among our subject population. Table III compares the two most sensitive subjects to the two subjects least affected by O_3. As can be observed, respiratory function and exercise ventilatory patterns were markedly impaired in less stressful protocols for two subjects (2 and 6). It must also be noted that these two subjects were unable to complete a full hour of exercise at 65% $\dot{V}O_2$ while breathing 0.30 ppm O_3.

Table III. Comparison of the Effects of O_3 Inhalation Upon Sensitive and Insensitive Subjects

| | O_3 Sensitive Subjects (2 & 6)* % $\dot{V}O_2$ max | | | | Insensitive Subjects (1 & 5)* % $\dot{V}O_2$ max | | | |
| | 45% | | 65% | | 45% | | 65% | |
Parameter	ppm O_3 0.15	ppm O_3 0.30	ppm O_3 0.15	ppm O_3 0.30	ppm O_3 0.15	ppm O_3 0.30	ppm O_3 0.15	ppm O_3 0.30
Residual volume	115.3‡	112.2	108.4	105.5	98.6	100.2	95.8·	97.4
Vital capacity	97.3	86.1	88.9	77.3	100.5	105.1	104.0	98.6
Forced expired volume – 1.0 sec	99.4	88.4	90.7	76.6	92.6	106.4	98.7	92.3
Mid-maximal flow rate	101.0	94.3	100.9	73.2	92.5	106.3	94.7	87.4
Respiratory+ frequency	89.9	136.1	157.5	173.2	82.4	86.5	104.9	99.9
Tidal volume+	110.6	85.3	71.6	54.1	106.9	96.1	98.0	92.4
Minute+ ventilation	98.1	108.8	110.7	115.1	100.2	93.3	96.7	93.2

*Mean values obtained for two subjects.
+Measurement taken at 60 min.
‡Values given are percent of pre-exposure value for pulmonary function measurements; with other parameters the values represent percent of control (filtered air inhalation).

Discussion

The present study is one of the first to incorporate exercise as a synergist in the enhancement of O_3 toxicity and, as well, measure exercise performance during exposure. Our results, in contrast to those of Bates et al and Hazucha et al, demonstrated no alteration in pulmonary function with resting or 25% $\dot{V}O_2$ max protocols. This may be somewhat unexpected, since our subjects were forced to inspire all their ventilatory volume through the mouth, bypassing the gas absorptive surfaces of the nose. Similar insensitivity of the subjects in the studies of Hackney et al was attributed to possible oxidant tolerance, but for our subjects this was unlikely.

The higher workloads required in our study, 45% and 65% $\dot{V}O_2$ max, resulted in four- and sixfold increase in $\dot{V}_E$ over resting. Using a formula presented by Folinsbee in a recent discussion of exercise potentiation of O_3 toxicity, we have calculated that the greater ventilatory demands of exercise may raise effective O_3 dose 2.5 and 3.5 times normal for a simple resting experiment (Table IV). When multiplying our dosage by these factors of 2.5 and 3.5, it can be seen that effective exposures of the lung may have been more comparable to those of other studies involving .25 to 1.0 ppm O_3 and one to four hour exposures.

Though this and other studies have not detected differences in $\dot{V}O_2$ with O_3 inhalation, it is apparent that other factors are involved in limiting performance when the lower respiratory tract is exposed to toxic gases. Though it is possible that exertional dyspnea may result from increased dead space, more studies will be required to answer questions regarding the mechanisms by which O_3 can limit human performance in more severe cases of acute intoxication.

Table IV. Exercise-Mediated Augmentation
of O_3 Delivery to the Lung

$$\text{Relative increase } O_3 \text{ delivery} = 1 + \cfrac{\cfrac{\dot{V}_E \text{ exercise*}}{\dot{V}_E \text{ rest}}}{2}$$

Workload (% $\dot{V}O_2$ max)	$\dfrac{\dot{V}_E \text{ Exercise}}{\dot{V}_E \text{ Rest}}$	Relative Increase O_3 Delivery
25%	2.6	1.8
45%	4.0	2.5
65%	6.1	3.5

*Folinsbee et al: *J. Appl. Physiol.* 38:996, 1001, 1975.

Cardiorespiratory Responses to Optimal Speed of Walking and to "Metabolic Intersection" Speed of Walking and Running

Hirohiko Kagaya

Introduction

Walking is one of the most fundamental movements of the body and has been studied by many authors from physiological aspects. Some researchers tried to determine the relation between energy expenditure and speed of walking since early in this century. Ralston [5] investigated the energy expenditure during walking at various speeds and found that a "natural" or "comfortable" speed of walking corresponded to an optimal speed which required minimum energy per unit distance walked. Furusawa et al [1] and Ogasawara [4] observed energy expenditure was greater for walking at high speed than for running. Recently, Noble et al [3] published a paper dealing with mode and metabolic changes from walking to running with special reference to perceived exertion.

The present author intended to measure energy expenditure of walking and running at various speeds in healthy male subjects and to determine an optimal walking speed as well as "metabolic intersection" speed defined as speed at which energy expenditure was equal for walking and running. The present study is also concerned with physiological intensities of these optimal and "metabolic intersection" speeds of walking.

Methods

Energy expenditure during level walking and running was studied on nine male students aged 16 to 22. Their physical characteristics are shown in Table I.

Subjects walked and ran for ten minutes on a motor-driven treadmill at a given speed ranging from 50 to 140 m/min for walking

Hirohiko Kagaya, Faculty of Education, Saitama University, Japan.

Table I. Physical Characteristics of Subjects (N = 9)

Variable	Average	Range
Age (years)	18.7	16.0-22.0
Height (cm)	171.3	163.2-176.7
Weight (kg)	62.3	53.0-72.4
$\dot{V}O_2$ max (l/min)	2.8	2.0-4.1
$\dot{V}O_2$ max (ml/kg/min)	45.0	36.8-58.3

and from 100 to 160 m/min for running. Several trials were requested of each subject. In each trial, two or three kinds of speeds were presented randomly with 15 to 30 minute intervals. All subjects were well accustomed to the apparatus and experimental procedure.

Electrocardiograms were recorded continuously all through the trial. Expired air was collected in Douglas bags during and after exercise. Aliquots of expired air for the first five minutes, second four minutes and the last one minute of exercise as well as 15-30 minutes of recovery period were analyzed for oxygen by means of the expired gas analyzer (IH 02-2,SANEI), periodically checked against a Scholander microanalyzer.

For the determination of optimal and "metabolic intersection" speed, oxygen requirement for a unit distance of walking or running was calculated per body weight and plotted against speed. Optimal speed of walking was defined as the speed at which subjects required minimum energy for a unit distance walking. Metabolic intersection speed was defined as the speed at which energy expenditure for walking and running was equal.

Results and Discussion

As shown in Figure 1, oxygen requirement per body weight was minimum at a certain speed when expressed per unit distance walked. It averaged 68.9 m/min (S.D. = 7.82) for nine subjects. Oxygen requirement at this speed was 0.087 ml/meter/kg (S.D. = 0.014). Ralston [5] indicated that energy expenditure was a linear function of the square of the speed during level walking. According to him, the relation was $\dot{E}w = 29 + 0.0053 V_2$ ($\dot{E}w$; cal/min/kg, V; speed in meter/min). Dividing the above equation by V:

$$\frac{\dot{E}w}{V} = Em = \frac{29}{V} + 0.0053 V \quad (Em; cal/meter/kg).$$

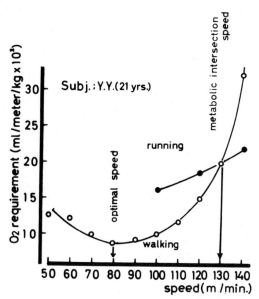

FIG. 1. Oxygen requirement of walking and running related to speed.

This equation was minimum when V = 74 m/min. Furthermore, Ralston suggested that a "natural" or "comfortable" speed of walking corresponded to a minimum value of the energy expenditure, that is, an optimal speed.

Oxygen requirement — speed curve for running was different from that for walking. Two curves intersected at a certain speed (Fig. 1), which is called "metabolic intersection" speed in this study. "Metabolic intersection" speeds for the present subjects averaged 128.9 m/min (S.D. = 6.01) and oxygen requirement was 0.184 ml/meter/kg (S.D. = 0.032). At higher speed, more energy was required for walking, while at lower speed the reverse was observed. Furusawa et al [1] and Ogasawara [4] suggested that at speeds higher than 120 m/min, oxygen requirement for walking was greater than for running. The metabolic intersection point investigated by Noble et al [3] was 4.92 mph (132 m/min) when heart rate was used as an indicator of metabolism. These results will suggest "metabolic intersection" speed may lie in the 120 to 140 m/min range for ordinary male subjects.

In order to show the relative physiological intensity of exercise, oxygen intake during the ninth to the tenth minute of exercise was expressed in percent of $\dot{V}O_2$ max in Figure 2. In Figure 3, heart rate at the end of exercise was plotted against speeds. Table II

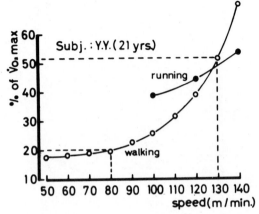

FIG. 2. Relation between oxygen intake during exercise and speed. Arrow indicates optimal and "metabolic intersection" speed.

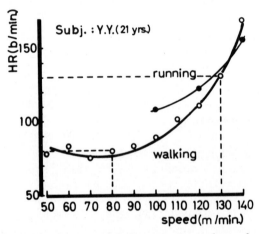

FIG. 3. Relation between heart rate during exercise and speed. Arrow indicates optimal and "metabolic intersection" speed.

summarized the mean and standard deviation of oxygen intake and heart rate during walking at optimal or "metabolic intersection" speed. It was found that oxygen intake during walking at optimal speed corresponded to 22.0% of $\dot{V}O_2$ max and heart rate was 95.1 beats/min. Responses to walking at "metabolic intersection" speed were 64.9% of $\dot{V}O_2$ max for oxygen intake and 157.0 beats/min for heart rate.

How to improve cardiorespiratory endurance of sedentary people is a very important problem and many investigations have been made

Table II. Mean and Standard Deviation of Oxygen Intake and Heart Rate
During Walking at Optimal or "Metabolic Intersection" Speed

| | Optimal Speed (N = 9) | | | Metabolic Intersection Speed (N = 9) | | |
	Speed (m/min)	$\dot{V}O_2$ (% $\dot{V}O_2$ max)	HR (beats/min)	Speed (m/min)	$\dot{V}O_2$ (% $\dot{V}O_2$ max)	HR (beats/min)
$\bar{X}$	68.90	22.00	95.10	128.90	64.90	157.00
S.D.	7.82	2.33	10.67	6.01	11.08	17.76

on this subject. Shephard [7] indicated in his paper that intensity of exercise was the most important factor to decide training effects. From the findings of Sharkey and Hollman [6], Kilbom [2] and others, physical training with an intensity corresponding to 50% to 60% of $\dot{V}O_2$ max or heart rate of 150 beats/min may give a training effect in healthy untrained men and women. It is suggested from these results that walking at "metabolic intersection" speed will be a useful exercise for the improvement of the physical work capacity of ordinary people.

Summary

Energy expenditure and heart rate were measured during walking and running at various speeds on a motor-driven treadmill in nine male students. Optimal walking speed averaged 68.9 m/min for these subjects. "Metabolic intersection" speed of walking and running was 128.9 m/min on average. Heart rate during walking at optimal speed was 95.1 beats/min and 157.0 beats/min at "metabolic intersection" speed. During walking at optimal speed and "metabolic intersection" speed, oxygen intake corresponded to 22.0% and 64.9% of $\dot{V}O_2$ max, respectively.

References

1. Furusawa, K., Hill, A.V. and Lupton, H.: Muscular exercise, lactic acid and oxygen. VIII. Muscular exercise and oxygen requirement. Proc. Roy. Soc. B. 97:167-176, 1924.
2. Kilbom, A.: Effect on women of physical training with low intensities. Scand. J. Clin. Invest. 28:345-352, 1971.
3. Noble, B.J., Metz, K.F., Pandolf, K.B. et al: Perceived exertion during walking and running. II. Med. Sci. Sports 5(2):116-120, 1973.
4. Ogasawara, M.: Energy expenditure in walking and running. J. Physiol. 81:255-264, 1934.
5. Ralston, H.J.: Energy-speed relation and optimal speed during level walking. Int. Z. Angew. Physiol. Einschl. Arbeitsphysiol. 17:277-283, 1958.
6. Sharkey, B.J. and Hollman, J.P.: Cardiorespiratory adaptation to training at specified intensities. Res. Q. 38:698-704, 1967.
7. Shephard, R.J.: Intensity, duration and frequency of exercise as determinants of the response to a training regime. Int. Z. Angew. Physiol. Einschl. Arbeitsphysiol. 26:272-278, 1968.

Physiological Adjustments to Continuous and Interval Running Training

F. S. Pyke, A. S. Ewing and A. D. Roberts

Introduction

Coaches of many sports which involve a large amount of running are using a wide range of training methods to improve the performance capacity of their athletes. These methods can be basically categorized as continuous or interval training. Continuous training involves running at a constant pace for extended periods of time, that is, 15 to 60 minutes, while interval training consists of repeating short periods of intensive running (usually less than three minutes) interspersed with periods of recovery. Interval training with short running efforts (< 30 sec) is referred to as spurt training, while longer running effort (30 to 60 sec) with longer recovery periods (150 to 500 sec) is termed repetition training. The relative effectiveness of these methods is not well understood. It is the purpose of this study to investigate (1) the responses of men to individual sessions of continuous and interval (spurt and repetition) running training and (2) their improvements after one month of participation in these different training regimens.

Study 1
Responses to Individual Sessions of Continuous, Spurt and Repetition Training

Methods

Five moderately active men, aged 24-28 years, were exposed to 20-minute sessions of intensive continuous running, spurt running (5 sec run, 15 sec recovery) and repetition running (30 sec run, 150 sec

F. S. Pyke, A. S. Ewing and A. D. Roberts, Department of Physical Education and Recreation, University of Western Australia.

This research was supported by a grant from the Community Recreation Council of Western Australia.

recovery). The men underwent the different sessions in random order at intervals of approximately 48 hours.

Before and after each session the men were weighed on Avery precision scales and their rectal temperature was measured with a clinical thermometer. Heart rate was monitored throughout with a Sieman's telemetry system. During the continuous and spurt regimens HR was recorded during the last ten seconds of every second minute and during the repetition regimen near the end of the work period and midway through and near the end of the recovery period. A blood sample was drawn from an arm vein five minutes after each session and analyzed for lactate by the enzymatic method [6].

All training sessions were conducted outdoors on a 400-meter grass track. Black bulb, dry bulb and wet bulb temperatures were recorded at intervals throughout the sessions, enabling a WBGT index to be calculated. The random assignment of subjects to training times resulted in the group being exposed to similar climatic conditions (WBGT index 21 to 23 C) while undertaking each type of training.

During continuous running the men were requested to run at a pace which they found quite comfortable for the entire session and which produced a HR 20 to 30 bpm below each individual's maximum. During both spurt and repetition running they were asked to cover as much distance as possible during the training session. This distance was measured by having them drop a bean bag in response to a whistle blown to indicate the end of each work period. The bag was then picked up prior to the next work period.

At a final test session it was determined how far the men could run from a standing start in 5 seconds, 30 seconds and 15 minutes, the mean distance in each case being 30.8, 198.6 and 3716 meters. This permitted some estimation of the intensity of effort being experienced in each work period of the training sessions. The latter distance corresponds to a predicted $\dot{V}O_2$ max of 53.0 ml/kg/min [2].

Results and Discussion

A summary of results is presented in Table I and Figure 1. It can be seen that in continuous running the men averaged 90% of their maximum speed for the distance. The energy for this effort was provided mainly by oxidative processes as indicated from an average HR of 184 bpm and the low level of lactic acid in the blood (4.7 mM/l). Spurt training produced a slightly lower HR (181 bpm) and a higher blood lactate accumulation (5.5 mM/l). Both regimens

Table I. Responses to 20-Minute Sessions of Continuous,
Spurt or Repetition Training

	Continuous	Spurt	Repetition
Number of work periods	1	60	7
Duration of work period (sec)	1200	5	30
Duration of recovery period (sec)	–	15	150
Work/recovery ratio	–	1:3	1:5
Total distance covered in session (M)	4451 ± 86	1660 ± 32	1311 ± 40
Average speed in work period (m/min)	222.4 ± 4.3	332.0 ± 6.5	374.6 ± 11.2
Percent of maximum speed for work period	89.9 ± 3.4	89.7 ± 2.1	94.3 ± 3.3
Weight loss (kg)	.58 ± .09	.55 ± .01	.36 ± .04*
Rectal temperature increase (°C)	1.7 ± .24	1.8 ± .08	1.3 ± .10*
Average heart rate (bpm) (average maximum = 204 bpm)	184 ± 6.8	181 ± 3.1	150 ± 4.8*
Post session blood lactate (mM/L)	4.7 ± .91	5.5 ± .18	8.5 ± .93*

Values given are means ± standard deviation.
*Significantly different from other group means ($p < .05$)

elevated rectal temperature to 39 C and elicited equivalent sweating rates.

Repetition running involved the glycolytic energy pathways to a significantly greater extent than either continuous or spurt running. This is undoubtedly the result of increasing the duration of each interval run from 5 to 30 seconds. It appears that the energy required for the short work periods (<10 sec) of spurt training was provided by alactic sources that were replenished in a short recovery period (<30 sec) and then reutilized in the next work period [1, 9]. In this way the involvement of the glycolytic energy pathway and lactic acid accumulation is minimized. The longer recovery periods of the repetition training regimen lessened the overall load on the cardiovascular system (mean HR 150 bpm) and, while the speed of running was faster than in the other regimens, the total work output

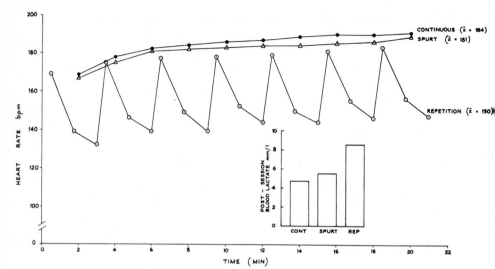

FIG. 1. Heart rate and blood lactic acid measured in 20-minute sessions of
continuous, spurt and repetition training.

was not high enough to produce equivalent increases in rectal
temperature and sweating rate.

Conclusion

It was concluded that continuous training requires
predominantly aerobic energy release while repetition training places
greatest emphasis on the lactacid anaerobic energy system. Spurt
training has both a high aerobic and alactic energy component and
places a moderate demand on the glycolytic energy system.

It is now of interest to observe the adjustments made to a period
of training using continuous, spurt or repetition methods.

Study 2

Adjustments to a Period of Continuous, Spurt
or Repetition Training

Methods

Three groups of five moderately active men, aged 18-26 years,
were matched on the basis of $\dot{V}O_2$ max, before completing 16
sessions of continuous, spurt or repetition training within a period of
one month.

Before and after the period of training the men reported to the
laboratory for testing on three separate occasions.

During the first test session the men undertook a ten-minute submaximal run at 11.3 km/hr on a level treadmill. $\dot{V}O_2$ was determined in the last three minutes of the run from measurements of respiratory gas exchange using a Triple J respiratory valve and a chain-compensated Tissot gasometer. Gas samples were analyzed for O_2 and CO_2 concentration by a Beckman E2 oxygen analyzer and a Godart capnograph CO_2 analyzer. HR was determined from electrocardiograms. Blood was drawn from an arm vein five minutes after the run for lactate analysis.

After a ten-minute recovery period each man performed a multistage treadmill test in which he ran at 11.3 km/hr up an increasing grade which gradually elevated $\dot{V}O_2$, HR and blood lactate to maximal levels. $\dot{V}O_2$ max was determined by drawing gas samples each minute from a mixing box and measuring gas volume with a Parkinson-Cowan dry gasmeter. HR and blood lactate were determined as for the ten-minute run.

During the second test session the men completed a five-minute interval effort alternating 5-second work periods and 15-second recovery periods at 13.7 km/hr up a 20% treadmill grade. A venous blood sample for lactate analysis was taken five minutes after the routine.

A third test session included a 27.4-meter (30 yd) overground sprint from a running start. The men were permitted 9.1 meters (10 yds) to accelerate before being timed over the test distance with a photoelectric timing system. This was followed by a sustained sprint to exhaustion at 13.7 km/hr up a 20% treadmill grade. The men were timed for the period that they could run without supporting themselves by the railing around the treadmill.

Differences between pre- and posttraining values obtained within each group were evaluated by t tests for related groups. Differences between groups were assessed by analysis of variance and covariance techniques.

Results and Discussion

Training. Between sessions 1 and 16 the men involved in each training regimen improved the distance that they could cover in a 20-minute session. The continuous group increased the mean distance run from 4369 to 4722 meters (8.1%), the spurt group improved from 1699 to 1807 meters (6.4%) and the repetition group from 1209 to 1316 meters (8.9%).

Submaximal run. A summary of results is presented in Table II. The oxygen consumed during the ten-minute submaximal run was not altered by any of the training methods. Such improvements in

Table II. The Effects of Training on Responses to Sprint, Interval and Endurance Running Performances

	Continuous			Spurt			Repetition		
	Pre	Post	P	Pre	Post	P	Pre	Post	P
Weight (kg)	66.1 ± 9.1	65.7 ± 8.9	NS	74.1 ± 8.0	73.3 ± 7.6	NS	66.3 ± 6.3	66.3 ± 6.2	NS
Submaximal Treadmill Run (11.3 km/hr, 0% Grade, 10 min)									
$\dot{V}O_2$ (L/min)	2.50 ± .20	2.38 ± .26	NS	2.81 ± .38	2.81 ± .34	NS	2.54 ± .32	2.51 ± .25	NS
$\dot{V}O_2$ (ml/kg/min)	38.1 ± 3.0	36.3 ± 1.9	NS	37.8 ± 1.2	38.3 ± 1.2	NS	38.2 ± 2.3	37.9 ± 2.5	NS
HR (bpm)	179.2 ± 12.7	166.8 ± 10.3	.05>p>.01	174.2 ± 11.4	169.4 ± 11.9	NS	172.0 ± 6.8	169.0 ± 14.8	NS
Blood Lactate (mM/L)	3.2 ± 1.4	2.5 ± 1.0	.05>p>.01	3.8 ± 1.9	3.1 ± 0.8	NS	2.1 ± 1.7	2.0 ± 1.3	NS
Maximal Treadmill Run (11.3 km/hr, Increasing Grade)									
Run Time (min)	7.3 ± 1.1	9.0 ± 0.9	<.01	7.0 ± 1.2	7.9 ± 1.8	.10>p>.05	7.1 ± 1.0	7.8 ± 1.5	NS
$\dot{V}O_2$ (L/min)	3.20 ± .55	3.54 ± .50	<.01	3.57 ± .56	3.78 ± .56	.05>p>.01	3.24 ± .46	3.40 ± .37	.10>p>.05
$\dot{V}O_2$ (ml/kg/min)	48.3 ± 4.2	53.8 ± 2.1	<.01	48.2 ± 4.6	51.5 ± 5.1	.05>p>.01	48.8 ± 4.9	51.4 ± 3.7	.10>p>.05
HR (bpm)	204.2 ± 8.0	199.2 ± 4.9	NS	200.4 ± 8.4	196.4 ± 10.7	NS	197.0 ± 4.8	195.6 ± 6.7	NS
Blood Lactate (mM/L)	11.5 ± 0.9	11.4 ± 0.6	NS	11.2 ± 1.2	11.2 ± 1.6	NS	10.6 ± 1.3	10.7 ± 0.8	NS
Interval Treadmill Run (5 sec work, 15 sec recovery at 13.7 km/hr, 20% Grade, 5 min)									
Blood Lactate (mM/L)	4.9 ± 1.1	3.5 ± 0.4	.05>p>.01	5.2 ± 1.0	3.4 ± 1.0	<.01	4.4 ± 1.7	2.8 ± 0.6	.10>p>.05
Sustained Treadmill Sprint (13.7 km/hr, 20% Grade)									
Run Time (sec)	44.1 ± 7.1	53.4 ± 8.4	<.01	49.5 ± 9.4	59.2 ± 11.1	.05>p>.01	48.5 ± 9.9	59.5 ± 11.8	<.01
Work Done (kgm)	2184 ± 255	2651 ± 484	<.01	2750 ± 372	3282 ± 607	.05>p>.01	2460 ± 635	3025 ± 793	.05>p>.01
Short Overground Sprint (27.4 m Running Start)									
Run Time (sec)	3.47 ± .10	3.45 ± .07	NS	3.36 ± .18	3.40 ± .20	NS	3.44 ± .17	3.46 ± .21	NS

Values given are Means ± Standard Deviation.
Differences between groups are not statistically significant = NS.

efficiency may require a program of much longer duration. Continuous training produced significant decreases in both HR and blood lactate, neither of which was evident in the other groups. The decrease in HR is a well-established physiological change which has been attributed to an improved stroke volume of the heart [2]. The decrease in submaximal HR with interval training is nonsignificant and less than that reported in other studies [5, 11]. This makes it interesting to speculate that the increases in maximal $\dot{V}O_2$ observed in spurt and repetition training are due more to peripheral than central adaptations.

Before starting to train, the men utilized about 78% $\dot{V}O_2$ max during the run without producing lactate levels substantially above those normally obtained during rest. However, the continuous group, by elevating their $\dot{V}O_2$ max by 11.4%, were able to work at less than 67% $\dot{V}O_2$ max in the submaximal run after training and became less dependent on energy from nonoxidative sources.

Maximal run. To match their submaximal performance improvements the continuous group also made the greatest gains during the maximal run. The average $\dot{V}O_2$ max of this group improved by 11.4% compared to 6.8% by the spurt group and 5.3% by the repetition group, although the differences between groups were not statistically significant. A similar magnitude of change was evident when $\dot{V}O_2$ was expressed in liters per minute or milliliters per kilogram per minute as weight was not altered by any form of training. These increases are comparable to those reported in other studies [3, 5] particularly when the short duration of the present study is considered. It should be understood that the apparent superiority of the continuous training regimen may be due to the trainability of the subjects concerned rather than being a true reflection of the effectiveness of this type of training. Maximal HR was reduced slightly by training, but this was not significant. Maximal blood lactate, reflecting access to glycolytic energy pathways, remained essentially unchanged. This supports the findings of other investigators [4, 7].

Interval run. All groups significantly reduced the blood lactate accumulated during the five-minute interval effort. There was no significant difference between the groups. However, using such a gross indicator of anaerobic energy release poses explanatory problems. It may be that training induced an increase in the oxidative capacity of the fast twitch muscle fibers [8] which can therefore function less anaerobically when recruited during such high intensity work. The finding may also reflect an increase in the availability of an alternative energy source in the muscle (oxygen bound to myoglobin) [1, 10, 13] which reduces the dependence upon energy release from the splitting of glycogen to lactic acid. However, circulatory factors contributing to acceleration of oxygen transport at the onset of work and to faster removal of lactate during recovery from work could also account for the observed result.

Sprint performance tests. All groups improved their performance time and work output in a sustained sprint up a steep treadmill grade. There was no significant difference between the groups. Realizing that the capacity for glycolysis as measured in the maximal run was unchanged with training, it may be that the performance improvements in a sustained sprint can be attributed to an increased capacity of the alactacid oxygen debt mechanism [4]. The release of energy by glycolytic mechanisms is consequently delayed until late in the run. However, psychological reasons for the observed improvement cannot be overlooked.

The time for a short overground sprint was not improved by any type of training. It seems that stamina training is incompatible with speed improvements [11, 14].

Conclusion

While the results do not statistically favor continuous training ahead of the two different forms of interval training, this regimen does seem to represent the best value for inducing change in variables related to stamina running performance.

However, with men possessing a moderate level of endurance fitness, the stimulus for improvement of aerobic power is present in any of the described continuous and interval running training programs. Such an improvement seemingly places less reliance on lactacid anaerobic energy release in sprint, interval and endurance running performances.

References

1. Astrand, I., Astrand, P.O., Christensen, E.H. and Hedman, R.: Myohemoglobin as an oxygen store in man. Acta Physiol. Scand. 48:454-460, 1960.
2. Balke, B.: A simple field test for the assessment of physical fitness. U.S. Civil Aeromed. Res. Inst. Rep. 6:1-8, 1963.
3. Ekblom, B., Astrand, P.O., Saltin, B. et al: Effect of training on circulatory response to exercise. J. Appl. Physiol. 24:518-528, 1968.
4. Fox, E.L.: Differences in metabolic alterations with sprint versus endurance interval training programmes. Second International Symposium on Biochemistry of Exercise, Magglingen, 1974 (Abstract).
5. Fox, E.L., Bartels, R.L., Billings, C.E. et al: Intensity and distance of interval training and changes in aerobic power. Med. Sci. Sports 5:18-22, 1973.

6. Gerken, G.: Die quantitative enzymatische Dehydrierung von L(+) lactat fur die Microanalyze. Z. Physiol. Chem. 320:180-186, 1960.

7. Gollnick, P.D.: Cellular adaptations to exercise. *In* Shephard, R.J. (ed.): Frontiers of Fitness. Springfield, Ill.:Charles C Thomas, 1971, pp. 112-126.

8. Gollnick, P.D., Armstrong, R.B., Saltin, B. et al: Effect of training on enzyme activity and fibre composition of skeletal muscle. J. Appl. Physiol. 34:107-111, 1973.

9. Margaria, R., Oliva, R.D., di Prampero, P.E. and Cerretelli, P.: Energy utilization in intermittent exercise of supramaximal intensity. J. Appl. Physiol. 26:752-756, 1969.

10. Pattengale, P.K. and Holloszy, J.J.: Augmentation of skeletal muscle myoglobin by a programme of treadmill running. Am. J. Physiol. 213:783-785, 1967.

11. Pyke, F.S., Elliott, B.C., Morton, A.R. and Roberts, A.D.: Physiological adjustments to intensive interval training. Br. J. Sports Med. 8:163-170, 1974.

12. Saltin, B., Blomqvist, G., Mitchell, J.H. et al: Response to submaximal and maximal exercise after bed rest and training. Circulation 38:(Suppl. 7), 1968.

13. Saltin, B. and Essen, B.: Muscle glycogen, lactate, ATP and CP in intermittent exercise. *In* Pernow, B. and Saltin, B. (eds.): Muscle Metabolism During Exercise. New York:Plenum Press, 1971, pp. 419-424.

14. Thorstennson, A., Sjodin and Karlsson, J.: Enzyme activities and muscle strength after sprint training in man. Acta Physiol. Scand. 94:313-318, 1975.

The Effect of High Intensity Weight Training on Cardiovascular Function

James A. Peterson

Introduction

Coaches, athletes and sport scientists have long ascribed to the opinion that weight training is an anaerobic activity which will, under certain conditions, improve muscular fitness, but will not, under those same conditions, appreciably affect cardiovascular efficiency. Such a premise is undoubtedly valid given the traditional modes of weight training, the traditional techniques employed in weight training and the equipment traditionally used by individuals engaged in weight training. In light of recent technological advances in isokinetic weight training equipment — most notably in the Nautilus Sports/Medical Industries machines — what would be the consequences of a weight training program which was not based on traditional practices? As part of a larger study which was designated as "Project Total Conditioning," the present investigation attempted to determine the effect on cardiovascular function of a high intensity weight training program — a program in which the individual is given minimal opportunity to rest between exercises and is forced both by the mechanical design of the equipment and by close supervision to perform each exercise in correct form to a point of almost complete exhaustion.

Methods

Thirty-two male volunteers, members of the Corps of Cadets, participated in the study. The subjects, all members of the intercollegiate varsity football team, were assigned to two matched groups: an experimental group and a control group. The experimental treatment consisted of three days of weight training per week on alternate days, with two days of rest after the third workout, for a period of eight weeks.

James A. Peterson, United States Military Academy, West Point, New York, U.S.A.

Contrary to traditional practices, each workout was relatively brief in duration, lasting only approximately 30 minutes. For all practical purposes, the intensity of the workouts was so severe that it would have been impossible to appreciably extend them. During their initial workouts, for example, several of the subjects became nauseated. Eventually, however, the subjects adapted to the intensity of the training to a point where not only did such negative reaction entirely disappear, but the average time to complete a comparable workout was considerably lessened.

Each experimental workout consisted of ten basic exercises. In addition, twice a week, the workouts included six exercises designed to strengthen the neck. Table I lists the exercises and the required equipment which, in varying combinations, constituted the experimental training program.

Three different methods of performing an exercise were prescribed. In the first type of training, an exercise was done in normal fashion. The subject lifted and lowered the resistance under his own power. In the second method, an exercise was performed in a negative-accentuated fashion: the subject lifted the weight with two limbs and lowered the weight using only one limb. In effect, negative-accentuated training (as opposed to "normal" work)

Table I. Exercises and Machines Used in "Project Total Conditioning"

Exercise	Machine*
1. Leg extension	Compound leg
2. Leg press	Compound leg
3. Squat	Leg and back
4. Hip and back	Super hip and back; Duo-Poly hip and back
5. Leg curl	Leg curl
6. Pullover	Pullover
7. Bench press	Infimetric bench; Omni bench
8. Chins	Multi-exercise
9. Dips	Multi-exercise
10. Torso arm pulldown	Torso arm
11. Seated press	Duo-shoulder
12. Double chest	Double chest
13. Decline press	Double chest
14. Biceps curl	Curl-triceps; Duo-Poly curl
15. Triceps curl	Curl-triceps; Duo-Poly triceps
16. Neck extension	4-Way neck
17. Neck flexion	4-Way neck
18. Bi-lateral neck flexion	4-Way neck
19. Shoulder shrug	Neck and shoulder
20. Rotary neck	Rotary neck

*All machines – Nautilus Sports/Medical Industries machines.

doubles the amount of resistance which one limb must accommodate in the eccentric contraction phase. The third (and perhaps most strenuous) way of weight training involved exercising in a negative-only fashion. In this method, experimenter personnel lifted the resistance to the contracted (concentric) position for the subject who in turn was required to lower the weight at a controlled pace through the eccentric contraction phase. The primary advantage of negative-only exercising is that it greatly increases the amount of resistance placed on a specific muscle or muscle group. Quite obviously, an individual can lower more weight than he can raise. In a program designed to exercise only in a "normal" fashion, the resistance in the eccentric contraction is by definition limited to the amount of weight lifted in the concentric phase of muscle contraction.

Another critical aspect of the experimental training was the strict requirement that each subject do as many repetitions as he could perform in proper form of every exercise in his workout. The amount of resistance for each exercise was periodically arbitrarily adjusted in an attempt to maintain the probable range of repetitions to a minimum of 5 and a maximum of 12. A workout consisted of a single set of each exercise. All training was conducted on a one-to-one (subject-to-supervisor) basis, with Nautilus Sports/Medical Industries personnel supervising the workouts and United States Military Academy officials providing overall project coordination.

After the experimental group had trained for two weeks,* all subjects were pretested on the following criteria: selected anthropometric measurements; physical fitness factors (strength, flexibility, body composition and cardiovascular fitness); and physical performance tasks (40-yard dash and vertical jump). At the end of six additional weeks of training by the experimental group, all subjects were retested on the pretest measures.

The tests for cardiovascular function consisted of a rest period (sitting on a bicycle ergometer); a continuous, progressive bicycle ergometer ride with increasing workloads (360 kpm/min for the first three steps, then 180 kpm/min increase every two minutes) until the subject could no longer keep the rate (60 rpm) or wanted to stop. This was followed by two minutes at a light workload (360 kpm/min which was also the initial workload), then three minutes of rest (sitting on the bike). Heart rate (HR), systolic (SBP) and diastolic (DBP) blood pressures, systolic tension time index $(STTI = HR \times SBP)$ and a subjective rating by the subject of the

---

*An arbitrary period of time allocated for the "learning effect."

perceived exertion (RPE, from 6 to 20) were obtained at each condition. In addition, total ride time was recorded. Since the same protocol was used for each subject, total ride time reflects the total work done by the subject and includes aerobic capacity, anaerobic capacity and motivation to continue work (an important element in this type of all-out performance). The work level necessary to achieve a heart rate of 170 (physical working capacity, PWC-170) and STTI of 25,000 was calculated by interpolating to determine the work level for each of these values. These measures reflect primarily the individual's submaximal aerobic efficiency and are not influenced by the subject's motivation to do all-out work. Maximal aerobic efficiency was assessed by a subject's performance on the 2-mile run, a standard event in the West Point and Army-wide physical ability testing programs.

Results

The group means and the standard error of the means for the cardiovascular measurements are presented in Table II. Differences on the initial test data were determined by a t-test on each variable. If there were no differences at an elevated significance level (.20) then a t-test was used on the final testing data to determine the effects of the training (.05 level). If there were initial differences, then analysis of covariance was used to determine if significantly different changes had occurred between the groups with the final test variable being the criterion measure and the initial variable being the covariate (.05 level).

The following significant differences (.05 level) resulted from the experimental training: lower HR at 360, 1080, 1260, 1620, and 1800 kpm/min; lower STTI at 360; RPE at 1260; longer ride time; a higher PWC-170; and a lower 2-mile run time. In almost every case, the experimental group performed better on the final testing period (or the change from initial to final) than did the control group.

The experimental group also experienced an apparent substantial improvement in muscular fitness. This change is reflected in the mean values for selected workout variables which are presented in Table III. After six weeks of training, the experimental subjects increased the amount of resistance used per exercise in a workout by 58.54% and 43.06%, respectively, for two sets of identical workouts (the 1st and 17th; and the 2nd and 16th).* In addition, the mean time to complete an identical workout decreased substantially.

---

*The variance in the values for the two "sets" of workouts is primarily attributable to the fact that each set of workouts employed a different set of exercises and a different combination of training methods.

Table II. Pre- and Posttest Mean Values for Cardiovascular Function Measurements

Variable	Initial Test* Exp. (18)	Con. (14)	P	Final Test* Exp.	Con.	P	Initial to Final† Exp.	Con.	P
Rest									
Heart rate (b/min)	76.6 1.5	73.9 2.8	.37	75.9 2.0	75.0 2.8	.81			–
Systolic BP (mm Hg)	131 3.7	127 2.8	.45	132 2.1	133 2.8	.97			–
Diastolic BP (mm Hg)	85 2.5	82 2.2	.41	89 2.1	86 2.6	.33			–
Systolic tension Time I	10036 339	9405 414	.24	10036 288	9952 497	.88			–
360 Kpm Workload									
Rating-perceived exert.	7.2 .31	7.1 .23	.85	6.4 .20	6.6 .23	.52			–
HR	105 2.2	100 2.3	.07	100 3.1	103 2.4	–	98	106	.02
SBP	145 5.0	144 3.6	.91	143 2.3	143 3.8	.89			–
DBP	81 2.5	76 2.5	.20	82 1.9	77 2.5	.12			–
STTI	15413 718	14470 466	.28	14426 524	14738 515	.50			–
720 Kpm Workload									
RPE	10.6 .37	11.0 .45	.50	8.9 .30	9.5 .33	.18			–
HR	121 2.8	121 1.9	.96	116 2.8	124 2.2	.06			–
SBP	157 5.3	159 4.9	.76	154 3.8	164 4.9	.12			–
DBP	78 2.4	76 2.4	.53	80 2.1	76 2.7	.21			–
STTI	19046 896	19267 742	.86	17979 650	20373 867	.03			–
1080 Kpm Workload									
RPE	13.2 .40	14.0 .38	.15	11.7 .36	12.9 .42	–	11.9	12.6	.17
HR	140 3.1	144 2.2	.34	134 3.1	144 1.8	.01			–

Table II. Pre- and Posttest Mean Values for
Cardiovascular Function Measurements (continued)

Variable	Initial Test* Exp. (18)	Con. (14)	P	Final Test* Exp.	Con.	P	Initial to Final† Exp.	Con.	P
SBP	171 5.9	188 5.0	.04	171 4.4	185 5.3	–	175	180	.38
DBP	75 2.9	75 3.5	.95	76 2.3	75 2.4	.74			–
STTI	24038 1111	27163 820	.04	23017 948	26742 845	–	23754	25796	.09
1260 Kpm Workload									
RPE	15.1 .44	15.9 .50	.24	13.8 .39	15.6 .50	.01			–
HR	151	156	.34	147	157	.03			–
1440 Kpm Workload									
RPE	16.7 .44	17.7 .44	.11	16.2 .47	17.4 .49	–	16.5	17.0	.39
HR	163 2.8	167 1.9	.26	158 3.0	165 1.9	.09			
SBP	192 5.5	205 5.6	.11	194 5.2	208 7.1	–	198	203	.44
DBP	73 3.1	74 2.6	.82	71 2.6	71 3.1	.96			–
STTI	31203 1051	34104 924	.05	30486 1145	34325 1162	–	31612	33182	.23
1620 Kpm Workload									
RPE	17.9 .38	18.8 .37	.11	18.1 .38	19.0 .36	–	18.4	18.6	.56
HR	172 2.3	174 2.0	.55	168 2.8	176 2.0	.05	–	–	–
1800 Kpm Workload									
RPE	18.9 .22	18.8 .48	.84	19.0 .23	19.5 .34	.25			–
HR	177 2.4	181 4.0	.40	171 1.8	181 3.8	.01			–
SBP	203 6.5	199 5.5	.75	204 6.3	208 11.5	.75			–
DBP	69 3.5	73 1.8	.53	65 3.5	65 3.5	.99			–

Table II. Pre- and Posttest Mean Values for
Cardiovascular Function Measurements (continued)

Variable	Initial Test* Exp. (18)	Con. (14)	P	Final Test* Exp.	Con.	P	Initial to Final† Exp.	Con.	P
STTI	35872	35948	.97	34964	37518	.28			–
	1264	777		1239	1920				
Max. Work									
RPE	19.6	19.6	.94	19.7	19.6	.92			–
	.12	.17		.11	.23				
HR	181	180	.57	180	180	.87			–
	2.0	2.1		1.8	2.3				
SBP	206	213	.44	208	218	.25			–
	6.2	5.0		4.7	6.7				
DBP	73	76	.46	70	71	.95			–
	3.0	2.7		2.9	2.7				
STTI	37319	38279	.52	37470	38758	.39			–
	1104	819		817	1321				
Recovery – 360									
RPE	7.3	8.2	.21	6.6	7.2	.11			–
	.45	.55		.38	.12				
HR	139	140	.70	138	143	.31			–
	2.8	2.4		3.2	3.4				
SBP	178	180	.90	182	185	.73			–
	5.8	7.0		6.9	5.1				
DBP	68	68	.95	63	62	.85			–
	3.2	2.9		3.1	2.5				
STTI	24978	25075	.93	25481	26491	.49			–
	695	827		1080	665				
Rec – Rest – 3									
HR	118	122	.26	113	120	.16			–
	2.1	3.2		3.1	3.7				
SBP	156	161	.54	170	168	.77			–
	5.2	6.1		4.6	5.8				
DBP	71	67	.37	67	67	.99			–
	3.1	2.9		2.6	2.5				
STTI	18288	19574	.27	19216	20070	.44			–
	710	933		728	803				
Recovery – 5									
HR	107	107	.96	104	107	.37			–
	2.3	2.5		2.2	3.6				

Table II. Pre- and Posttest Mean Values for Cardiovascular Function Measurements (continued)

Variable	Initial Test* Exp. (18)	Con. (14)	P	Final Test* Exp.	Con.	P	Initial to Final† Exp.	Con.	P
SBP	141 4.5	141 4.5	.94	147 2.7	151 4.8	.44			–
DBP	80 2.4	72 3.3	.04	78 1.8	74 3.0	–	76	76	.83
STTI	15045 628	16000 914	.38	15212 445	16219 814	.26			–
Total ride time (min)	14.4 .45	13.3 .60	.16	14.8 .45	12.8 .60	–	14.5	13.5	.03
Physical work capacity-170	1571 49	1532 34	.53	1672 55	1498 37	.02			–
STTI-25,000 work level	1117 63	1006 39	.18	1177 55	988 51	–	1145	1029	.06
10 Sec Post Max (at 360)									
HR	164	168	.37	165	169	.26			–
STTI	29501 779	31136 1155	.41	30313 1307	31940 865	.35			–
2-mile run time	13:08	13:04	.95	11:50	12:44	.01			
Age	19.3	20.1	.04						
Height	74.6	72.7	.01						
Weight	210 4.9	197 4.2	.05	210	195				

*Group mean and standard error of mean reported for each variable. Difference determined by t-test. Significant differences, P < .05.

†Adjusted means reported. Group differences determined by analysis of covariance with final test variable being criterion variable and initial test variable being covariate.

Table III. Mean Values of Selected Workout Variables

	Workout "A" Session #1	Session #17	%	Workout "B" Session #2	Session #16	%
Amount of resistance	93.8#	146.8#	+58.54	72.7#	103.9#	+43.06
Number of repetitions	9.1	9.7	+ 6.59	12.5	12.6	+ 0.8
Duration of the workout	37.7 min	28.6 min	−24.09	27.9 min	23.2 min	−16.94

Discussion and Conclusions

In the present study, by maintaining the intensity of the training at a high level, substantial improvement was achieved in both the level of muscular fitness and the cardiovascular condition of the experimental subjects. In addition to enabling the subjects to accommodate more resistance in a shorter period of time, the training caused the experimental group to work more efficiently (lower HR) at light, moderate and near-maximal levels. The subjects could also do more work before reaching a set heart rate (170), as well as do more total work. The similarity of their response to maximal work indicates that they appeared to be stressed to similar maximal levels. Accordingly, the differences in total work appear to have resulted from changes in cardiovascular condition, not from different levels of subject motivation.

The results of this study support the conclusion that the consequences of a weight training program are directly related to the methods and equipment used in the program. Obviously, the methods and procedures followed in the experimental training, in concert with the mechanical and design advantages of the Nautilus machines, affected more than merely the muscular fitness of the subjects.

Unfortunately, the misinformation and speculation attendant to many of the traditional practices in weight training have hampered the search for insight and clarification into the proper ways to train and the benefits of such training. One of the most lamentable byproducts of such a state of affairs is that many questions concerning weight training remain unanswered. Hopefully, the results of "Project Total Conditioning" will contribute, not only a partial solution to many of the enigmas associated with weight training, but also the impetus for additional scientific inquiry into this area.

Impact of Yogic Exercises on the Indian Field Hockey Team — Winners of the Third World Cup, 1975

S. Mookerjee, K. S. Chahal
and C. Giri

The "Pre-start Phenomenon" based on Pavlov's doctrine of higher nervous activity may elucidate the stressful effects of competitive situations by the conditioned reflex regulation of body functions. Morehouse suggests that a competitive setting influences the state of the organism before the start and also affects its activity during the period of the effort and in the restorative period after it is over [4].

During intensive training under high emotional tension the nonspecific natural resistance to stress is lost first. The vegetative functions deteriorate next, and finally the motor coordinations are affected resulting in poor performance. Since in severe competition the hard physical work with emotional tensions is bound to be present, several ways of meeting these stresses are sought by diet, physiotherapeutic means, improved routines of training and, finally, by relaxation [2].

It is now an accepted practice in countries leading in various sports to emphasize relaxation before an important competition. Jacobson and Rathbone had introduced and established specific techniques for relaxation to release tension [5]. Too much tension results in hypertonus which is detrimental to the individual's performance [6]. Also it disturbs his other important physiological functions like digestion, circulation, excretion and sleep.

The decisive role played by the mind in promoting success or failure is a well-recognized factor and much careful attention is nowadays given to the psychological attitude of team members especially during their precompetition training program. According to Michielli there is evidence that emotional and psychological stress causes specific physiological changes in the body. It has been shown

---

S. Mookerjee and K. S. Chahal, Department of Physiology, Christian Medical College, Ludhiana and C. Giri, State Yoga Organizer, Chandigarh, India.

that daily emotional stress may be sufficient to impair total body efficiency [3]. Precompetition tension creates various types of emotional problems since each individual in a team is temperamentally different, coming from different backgrounds. A well-knit team being encouraged to be fairly confident of its success tries to do its best, but the moment there are differences and emotional problems among the team members chiefly arising due to tension and stress, the team is very likely doomed to failure. The building of team spirit involves influencing the mental set of the team members to stay together and work together to the best of their abilities for the common cause and motivation, so that they may bring honor to their team and country. Besides the physical fitness of a team this team spirit produces the psyche which is another very important factor in promoting success.

While the Indian National Hockey Team was undergoing training at Panjab University, Chandigarh, before the Third World Cup Hockey tournament at Kuala Lumpur, tests were conducted by us to study their physical fitness. We wanted to insure their deep relaxation to promote improved performance. It was decided to follow our Indian method, so yogic exercises were introduced. The beneficial role of isometric and deep relaxation exercises is now well accepted and yogic exercises (Asanas) fall in this category. It was not possible to follow all the steps of "Astanga Yoga" of Maharashi Patanjali and only part of "Bahiranga Yoga" could be attempted in the daily routine of the coaching camp with strict discipline. Every morning a few asanas were practiced by all the players for some time to promote flexibility of the body, followed by "Shavasana" which was emphasized to insure concentration and deep relaxation. There was definite indication of reduction of tension and stress as the trainees continued developing a less tense attitude and there were no sleep disturbances or any other complaints arising due to stress. Yogic exercises had significantly helped in reducing tension and the players exhibited a relaxed state, which slowly and steadily improved their performance in the field. Some of the significant physiological parameters are presented (Figs. 1-10).

All these changes cannot be attributed to the yogic exercises alone and could be also due to the regular hard physical training. However, the decrease of pulse rate, blood pressure and resting metabolism and also some of the lung parameters showing significant changes and improvement is suggestive of reduction of tension [1]. Subsequently, players under great stress during the tournament trailing behind in crucial matches could remain calm and steady, not

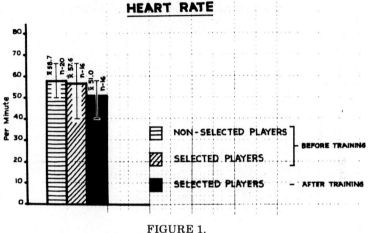

FIGURE 1.

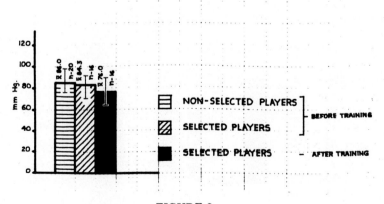

FIGURE 2.

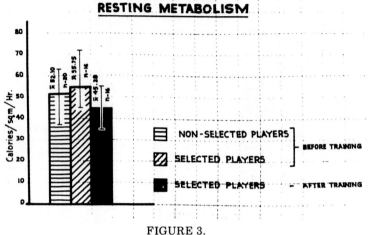

FIGURE 3.

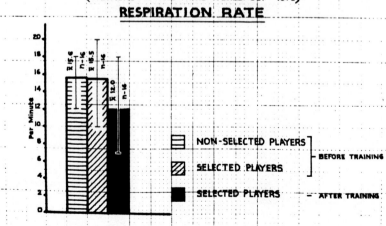

FIGURE 4.

SOME PHYSIOLOGICAL PARAMETERS OF THE NATIONAL HOCKEY TEAM OF INDIA
(WINNERS OF THE THIRD WORLD CUP - 1975)
VENTILATION EQUIVALENT

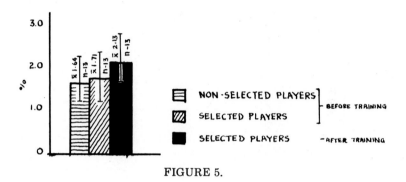

FIGURE 5.

SOME PHYSIOLOGICAL PARAMETERS OF THE NATIONAL HOCKEY TEAM OF INDIA
(WINNERS OF THE THIRD WORLD CUP — 1975)
TIDAL VOLUME

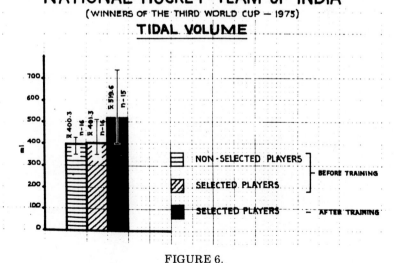

FIGURE 6.

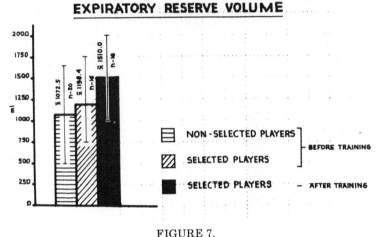

FIGURE 7.

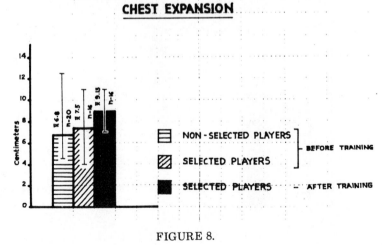

FIGURE 8.

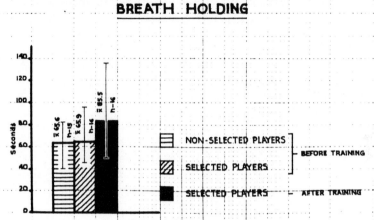

FIGURE 9.

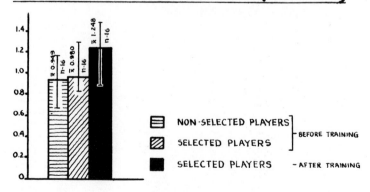

FIGURE 10.

only equalizing but winning eventually. This steadiness could be attributed to improved mental fitness along with physical fitness. Adequate yogic training leads the mind to such a tranquil equilibrium that the person automatically performs his task to the best of his ability without unduly worrying about the consequences or rewards. The introduction of yogic exercises in the coaching camp seemed to be one of the deciding factors in the ultimate success of our hockey team against apparently physically superior formidable opponents, supporting the statement: "They succeed who believe they can." Yogic training promotes this self-confidence.

Acknowledgment

Our grateful appreciation to all those who have assisted and labored to make this study worthwhile, especially the players, who cooperated with us throughout, have certainly earned our sincere gratitude.

References

1. Baumann, R. et al: Influence of acute psychic stress situation on biochemical and vegetative parameters of essential hypertension at early stages of disease. Psychother. Psychosom. 22:131-140, 1973.
2. Karpovitch, P.: Physiology of Muscular Activity, ed. 6. Philadelphia and London:W. B. Saunders Company, 1965.
3. Michielli, W.: Stresses. Encyclopedia of Sports Science and Medicine. New York:MacMillan Company, VII (B) 12, 1971, p. 1408.
4. Morehouse, L. and Miller, A.: Physiology of Exercise, ed. 6. St. Louis:The C. V. Mosby Company, 1971.
5. Rathbone, J.L.: Relaxation. Philadelphia:Lea & Febiger, 1969, pp. 92-103.
6. Sainbury, P. and Gibson, J.J.: Symptoms of anxiety and tension and the accompanying physiological changes in the muscular system. J. Neurol. Neurosurg. Psychiat. 17:216-224, 1954.

The Physiological Responses During Kendo (Japanese Fencing) Practice on Japanese Men 6 to 73 Years of Age

Noboru Niwa

Introduction

The purpose of the present study was to investigate the relative metabolic rate, calorie requirement, ventilation, heart rate, ratio of oxygen uptake during exercise to maximum oxygen uptake and oxygen debt to oxygen requirement in Kendo practice.

Kendo, a traditional Japanese sport, is gaining worldwide popularity as a good training sport for body and mind regardless of age or sex. In Japan a man of 89 years still enjoys practicing, not to mention men in their sixties or seventies. From the view of kinetics, blow striking is a major exercise.

Methods

The subjects were 26 males, aged 6 to 73, who have continually practiced Kendo (Table I). The subject was connected to a Douglas bag through a face mask and a suitable length of tubing (Fig. 1). A transmitter of telemeter was put at the back of the waist. Expired gas was collected during 10-minute rest, 5-minute exercise and 30-minute recovery. The test to measure maximum oxygen uptake on a Monark bicycle ergometer was based on the method that is described in IBP Handbook No. 9 *Human Biology*. The bicycle test was a progressive work test on the bicycle ergometer which was designed to exhaust the subject in approximately six to seven minutes. Pedal frequency was maintained as closely as possible to 60 rpm with the aid of a metronome. The initial workload was 90 to 720 kpm/min. The workload was generally increased at a rate of 180 kpm at a 2-minute interval, until the subjects could no longer perform at the prescribed cadence. The subjects in their seventies

Noboru Niwa, Department of Health and Physical Education, Tokyo Gakugei University, Tokyo, Japan.

Table I. Characteristics of Subjects

Subject No.	Age yr	Height cm	Weight kg	BSA, m^2	$\dot{V}O_2$ max, ml/kg/min
1	6	115	21	0.82	40.0
2	7	120	21	0.85	49.6
3	8	128	25	0.96	54.2
4	8	128	28	1.00	39.6
5	10	138	35	1.17	45.2
6	10	133	28	1.04	42.1
7	12	158	45	1.43	39.2
8	12	155	40	1.33	48.6
9	14	163	56	1.61	43.3
10	14	160	51	1.53	44.0
11	16	164	62	1.69	42.3
12	16	160	48	1.49	40.4
13	19	169	64	1.75	42.3
14	20	164	58	1.64	46.4
15	21	165	61	1.69	45.8
16	23	163	57	1.63	44.8
17	30	170	62	1.74	43.7
18	35	157	59	1.60	42.4
19	46	176	80	1.98	31.4
20	47	171	71	1.85	35.1
21	56	160	55	1.58	33.3
22	57	163	61	1.78	29.8
23	64	164	68	1.76	26.5
24	65	162	63	1.69	25.5
25	71	165	55	1.61	29.1
26	73	165	56	1.62	31.1

walked on the treadmill, because they were strikingly weak and, at the same time, to avoid risk. This treadmill test was a progressive work test designed to be started at the horizontal walking grade and to exhaust the subject at 15%. Walking speed was set to be 70 meters/min.

Time (min)	w-up (2')	start	1 min	2 min	3 min	4 min	5 min
Grade %	0	0	5	10	12.5	15	15

Expired gas was collected at every minute for four minutes from the start and collected gas at two times, at the last minute to exhaustion and at two minutes before the last was analyzed. The larger figure was taken as the maximum oxygen uptake. The gas samples were analyzed by the Scholander Micro Gas Analyzer. Basal metabolism was calculated from body surface area according to the formula of Takahira. Heart rate was measured by a one-channel telemeter and

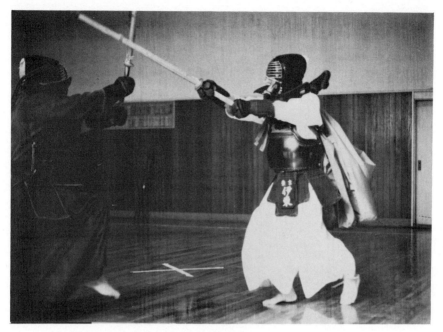

FIG. 1. Kendo subject, age 73, during five-minute exercise.

recorded on an oscillograph. Striking times and movements of each subject during exercise were recorded on 8 mm film. These measurements were done from April 1974 to December 1975 at the laboratory of our University.

Results

Tables II and III show relative metabolic rate, calorie requirement, ventilation, heart rate, ratio of oxygen uptake during exercise to maximum oxygen uptake and oxygen debt to oxygen requirement of each subject in match practice. Each measurement value was as follows: the relative metabolic rate (RMR) was 2.7 to 13.6 and the mean was 8.8 ± 3.1; the calorie requirement (cal. req.) was 5.5 to 16.6 cal/kg/hr and the mean 10.5 cal/kg/hr $\pm$ 3.0; the ventilation ($\dot{V}_E \cdot$ BTPS) was 44 to 173 liters/min and the mean 115 liters/min $\pm$ 35; the ratio of oxygen uptake ($\dot{V}O_2$) during exercise to maximum oxygen uptake ($\dot{V}O_2$ max) was approximately 45% to 90% and the mean 72.4% $\pm$ 11.5; the heart rate (HR) during exercise was 115 to 176 beats/min after three minutes from the start of exercise and the mean 153 beats/min $\pm$ 16; the heart rate after five minutes at the end of the exercise period was 118 to 185 beats/min

Table II. RMR, Calorie Requirement, $\dot{V}_E$, and $\dot{V}O_2/\dot{V}O_2$ max
in Kendo Practice

Subject	RMR	Cal. Req. (Cal/kg/hr)	$\dot{V}_E$ (l/min, BTPS)	VO_2/VO_2 max (%)
1	3.2	6.5	44	61.3
2	2.7	5.5	47	46.6
3	3.3	6.2	52	45.2
4	5.5	10.0	71	73.0
5	6.7	10.4	94	68.8
6	5.1	8.9	77	66.3
7	9.7	13.9	152	85.7
8	10.0	15.1	126	81.3
9	11.0	13.0	130	81.3
10	8.0	9.9	100	62.3
11	11.1	12.1	109	68.3
12	9.0	16.6	108	75.5
13	12.3	13.1	156	83.2
14	10.1	10.9	111	73.9
15	9.8	10.3	131	64.8
16	12.4	13.5	151	77.7
17	13.6	14.4	173	88.1
18	13.2	13.4	153	89.9
19	10.8	9.8	145	79.9
20	10.7	10.2	134	77.5
21	7.9	8.1	105	70.3
22	7.3	7.5	100	72.1
23	9.3	8.0	145	83.8
24	9.5	9.2	142	74.5
25	6.8	6.9	116	56.7
26	9.7	9.1	106	75.2
Mean	8.8	10.5	115	72.4
SD	3.1	3.0	35	11.5

and the mean 159 beats/min ± 18; the ratio of oxygen debt to oxygen requirement was 10.8% to 45.7% and the mean 29.1% ± 8.5.

Discussion

Match practice in the present study is an exercise which is largely influenced by the partner. Figure 2 shows the heart rate of a subject aged 51 when he performed almost continually five exercise matches with five partners who had different ranks. (The ranks are divided from 1 to 10 and the larger number means the better player. The ninth and tenth are the supreme and honorary grades.) The five partners' ranks were as follows: A and E had the third rank; C, second; B and D had no rank. The heart rate increased as the rank of

Table III. HR and O_2 Debt/O_2 Requirement in Kendo Practice

Subject	HR (beats/min)		O_2 Debt/O_2 Requirement (%)
	3 min	5 min	
1	153	171	18.1
2	160	164	10.8
3	141	153	12.0
4	150	160	31.0
5	167	171	25.4
6	133	125	26.9
7	167	180	37.5
8	176	185	32.2
9	176	176	28.2
10	147	169	29.4
11	153	160	37.7
12	167	169	40.6
13	160	171	26.5
14	144	147	17.6
15	144	152	25.3
16	164	176	30.7
17	169	180	27.7
18	157	169	23.0
19	164	160	33.4
20	160	165	30.0
21	129	129	27.0
22	133	138	28.8
23	137	137	45.7
24	164	167	34.4
25	115	118	42.8
26	138	145	34.7
Mean	153	159	29.1
SD	16	18	8.5

the partner improved. This is ascertained by my other experiments and the investigation by Ogawa reports the same result. Besides, the intensity of exercise can be adjusted in this match practice. It was observed that the increasing curve around the upward mark ($\uparrow$) resulted from the aggressive blows of the subject against partner D when he was tired and did not try to strike.

In order to know whether the match practice of kendo has training effects, Katsuta examined the physical fitness of men aged 45 to 55 who had exercised more than 25 years and still had at least one training a week and who had not had any training since their young days. The subjects were kendo men, track and field sportsmen, ballgame players and those who did not have any

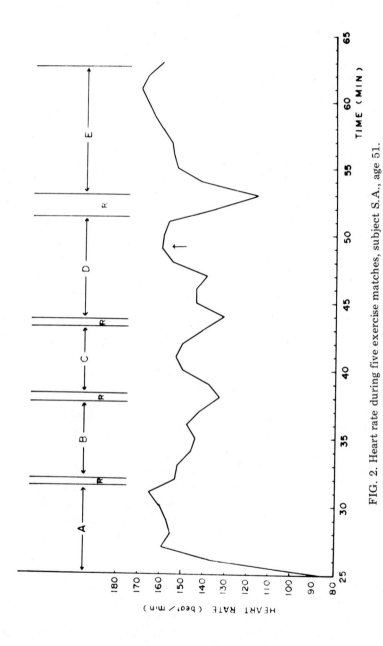

FIG. 2. Heart rate during five exercise matches, subject S.A., age 51.

Table IV. Physical Fitness of Four Groups Aged 45 to 55 (Mean)

Group	N	Height, cm	Weight kg	Back Strength kg	Vital Capacity ml	Step Test Score	Reaction Time msec (light)
Kendo	8	168.5	67.8	142	4009	64.4	383
Track and field sports	5	169.3	71.8	173	4330	52.8	338
Ball game	5	167.5	68.9	133	4020	56.8	341
Control	14	160.0	58.7	132	3306	52.4	393

particular sport. Table IV shows the results. Kendo men showed the best result in the step test, which means that kendo practice has endurance training effect. As the results showed, the ratio in our experiments of oxygen uptake during exercise to maximum oxygen uptake was approximately 45% to 90% and the mean 72.4 ± 11.5. In kendo, exercise of this intensity which lasts approximately five minutes is usually repeated several times. Therefore, not to speak of maintenance of physical fitness, training effect of physical fitness can be enough expected. But as the studies of Hermansen, Saltin and others show, it should be taken into consideration that measurement values on the bicycle ergometer are a bit smaller than the values on the treadmill.

Evaluation de l'aptitude physique d'une sélection de nageurs ivoiriens

G. Danon, Y. Dosso,
F. Boutros-Toni et J. M. Kanga

Introduction

La pratique de la natation est très peu répandue dans un certain nombre de pays africains contrairement à ce que l'on pourrait penser. En 1972, à la Faculté de médecine d'Abidjan, une enquête sur environ une centaine d'étudiants de deuxième année a permis de constater qu'aucun des étudiants africains ne savait nager.

D'autre part, en comparent les résultats spirographiques de ces étudiants à ceux des sujets européens du même âge on mettait en évidence que la capacité vitale représentait 77% environ en moyenne des valeurs théoriques moyennes utilisées en France* Danon [8]. Ces résultats sont en accord avec ceux obtenus sur des populations d'origine africaine, en particulier, parmi les plus récents, aux Etats Unis Abramowitz et coll. [1], Miller et coll. [16], au Nigéria Femi-Pearse et Elebute 1971 [11], et en Afrique du Sud, Johansen et Erasmus [12].

Une étude biométrique comparée entre deux populations homogènes ivoirienne et caucasienne fait apparaître que, lorsqu'on considère deux sujets de même taille, l'ivoirien a les membres inférieurs plus longs et donc le thorax plus court (et aussi plus étroit) que l'européen. C'est donc vraisemblablement parce qu'il a un volume thoracique plus faible que l'africain a une capacité vitale moindre.

Depuis quelques années, le Ministère de la Jeunesse et des Sports a fait de sérieux efforts pour promouvoir la pratique de la natation par les enfants. Dans le cadre d'un programme de recherche portant sur "l'évaluation de l'aptitude physique de la population ivoirienne et de ses relations avec le développement,"† il a semblé intéressant

---

G. Danon, Y. Dosso, F. Boutros-Toni et J. M. Kanga, Laboratoires de physiologie-explorations fonctionnelles, Faculté de médecine, Abidjan, Côte d'Ivoire.

*Valeurs théoriques de la C.E.C.A.

†Programme F.M. N° 3506 subventionné par le Ministère de la Recherche Scientifique de Côte d'Ivoire (Professeur agrégé G. Danon).

d'étudier des enfants nageurs et, en les comparant à des enfants non nageurs de rechercher d'éventuelles modifications morphologiques et physiologiques.

Les sportifs des équipes nationales et principalement les membres de l'équipe de natation ont également été examinés. Les résultats rapportés concernent une sélection de ces nageurs. Le but de cette étude était d'évaluer leur aptitude physique et de comparer les divers paramètres mesurés à la fois aux valeurs de la population ivoirienne et aux résultats de la littérature.

Sujets et méthodes

Tous les examens ont été pratiqués au laboratoire en atmosphère climatisée ($22°C$, 55% d'humidité, environ).

Il y avait 20 nageurs de sexe masculin âgés de 11 à 26 ans lors du premier examen (13 à 30 ans en 1976). Parmi eux certains ont été suivis depuis 1972. On a pris comme population de référence, ne sachant pas nager, des enfants de même provenance socio-économique, et, pour les adultes, essentiellement des étudiants en médecine de 2ème année.

Méthodes

1. *Mesures anthropométriques:* on a mesuré poids, taille debout, taille assis, longueur des membres, les diamètres (thoraciques et osseux), les périmètres (du thorax et des membres). Le poids maigre a été calculé à partir de la somme de quatre plis cutanés d'après Durnin et Rahaman [9].

2. *Spirographie:* on a mesuré les divers volumes et débits pulmonaires. Le volume résiduel a été déterminé par la méthode de dilution à l'hélium (appareillage Morgan). Tous les résultats ont été exprimés dans les conditions BTPS et comparés (à l'exception du volume résiduel) aux valeurs de référence de la population ivoirienne établies à partir de la thèse de Kounandi Coulibaly [13].

3. *La capacité de diffusion* pulmonaire de l'oxyde de carbone a été déterminée en régime stable et en apnée par le "Transfert Test Morgan."

Les résultats en apnée ont été comparés aux valeurs de référence ivoiriennes ainsi qu'aux valeurs rapportées par Cotes [5] sur les enfants et les adultes caucasiens.

4. *La consommation maximale d'oxygène* ($\dot{V}O_2$ max) a été estimée par le step-test d'Astrand-Ryhming [4]. On a enregistré la

fréquence cardiaque sur un physiographe (Narco Biosystem), à partir de deux électrodes transthoraciques. Pour les enfants, le nomogramme utilisé pour les adultes a été extrapolé selon des indications de Shephard [20] et il a été tenu compte de la correction pour la fréquence cardiaque.

5. *La capacité de travail* correspondant à 170 pulsations cardiaques (CT 170) a été mesurée graphiquement à partir de trois exercices sous-maximaux sur bicyclette ergométrique.

6. *Le volume cardiaque* a été mesuré en décubitus ventral par la méthode radiographique décrite par Reindell [19].

Résultats

1. *Anthropométrie:* En ce qui concerne la taille debout, dans toutes les tranches d'âge considérées, enfants, adolescents, adultes, on constate que les nageurs sont en moyenne plus grands que les témoins. Les dimensions du thorax sont aussi significativement supérieures à celles des témoins du même âge (Tableau I). Ces différences persistent quand on corrige les résultats pour tenir compte de la taille debout.

Le rapport poids maigre/poids total est significativement plus grand chez les nageurs.

2. *Spirographie* (Figs. 1 et 2): Pour chacun des nageurs, la capacité vitale est supérieure à la valeur théorique moyenne ivoirienne. Les différences sont significatives quelle que soit la tranche d'âge considérée.

Tableau I. Comparaison entre des paramètres biométriques de nageurs et non-nageurs (adultes de 18 à 30 ans)

	Nageurs (N = 10) moyenne ± écart-type (cm)	Etudiants (N = 59) moyenne ± écart-type (cm)	Test t
Taille debout	172.9 ± 4.75	170.2 ± 6.01	NS
Taille assis	87.5 ± 3.50	85.9 ± 3.02	NS
Circonférence poitrine	92.9 ± 4.14	85 ± 4.28	TS
Diamètre thoracique transverse	34.7 ± 2.70	30.9 ± 1.73	TS
Diamètre thoracique antéro-postérieur	21.2 ± 1.13	19.6 ± 1.36	TS
Diamètre biacromial	37.4 ± 2.10	33.9 ± 1.58	TS

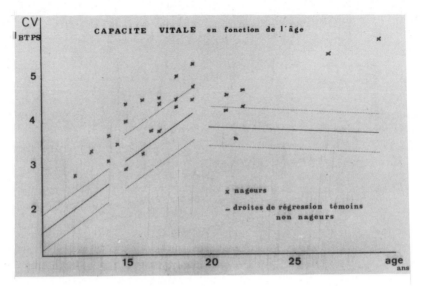

FIG. 1. Capacité vitale des nageurs en fonction de l'âge comparaison avec des valeurs de témoins ivoiriens non nageurs.

En ce qui concerne les sujets adultes (18 ans et plus), la capacité vitale représente en moyenne 93% des valeurs théoriques de la C.E.C.A. c'est-à-dire qu'elle est équivalente à celle des européens.

Le volume résiduel des nageurs adultes représente 108% des valeurs théoriques moyennes de la C.E.C.A. et il n'est pas significativement différent de celui de la population estudiantine de même âge. Il est donc à noter que le volume résiduel des africains n'est pas inférieur à celui des européens, contrairement aux autres volumes pulmonaires, du moins pour l'échantillonnage observé. Toutefois, comme le volume de réserve expiratoire est plus faible que celui de l'européen, la capacité résiduelle fonctionnelle est inférieure.

3. *La capacité de diffusion* pulmonaire mesurée par le transfert de l'oxyde de carbone en apnée (T_{CO}) est significativement supérieure aux valeurs théoriques (Fig. 3).

La plus grande valeur de T_{CO} a été obtenue chez un sujet de 19 ans (50.3 ml STPD torr^{-1}·min^{-1}). Elle est supérieure de 53% aux valeurs de Cotes. C'est un nageur de 14 ans et demi qui a la valeur la plus basse, 31.3 ml STPD min^{-1}·torr^{-1}, soit 112% de la valeur théorique.

Il n'a pas été tenu compte des résultats de la diffusion en régime stable qui sont apparus beaucoup moins reproductibles que ceux en apnée.

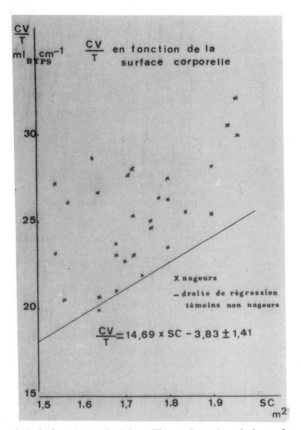

FIG. 2. Capacité vitale rapportée à la taille en fonction de la surface corporelle.

4. *Le volume cardiaque* des sujets varie entre 408 ml pour un jeune nageur de 13 ans et 950 ml à 26 ans. Rapportées au poids corporel, les valeurs sont comprises entre 9.5 et 12.8 ml·kg^{-1}. La figure 4 met an évidence que tous les volumes sont au dessus de la droite de régression établie sur la population témoin (enfants et adolescents). Lorsqu'on compare le volume cardiaque moyen pour l'ensemble des nageurs il est significativement supérieur à celui des témoins adultes de 20 à 30 ans bien que la moyenne d'âge soit significativement inférieure (561 ml ± 93 pour les témoins et 722 ml ± 96 pour les nageurs soit respectivement 8.88 ml·kg^{-1} ± 1.42 et 11.65 ml·kg^{-1} ± 0.88).

5. *La consommation maximale d'oxygène* est comprise entre 2.80 1 pour un enfant de 14 ans et 6.21 1 STPD min^{-1} pour le nageur le plus âgé (49.5 et 82.1 ml STPD min^{-1}·kg^{-1}). Il existe une corrélation linéaire entre la $\dot{V}O_2$ max et l'âge des nageurs (Fig. 5).

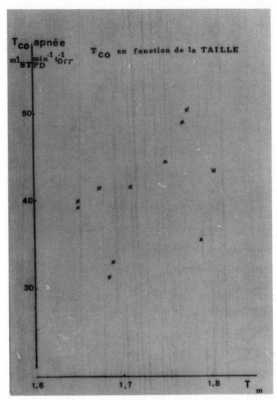

FIG. 3. Capacité de diffusion en apnée des nageurs en fonction de la taille.

La comparaison des moyennes de la $\dot{V}O_2$ max des nageurs et des témoins adultes met en évidence des différences très significatives ($p < 0.01$) (Tableau II).

Tableau II. Comparaison des moyennes des consommations
maximales d'oxygène

Paramètres	Nageurs (N = 14)	Etudiants (N = 27)	Test t
Age (ans)	17.9 ± 4.3	23.8 ± 6.6	TS
$\dot{V}O_2$ max (l STPD min⁻¹)	4.15 ± 0.99	3.07 ± 0.32	TS
$\dot{V}O_2$ (ml STPD min⁻¹ · kg⁻¹)	64.6 ± 9.9	46.3 ± 7.5	TS

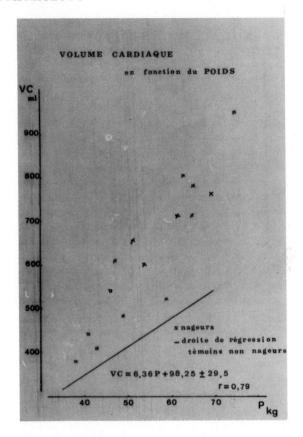

FIG. 4. Valeurs du volume cardiaque en fonction du poids des nageurs comparées à la ligne de regression des témoins non nageurs.

6. *La capacité de travail 170* des nageurs est très significative-ment supérieure à celle des étudiants. On a obtenu 1,113 kgm·min^{-1} pour les nageurs et 912 pour les étudiants soit 16.4 kgm·min^{-1}·kg^{-1} et 13.8, respectivement.

Discussion

Ces résultats mettent en évidence des différences morphologiques et physiologiques entre les nageurs et les témoins. Les modifications portent sur la taille, les dimensions du thorax, les volumes pul-monaires, la capacité de diffusion, le volume cardiaque, la consom-mation maximale d'oxygène, la capacité de travail 170.

Un certain nombre d'auteurs ont étudié des nageurs, dont Newman et coll. [18], Astrand et coll. [3], Magel et Faulkner [15],

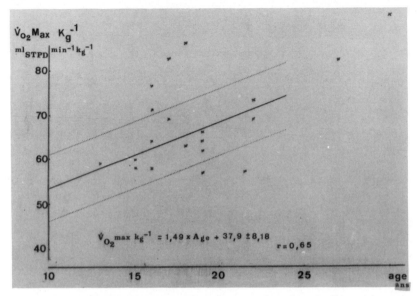

FIG. 5. Consommation maximale d'oxygène en fonction de l'âge des nageurs avec la ligne de régression correspondante.

Ekblom et coll. [10], Magel et Andersen [14] Sobolova et coll. [21], Andrew et coll. [2], et Cunningham et Eynon [6]. Ils ont également constaté de semblables différences dans les paramètres mesurés mais il s'agissait toujours de sujets d'origine caucasienne.

Pour les sujets africains, divers problèmes se posent dont l'un concerne la diffusion alvéolo-capillaire. Les nageurs ont généralement une capacité de diffusion élevée, comme Mostyn et coll. [17] l'ont bien montré, mais ils ont aussi de très grandes capacités vitales. Or, on constate que si la capacité vitale des nageurs ivoiriens, après plusieurs années d'entraînement, atteint la capacité vitale théorique moyenne de l'européen, la capacité de diffusion dépasse parfois de plus de 50% les valeurs théoriques moyennes. D'autre part, la capacité de diffusion de l'africain non entraîné est égale à celle du caucasien — Miller [16], Cotes [5], Danon et Dosso 1976 (non publié). Une étude plus approfondie avec la mesure du volume capillaire pulmonaire devrait permettre d'expliquer ces résultats.

Malgré les différences biométriques, l'africain a une $\dot{V}O_2$ max comparable à celle de l'européen lorsqu'on la rapporte au poids corporel — Wyndham et Heyns [23], Danon et coll. [8]. Toutefois sa moindre adiposité et sa plus faible capacité résiduelle fonctionnelle contribuent à une moins bonne flottabilité. Si, par l'entraînement, la diffusion et le transport de l'oxygène deviennent excellents il est possible que ces facteurs contrebalancent la moins bonne flottabilité. Il est d'ailleurs intéressant de constater qu'une étude faite sur des enfants de 4 à 16 ans a montré qu'après deux ans de pratique de la natation (en dehors de la compétition), le volume cardiaque de l'ivoirien était significativement supérieur à celui des témoins non nageurs Danon et coll. [7].

On ne connaît pas encore avec précision le rôle des facteurs acquis comme l'entraînement, la période de la vie où il est pratiqué, l'environnement, et des facteurs héréditaires dans l'amélioration des performances. L'analyse des résultats individuels fait apparaître que les effets de l'entraînement sont indépendants de l'âge de l'enfant et ils sont en accord avec les récents travaux de Weber et coll. [22] sur les jumeaux. Chez l'ivoirien, il existe une certaine homogénéité de quelques-uns des facteurs en cause (absence d'antécédents familiaux dans la pratique de la natation ou d'autres sports, même provenance socio-économique et environnement) et, des recherches dans un tel contexte devraient aider à une meilleure connaissance de ces problèmes.

Conclusion

Cette étude des nageurs ivoiriens met en évidence que la natation peut modifier d'une façon très significative les paramètres biométriques de l'africain en faisant disparaître des différences existant avec l'européen. Il est possible que la pratique de ce sport à un très jeune âge entraîne, avec l'augmentation du volume cardiaque et des volumes pulmonaires, non seulement une meilleure aptitude physique mais aussi une flottabilité comparable à celle des caucasiens.

Références

1. Abramowitz, S., Leiner, G.C., Lewis, W.A. and Small, M.T.: Vital capacity in the Negro. Am. Rev. Resp. 92:287-292, 1965.
2. Andrew, G.M., Becklake, M.R., Guleria, J.S. and Bates, D.V.: Heart and lung functions in swimmers and non athletes during growth. J. Appl. Physiol. 32:245-251, 1972.
3. Astrand, P.O., Engstrom, L., Erikson, B. et al: Girl swimmers with special reference to respiratory and circulatory adaptation and gynaecological and psychiatric aspects. Acta Paediatr. Suppl. 147, 1963.
4. Astrand, P.O. and Ryhming, I.: A nomogram for calculation of aerobic capacity from pulse rate during submaximal work. J. Appl. Physiol. 7:218, 1954.
5. Cotes, J.E.: Lung Function. Oxford:Blackwell Scientific Publications, 1975.

6. Cunningham, D.A. and Eynon, R.B.: The working capacity of young competitive swimmers 10-16 years of age. Med. Sci. Sports 5-4:227-231, 1973.

7. Danon, G. et Boutros-Toni, F.: Le volume cardiaque d'enfants de 6 à 14 ans vivant en Côte d'Ivoire. J. Physiol. (Paris) 69 — 2, 192A, 1974.

8. Danon, G., Carles, J., Marty, N. et Kounandi Coulibaly, F.: Etude de quelques paramètres biologiques des étudiants en médecine de la Faculté d'Abidjan. Ann. Univ. Abidjan Méd. 7:111-117, 1973.

9. Durnin, J.V. and Rahaman, M.M.: The assessment of the amount of fat in the human body from measurements of skinfold thickness. Br. J. Nutr. 21:681-689, 1967.

10. Ekblom, B.: Effect of physical training in adolescent boys. J. Appl. Physiol. 27:350-355, 1969.

11. Femi-Pearse, D. and Elebute, E.A.: Ventilatory function in healthy adult Nigerian. Clin. Sci. 41:203-211, 1971.

12. Johansen, Z.M. and Erasmus, L.D.: Clinical spirometry in normal Bantu. Am. Rev. Resp. Dis. 97:585-597, 1968.

13. Kounandi Coulibaly, F.: Contribution à l'étude des normes spirométriques et hémo-respiratoires de l'Africain en Côte d'Ivoire. Thèse Médecine — Abidjan, n° 63, 1975.

14. Magel, J.R. and Andersen, K.L.: Pulmonary diffusing capacity and cardiac output in young trained Norwegian swimmers and untrained subjects. Med. Sci. Sports 1:131-139, 1969.

15. Magel, J.R. and Faulkner, J.A.: Maximum oxygen uptake of college swimmers. J. Appl. Physiol. 22:929-933, 1967.

16. Miller, G.J., Cotes, J.E., Hall, A.M. et al: Lung function and exercise performance of healthy men and women of African ethnic origin. Q. J. Exp. Physiol. 57:325-341, 1972.

17. Mostyn, E.M., Helle, S., Gee, J.B.L. et al: Pulmonary diffusing capacity of athletes. J. Appl. Physiol. 18:687-695, 1963.

18. Newman, F., Smalley, B.F. and Thomson, M.L.: Comparison between body size and lung function of swimmers and normal school children. J. Physiol. London 156:9-10, 1961.

19. Reindell, H., König, K. and Roskamm, H.: Funktionsdiagnostik des gesunden und kranken Herzens. Stuttgart:Thieme Verlag, 1967.

20. Shephard, R.J.: Frontiers of fitness. Springfield, Ill.:Charles C Thomas Publisher, 1971.

21. Sobolova, V., Seliger, V., Grussova, D. et al: The influence of age and sport training in swimming on physical fitness. Acta Paediatr. Scand. Suppl. 217:63-67, 1971.

22. Weber, G., Kartodihardjo, W. and Klissouras, V.: Growth and physical training with reference to heredity. J. Appl. Physiol. 40:211-215, 1976.

23. Wyndham, C.H. and Heyns, A.J.: Determinants of oxygen consumption and maximum oxygen intake of Bantu and Caucasian males. Int. Z. Angew. Physiol. 27:51-75, 1969.

Cardiorespiratory Performance Testing in Children and Adolescent Competitive Swimmers: A Demographic Study

Douglas B. McKeag, Raymond Fuller and
Frederick W. Bakker-Arkema

Introduction

The advent of the multistage treadmill test has made possible a valid, reproducible way of measuring physical fitness. There is a paucity of data on this subject involving the 18 and under or adolescent-pre-adolescent age group. There are few longitudinal studies involving cardiorespiratory endurance and its correlation with supervised exercise programs. This study was attempted with the purpose of investigating the effects of measured exercise (competitive swimming) on the cardiorespiratory performance of adolescents and pre-adolescents — its measuring stick, the modified Bruce protocol multistage treadmill test.

Materials, Methods, Objectives

Ninety male and female competitive or beginning competitive swimmers and 21 control volunteers were tested. This group was held constant and no replacements were found for those who dropped the program. Each subject was asked to obtain both parental and medical permission prior to the series of tests. Each was screened with a health questionnaire which included pertinent physical statistics, previous swimming experience, past medical history and a cardio-respiratory review of systems. In addition, a cardiovascular physical exam was done. Each volunteer was also subjectively "rated" by his/her swimming coach.

Repeat multistage treadmill testing before, during and following the swimming season furnished the necessary data used for statistical

Douglas B. McKeag, Raymond Fuller and Frederick W. Bakker-Arkema, Blodgett Memorial Medical Center, Department of Medical Research and Grand Rapids Area Medical Education Center, Grand Rapids, Michigan, U.S.A.

415

analysis (Fig. 1). Height, weight and recent medical history, including medication intake, were recorded each time. Baseline electrocardiograms were obtained on each subject. Each youth was reminded of the test protocol prior to the testing itself. Each test was overseen by both a treadmill technician and a nurse with a resident either present or available. An arbitrary maximum heart rate of 200 beats/minute was designated the automatic stopping point; the subject could stop the test himself at any time. Blood pressure, heart rate and EKG lead V_5 were monitored continuously throughout the test and during recovery. Duration and length of recovery were measured and lead V_5 investigated for any repolarization, conduction or arrhythmia abnormalities. Duration of exercise ranged from 4½ to 24 minutes; recovery time ranged from 1 to 15 minutes. All information was then categorized and analysis of various parameters follows. Age group and sex distribution of project volunteers can be studied on Figure 2.

Results

Swimmers vs. Controls

No significant difference was noted in the duration of testing, although each group significantly lengthened their duration on subsequent treadmills. Recovery time was analyzed and revealed a difference between swimmers and controls. A decreasing quantity of time needed for recovery with each succeeding treadmill test for each group was observed. However, none of these differences were significant. Slopes of heart rate, diastolic blood pressure and systolic blood pressure rise and fall during the testing procedure were considered. While again it was evident that the heart rate rise of the swimmers and the nonswimmers decreased with each succeeding treadmill, no statistical difference was noted between the two groups. The negative slopes resulting from heart rate decrease during recovery did indicate that the swimmers recovered faster than the control group. No significance was noted in diastolic blood pressures, although, again in treadmill # 3, swimmers recovered faster than controls. The slope of systolic blood pressure changes revealed no difference between the groups.

An attempt was then made to eliminate faulty data due to lack of motivation or poor performance on the part of the subjects. All data from volunteers who did not attain a level of 90% maximal arbitrary heart rate prior to stopping the treadmill were eliminated. Swimmers and nonswimmers were again analyzed. Swimmers who

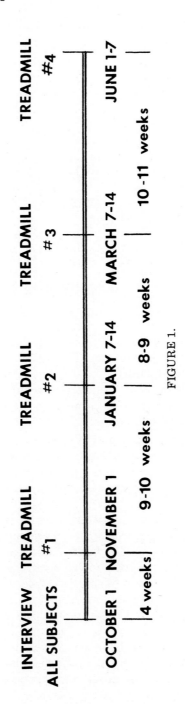

FIGURE 1.

AGE AND SEX DISTRIBUTION OF PROJECT

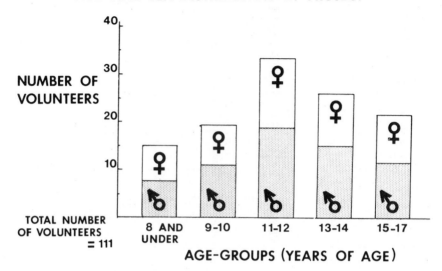

FIGURE 2.

achieved heart rates of 180/min and greater lasted longer and recovered sooner than controls. This trend, although constant, was not statistically significant.

Further analysis was conducted using various physiological parameters as subgroups and comparing the performances of swimmers and controls as seen below:

1. *Chronological age.* Analysis here was incomplete as a result of the small size of most of the groups. Where significant differences were present, they again reflected the same trend as previously stated — swimmers lasted longer and took less time recovering than controls.

2. *Age group* (arbitrarily determined on the basis of current U.S. competitive swimming age groups). Please refer again to Figure 2 for age group distribution. On the basis of all treadmills, the 9-10, 13-14, and 15-and-over age groups showed significant differences in either duration or recovery times (Table I). Also evident was the failure of the 8-and-under group to achieve a similar duration on the treadmill as the other age groups. Consequently, the recovery time was less than the others.

Examining all subjects in an age group and comparing differences by consecutive treadmills, the following can be noted:

a. The 8-and-under age group had shorter durations and recovery times than the remaining age groups.

Table I. Mean Duration and Recovery Analyzed by Age Groups

	Mean Duration (minutes)		Mean Recovery (minutes)	
	Swimmers	Control	Swimmers	Control
1) 8 and Under	12.0	12.3	3.4	2.5
2) 9 - 10	15.0	10.5	4.0	5.0
3) 11 - 12	14.3	13.9	4.8	3.5
4) 13 - 14	15.2	14.0	5.1	4.3
5) 15 and Over	14.4	14.4	5.2	7.2

b. All age groups had a shorter duration on treadmill # 1 than the other treadmills.

c. All four older age groups had similar duration values.

d. The 9-10, 11-12, 13-14 showed an increase in duration from T_1 to T_2, slight increase from T_2 to T_3, and a slight decrease from T_3 to T_4 in duration only.

e. 15-and-over subjects had highest mean duration with T_2, then showed decreases on the remaining treadmills.

f. Recovery time was consistently less for 8-and-under group and greater for 15-and-over group for all treadmills.

g. All age groups showed a decrease in recovery times with each succeeding treadmill with a significant drop for T_3 and T_4.

3. *Sex.* No differences between female swimmers and controls for duration or recovery time were noted. Male swimmers did last significantly longer and recovered faster than controls. It should be mentioned that females lasted longer and recovered quicker than males (Table II).

4. *Height and weight.* Changes in these parameters in volunteers on the average had no relation to treadmill performance.

5. *EKG findings.* On the basis of findings on the baseline electrocardiogram, two groups were formulated: those with normal EKGs and those with abnormal asymptomatic findings. No symptomatic patients were accepted for this project. No significance was

Table II. Mean Duration and Recovery Analyzed by Sex

	Mean Duration (minutes)		Mean Recovery (minutes)	
	Swimmers	Control	Swimmers	Control
1) Male	13.6	11.9	4.9	5.3
2) Female	14.8	15.1	4.2	4.4

found although the diastolic blood pressure fall appeared accentuated in the abnormal group.

6. *Cardiac rhythm.* Initial rhythm at the beginning of the testing each time was divided into normal sinus rhythm and sinus tachycardia groups with 55% and 45% of the total treadmills run, respectively. Sinus tachycardia was defined as those resting heart rates greater than 95 beats/min. Those volunteers in sinus rhythm at the start of the test lasted longer and recovered quicker than those who began in sinus tachycardia. Swimmers with sinus tachycardia had longer durations and less of a recovery time than controls with sinus tachycardia.

7. *Reasons for stopping test.* Approximately 50% of the subjects stopped their tests after requesting to do so. The remainder achieved our arbitrary maximal heart rate of 200 beats/min. Those who attained a maximal heart rate response lasted significantly longer on the treadmills and also took longer to recover. This percentage remained constant for each of the four treadmills.

Classification of these volunteers was also accomplished on the basis of nonphysiological groupings determined solely on the basis of medical history and other parameters. Again, the results are presented below:

1. *Positive medical history.* Approximately 33% of the subjects had positive past (or present) medical histories. Comparison of duration, recovery time and their respective slopes reveals no difference at all between those with positive histories and those without. The one exception appeared to be a slower, longer recovery by control subjects with a positive medical history.

2. *Competitive swimming experience.* The average number of years experience in competitive swimming for the swimmer of this project was 3.4 years with males averaging 3.9 years and females 2.8 years. Beginning swimmers without any experience were included, but controls were not. Those swimmers with greater than three years of experience had longer durations for progressive treadmills. However, they also had longer recovery times. It should be mentioned here that each succeeding treadmill recovery time became shorter with both groups.

3. *Rating* (prior to the start of the competitive season). As mentioned earlier, each volunteer was subjectively "rated" prior to the swimming season on the basis of past performance, overall ability and how this ability compared to *other competitive swimmers of the same age* for the State of Michigan. The key to each rating is as follows:

0 - control (nonswimmer)
1 - beginning swimmer (no previous record)
2 - below average swimmer
3 - average swimmer
4 - above average swimmer
5 - championship swimmer (record-holder)

From analysis of duration and recovery time by the rating system, the control group had the lowest performance of any of these groups with the beginning swimmers next (Table III). Groups 2 to 5 were closely bunched with 5-rated swimmers obviously showing the best performance and the below-average swimmers the worst performance of these four.

Discussion

This study has attempted to fill the void of information concerning the teenager and pre-teenager and his response to measured exercise. It was also able to look at various biological and epidemiological parameters and their relationship with exercise. Because of the size of this project, as well as physical and equipment limitations, actual respiratory performance was not measured. It does provide a unique look at longitudinal cardiorespiratory performance changes.

The study did show that competitive swimmers generally lasted longer on the treadmill and took less time recovering to a pretest cardiac level than controls (Fig. 3). However, these differences were not significant and mean values for these two groups were surprisingly close together. Each group improved treadmill performance — a function of two variables, I believe:

1. Acclimation to the treadmill testing procedure.

2. Improved physical endurance secondary to physical activities (training) and age.

Table III. Mean Duration and Recovery Analyzed by Rating

	Mean Duration (minutes)		Mean Recovery (minutes)	
	Swimmers	Control	Swimmers	Control
0		13.7		4.9
1	12.7		4.7	
2	14.9		5.2	
3	14.5		3.9	
4	13.8		4.5	
5	15.6		4.6	

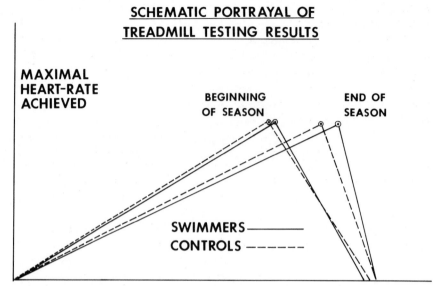

SCHEMATIC PORTRAYAL OF
TREADMILL TESTING RESULTS

MAXIMAL
HEART-RATE
ACHIEVED

BEGINNING
OF SEASON

END OF
SEASON

SWIMMERS ————
CONTROLS — — — — —

TREADMILL TESTING TIME — DURATION & RECOVERY
(MINUTES)

FIGURE 3.

A critical look at the control group reveals, perhaps, another reason for this group's performance. Almost all of the controls were the nonswimming siblings or friends of project swimmers and just as athletically active in their own respective sports as the swimmers were in their sport.

Age-group analysis considered not only duration and recovery time, but also the rate of increase and decrease of heart rate and blood pressures. It indicated that significant differences do exist between swimmers and controls in one or more of these parameters in all age groups except 8 and under. Unfortunately, this latter group lacks an appropriate number of control studies.

Examination of sex as a factor revealed a difference in performance between males and females with females performing better. Male and female swimmers outperformed their nonswimming counterparts. This is consistent with other studies.

No significant difference was noted between those subjects with "abnormal" electrocardiograms and those with normal EKGs. One child was discovered to have had rheumatic valvular disease and dropped out of the project. As might be expected, volunteers whose resting heart rate was in tachycardia did not perform as well as those who began the testing in sinus rhythm.

Significant medical history including physical deformities (such as scoliosis), allergic conditions, asthma, recurrent pneumonia, infectious mononucleosis, hypertension and corrective cardiac surgery (necessitating the use of digoxin) was considered. No significant change was seen and therefore should not have been a factor in treadmill performance.

Those swimmers with three or more years of competitive swimming experience showed better performance than those with less experience. While age and weight may have been factors here, remember, no age factor past 8 years old was demonstrated. The more experienced certainly are more acclimated to physical conditioning.

Analysis of the coach's subjective rating of each project volunteer reveals better performance by the better swimmers.

Summary

Treadmill testing can be successfully done on pre-adolescents and adolescents. Continuous exercise in a structured athletic program does show improved performances of those taking part. The above may not be true, however, for younger 8-year-olds and under. They may already be operating at peak efficiency, in which case no amount of exercise will have an effect on their performance. The "better" swimmers performed better, as did the more experienced. Females performed better than males.

Effects of Training on Cardiorespiratory Functions in Women

G. M. Andrew, S. Corneil and E. Watson

Introduction

The physiological effects on man of chronic and seasonal exercise programs have been the basis of many studies in recent years [4]. As a consequence, the changes which occur in humans with athletic training have been well documented. Workers are in agreement that training enhances the dimensions and functional capacities of the oxygen transport and utilization system [1, 7, 10]. In addition, training evidently is associated with improved regulation of circulatory and respiratory functions during exercise [2, 8].

For the most part, such studies on humans have been made on men of young adult age. In contrast, there is a relative paucity of reports in which adult women have been studied [6]. Moreover, the intensity and duration of training required to induce physiological changes have not been studied extensively [11]. Accordingly, the present study was proposed to examine some aspects of this topic.

Methods

Forty-three women aged 30-40 were selected from volunteers for the study. Following an interview, during which a detailed description of the 20-week program was given, a physical examination, including a 12-lead electrocardiogram and measurements of the static and dynamic lung functions were performed. These observations, combined with a support letter from the subject's personal physician, were used to insure no one with, overt cardiorespiratory problems was included in the study.

Subject screening and initial testing was performed during four visits to the laboratories; all tests were carried out under climate-controlled conditions. During the initial two visits, the physical

G. M. Andrew, S. Corneil and E. Watson, School of Physical and Health Education and Department of Physiology, Queen's University, Kingston, Ontario, Canada.

examination, blood and lung function measurements and orientation to the test apparatus were performed. On visit three, maximal oxygen uptake ($M\dot{V}O_2$) and associated functions were measured on the treadmill using a modified Balke test [5]; on the final visit, exercise was performed at approximately 40%, 60% and 80% of the subject's $M\dot{V}O_2$ on a bicycle ergometer during which oxygen uptake, cardiac output and related functions were measured using techniques previously described [9]. All exercise testing was repeated after 10 and 20 weeks of training. Subjects were divided into three groups using two criteria: (1) on the basis of their measured $M\dot{V}O_2$, into low (L), middle (M) and high (H) training groups; (2) by age to insure groups did not differ in this respect.

The groups followed a supervised training program of three one-hour sesions per week for ten-week periods according to the schedule indicated on Table I. Each training session included a warm-up period of 10 to 15 minutes, followed by an endurance component of up to 25 minutes of jog-walk exercise and terminated with warm-down exercise. In the preliminary data analysis, intergroup comparisons were made by student's t-test; intraindividual differences observed with training were tested by means of a paired t-test, each individual thus serving as her own control.

Results

Intergroup comparison at intake indicated no differences in respect to age, height, weight, hematocrit, hemoglobin, static and dynamic lung functions nor heart rate during maximal exercise. Only in respect to oxygen uptake ($M\dot{V}O_2$) and minute ventilation at maximal exercise (MV) were consistent differences observed, these

Table I. Schedule for Training Program

A: *Intensity and Duration*

Training Group	Intensity	
	0-10 Weeks	*11-20 Weeks*
L	low	low
M	low	medium
H	medium	high

B: *Target Heart Rate*

Intensity	*Heart Rate (b/min)*
low	130-140
medium	140-155
high	160-170

values being significantly lower in group L but not different between groups M and H.

In Figure 1, the intragroup mean maximal values for heart rate (MHR), minute ventilation, oxygen uptake and O_2 debt are shown for each group (L, M and H) before and after 10 and 20 weeks of training. MHR was unaffected by the exercise programs in all groups; similarly, the O_2 debt, as measured during 15 minutes of recovery and extrapolated to the measured preexercise level, was not affected by training, except in group H after ten weeks of high intensity training; nor were there any consistent significant intergroup differences between these variables (MHR and O_2 debt). In contrast, $M\dot{V}O_2$ was significantly increased over initial values in all groups after 20 weeks of training. In group L, the group with the lowest aerobic capacity, at intake low intensity training for ten weeks produced a highly significant increase in $M\dot{V}O_2$. A further ten weeks of training at the same target heart rate effected only a slight additional increase which was not found significant. In group M, ten weeks of low intensity training increased $M\dot{V}O_2$ by 3.2 ml/kg/min; a subsequent ten weeks of medium intensity exercise effected a comparable increase, resulting in a significant difference (P < .01) between the pre- and posttraining period of 20 weeks. Group H, with ten weeks of medium intensity training, displayed no change in $M\dot{V}O_2$; however, a further ten weeks of high intensity training increased the $M\dot{V}O_2$ by 6.2 ml and this change was highly significant (P < .05). The changes with training on pulmonary ventilation during maximal exercise essentially paralleled those observed in $M\dot{V}O_2$ except in group L where the increased MV was found significantly higher only after 20 weeks of low intensity training.

Figure 2 summarizes the results of the training on selected cardiorespiratory functions during submaximal exercise. Mean values are expressed as differences from the pretraining value after 10 and 20 weeks of training. Table II shows the level of significance of differences after 10 and 20 weeks of training for each group as indicated by a paired t-test. Oxygen uptake ($\dot{V}O_2$) during submaximal work was reduced after ten weeks of training but unchanged with additional training; likewise, minute ventilation ($\dot{V}$) was reduced after ten weeks and was further decreased with continued training. Cardiac output ($\dot{Q}c$) was reduced with training; this was consistently apparent after ten weeks of training, significantly so in groups L and M. This was further reduced with the additional training. The decrease in cardiac output was primarily the consequence of a reduced heart rate (HR) and to a lesser degree a

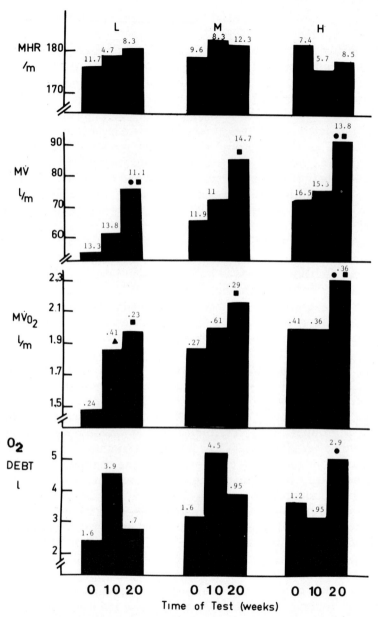

FIG.1. Intragroup comparison of mean maximal values measured at intake (0) after 10 and 20 weeks of training. MHR — maximal heart rate, MV̇ — maximal minute ventilation, MV̇O$_2$ — maximal oxygen uptake, O$_2$ Debt — recovery O$_2$ uptake. Level of significance of differences in means indicated for a P < .05 as follows: ▲ 0-10, ● 10-20, ■ 0-20. Numbers indicate ± 2 SD.

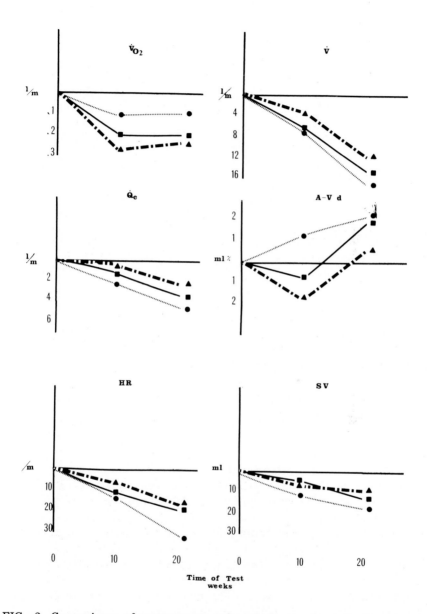

FIG. 2. Comparisons of responses to submaximal exercise tests for oxygen uptake ($\dot{V}O_2$), minute ventilation ($\dot{V}$), cardiac output ($\dot{Q}c$), arteriovenous oxygen difference (A-V d), heart rate (HR), stroke volume (SV), (legend: group L = •-----•, group M = ■————■, group H = ▲-----▲). Table II indicates level of significance of differences from intraindividual comparison.

Table II. Intragroup Differences During Submaximal Exercise

Group	Tests Comparison	$\dot{V}_{O_2}$	$\dot{V}$	$\dot{Q}c$	$(A\text{-}V)_{O_2}$	HR	SV
L	0-10	⊗	⊗	⊗	NS	⊗	×
	10-20	NS	⊗	NS	NS	⊗	NS
	0-20	⊗	⊗	⊗	NS	⊗	×
M	0-10	⊗	×	×	NS	⊗	NS
	10-20	NS	⊗	⊗	⊗	–	×
	0-20	⊗	⊗	⊗	NS	⊗	NS
H	0-10	⊗	NS	NS	⊗	×	NS
	10-20	NS	⊗	⊗	×	⊗	NS
	0-20	⊗	⊗	⊗	NS	⊗	NS

Statistical comparison within groups for oxygen uptake ($\dot{V}_{O_2}$), minute ventilation ($\dot{V}$), cardiac output ($\dot{Q}c$), arteriovenous O_2 difference ($(A\text{-}V) O_2$), heart rate (HR) and stroke volume (SV) between tests at intake (0), after 10 and 20 weeks of training. Level of significance: NS – P > .05

$$\times \; - \; P < .05$$
$$\otimes \; - \; P < .01$$

decrease in stroke volume (SV), especially in group L. The change in the calculated arteriovenous oxygen difference ($(A\text{-}v) O_2$) was inconsistant after ten weeks but showed a consistent widening after a further ten weeks of training.

Discussion

The changes observed with training in women are in general consistent with findings in adult males. The increase in $M\dot{V}O_2$, whether expressed in absolute values or as per unit of body weight, varied from 30% in those with lowest initial values (group L) to about 12% in the group with highest initial level. This observation clearly supports the view that the magnitude of the training effect is dependent upon the initial aerobic capacity [12]. Because aerobic capacity is such a good index of the level of fitness, it follows that the least fit will show greater change with training. It is noted that in group H, no change in aerobic capacity was observed with ten weeks of moderately intense training; only after an additional ten weeks of more intense training was this capacity increased. This suggests that for the relatively fit person moderate intensity exercise may be considered as an adequate maintenance training stimulus whereas, in this study at least, this same intensity training exercise was adequate to increase $M\dot{V}O_2$ in the other two less fit groups. These changes in $M\dot{V}O_2$ were accompanied by parallel changes in maximal minute ventilation (MV) and indicate the close correlation that prevails between these two functions. By contrast, oxygen debt is evidently not affected by a training program which is adequate to elicit an increase in aerobic capacity; the increase observed in group H seemingly is related to the intense bouts of exercise included in their training regimen.

The decreases with training in cardiorespiratory functions during submaximal exercise indicate an improved efficiency, not only in the mechanical sense, but also in regulation of other functions such as minute ventilaton, heart rate and cardiac output. These changes would suggest an economy of effort since the same absolute amount of work is performed with less stress on the oxygen delivery system. A surprising finding was the decrease observed in the calculated stroke volume. It has long been accepted that the highly trained person is characterized by a large stroke volume [3]. The present observation suggests that one of the early effects of training (i.e., training of short duration) is improved regulation of function and that the dimensional change associated with the stroke volume mechanism presumably requires training of greater duration [9].

Finally, an interesting observation which has practical significance is that low intensity training of short duration can improve the aerobic capacity and associated functions if the initial fitness level is low or even moderate. A common problem among adults starting exercise programs, and which often leads to their cessation of exercising, is the high incidence of soreness and injury. These effects are minimized by a less intense initial work level and may have been an important factor in maintaining the high participation and adherence rate of 87% in the present program.

References

1. Andrew, G.M., Becklake, M.R., Guleria, J.S. and Bates, D.V.: Heart and lung functions in swimmers and non-athletes during growth. J. Appl. Physiol. 32:245-251, 1972.
2. Andrew, G.M., Guzman, C.A. and Becklake, M.R.: Effects of training on exercise cardiac output. J. Appl. Physiol. 21:603-608, 1966.
3. Astrand, P.-O., Engstrom, L., Eriksson, B.O. et al: Girl swimmers. Acta Paed. Suppl. 147:3-75, 1963.
4. Astrand, P.-O. and Rodahl, K.: Textbook of Work Physiology. New York:McGraw-Hill, 1970, pp. 373-430.
5. Balke, B. and Ware, R.: An experimental study of physical fitness of air force personnel. U.S. Armed Forces Med. J. 10:675-683, 1959.
6. Drinkwater, B.L.: Physiological Responses of Women to Exercise. In Wilmore, J.W. (ed.): Exercise and Sport Sciences Review. Academic Press, 1973, Vol. 1, pp. 125-153.

7. Ekblom, B.: Effect of training on adolescent boys. J. Appl. Physiol. 27:350-355, 1969.
8. Ekblom, B., Astrand, P.-O., Saltin, B. et al: Effect of training on circulatory response to exercise. J. Appl. Physiol. 24:518-528, 1968.
9. Hamilton, P. and Andrew, G.M.: Influence of growth and athletic training on heart and lung functions. Europ. J. Appl. Physiol. 36:27-38, 1976.
10. Holmgren, A. and Astrand, P.-O.: D_L and the dimension and functional capacities of the O_2 transport system in humans. J. Appl. Physiol. 21:1463-1470, 1966.
11. Pollock, M.L.: The quantification of endurance training. *In* Wilmore, J.H. (ed.): Exercise Sport Sci. Rev. 1:155-188, 1973.
12. Shephard, R.J.: Intensity, duration and frequency of exercise as determinants of the response to a training regime. Int. Z. Angew. Physiol.

A Study on the Effect of Long-Term Physical Training of Adult Men

Hidetaro Shibayama and Hiroshi Ebashi

Introduction

The importance of improvement of health and physical fitness of the adult and prevention of early ageing is now attracting general attention because of the prolongation of the average human life span and the increase of elderly population. In general, the decline of the physiological functions due to ageing seems to be inevitable [1], and the question arises whether it is possible to slow down the decline or even to improve the functions by some measure. It is a well-known biological principle that the disuse or lack of stimulation results in atrophy [3], and the significance of repetitive stimulation by physical exercise as a countermeasure against ageing seems to be related to that principle.

The purpose of physical training in adult age is substantially different from that in childhood and adolescence which aims at promoting physical growth and development. It is repeatedly emphasized that the formation of exercise habit in daily life is especially important in the case of adult age [8], and there have been debates on the adequate intensity and duration of exercise as well as its frequency in a week [9]. In the present study, an attempt was made to follow up as long as possible the effect and its physiological mechanism of regular controlled physical exercise in adult men. Attention was especially paid to the time course of appearance of training effect and the pattern of changes in physiological functions.

Methods

The subjects were five healthy adult men, engaged in research work at the institute, whose age ranged from 30 to 47 years (Table I). Needless to say, medical checks were carefully made on them to ascertain that they had no abnormality, particularly in the respiro-

---

Hidetaro Shibayama and Hiroshi Ebashi, Department of Physiology, Physical Fitness Research Institute, Meiji Life Foundation of Health and Welfare, Tokyo, Japan.

Table I. Physical Characteristics of Subjects

Subjects	Age and Sex	Body Height (cm)	Body Weight (kg)	Chest Girth (cm)	Rohrer's Index	Skinfold Thickness Upper Arm (mm)	Back (mm)
H.E.	32, m	163.5	54.0	85.0	123.5	4.6	7.5
H.S.	38, m	165.8	59.1	86.8	129.3	4.5	10.0
Y.G.	30, m	162.5	58.7	89.5	136.8	6.5	7.8
T.T.	47, m	167.3	56.7	88.8	121.1	6.2	7.0
N.K.	39, m	174.3	54.7	85.2	103.3	2.6	5.7
Average	37.2	166.7	56.6	87.1	122.9	4.9	7.6

circulatory system. The exercise for training was treadmill running with a constant speed, which was regulated in each subject so that the intensity of work corresponded to two-thirds $\dot{V}O_2$ max [5,9]. The inclination of the running belt was $3°$. A bout of 20 minutes was imposed upon them five days a week except Saturday and Sunday. The period of observation was tentatively decided as three years (about 160 weeks). The condition of the exercise and the maximal exercise data in each subject are shown in Table II.

Results

Observations were made laying stress upon changes in respiro-circulatory functions. The heart rate at rest decreased by 5 to 6 beats per minute in 5 to 15 weeks, and the heart rate just after the daily exercise also decreased by about 10 beats per minute in 10 weeks (Fig. 1). Changes in results of blood tests became appreciable after about 20 weeks of training and the increase in red cell count and saturation index was rather marked (Fig. 1). The decrease in total cholesterol of the blood was noticed after 25 to 30 weeks (Fig. 2).

Table II. Maximal Exercise Data and Duration of Training

Subject	$\dot{V}O_2$ Max l/min	$\dot{V}O_2$ Max ml/kg/min	$\dot{V}_E$ l/min. STPD	HR Max beats/min	Training Load. m/min, speed	Duration of Training
H.E.	3.62	66.9	94.45	193	150	165 weeks, continued
H.S.	3.49	59.1	102.53	187	140	165 weeks, continued
Y.G.	3.50	59.7	110.89	185	140	161 weeks, continued
T.T.	2.97	52.4	87.15	162	130	19 weeks, discontinued
N.K.	2.98	54.6	87.88	181	130	43 weeks, interrupted
Average	3.31	58.5	96.58	181.6	138.0	

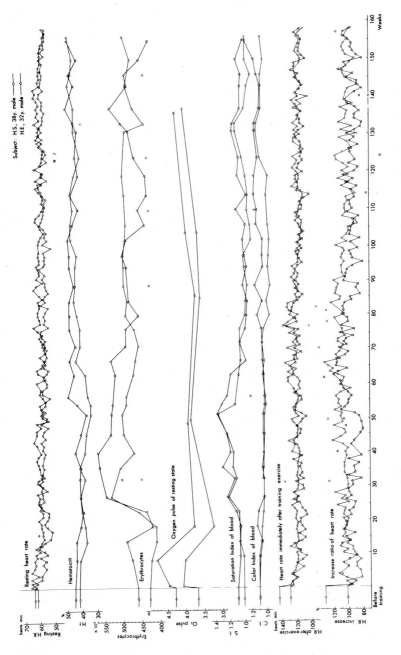

FIG. 1. Changes in the circulatory functions due to long-term physical training.

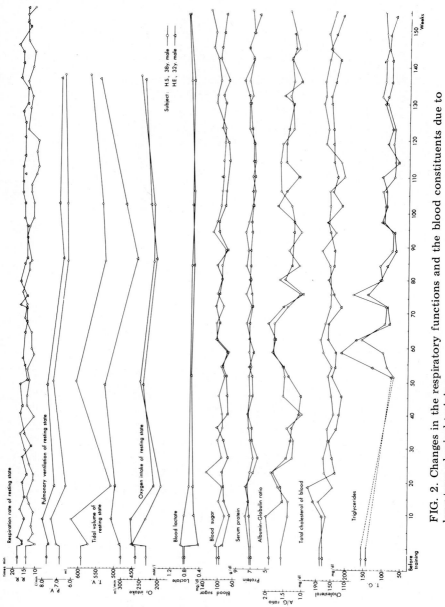

FIG. 2. Changes in the respiratory functions and the blood constituents due to long-term physical training.

The improvement of adaptation to the exercise became noticeable especially in respiratory functions, namely, the improvement of ventilatory efficiency became evident (Figs. 3 and 4), the oxygen intake corresponding to the same workload decreased (Fig. 3) and the lactate production due to exercise decreased in 10 to 15 weeks (Fig. 5). In 20 weeks of training, the respiration rate raised its

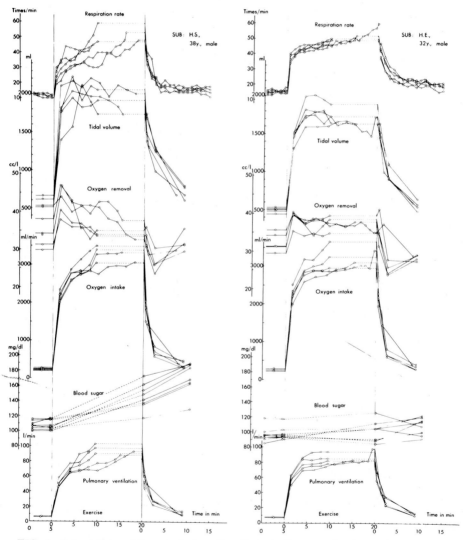

FIG. 3. Adaptation of the respiratory functions to the exercise due to long-term physical training.

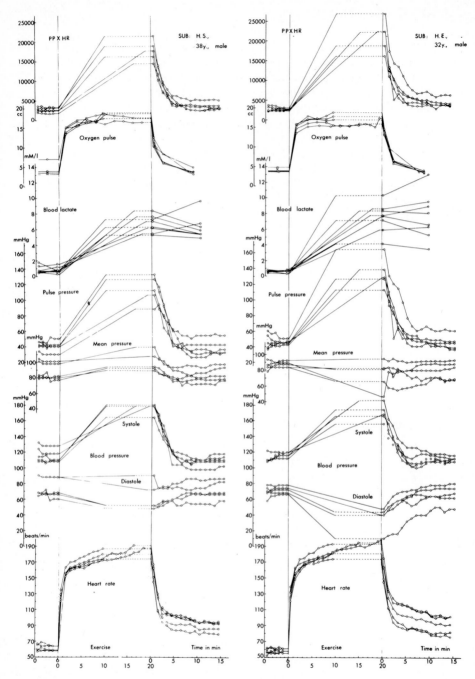

FIG. 4. Adaptation of the circulatory functions to the exercise due to long-term physical training.

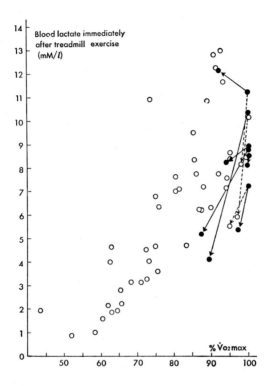

FIG. 5. Relation between % $\dot{V}O_2$ max and blood lactate.

stability (Fig. 6). The effect of training upon the heart rate during exercise could be noticed in rather an early state of training, and the exercise heart rate became stable in about ten weeks (Fig. 7). Thus, considerable physiological changes occurred in the first 20 weeks, but the changes seemed to slow down thereafter and most functions showed the tendency of remaining at the same level (Figs. 1 and 2). However, the hematocrit began to increase after 50 weeks (Fig. 1) and slight increases in the area of heart silhouette and cardiothoracic ratio were noticed after 85 weeks (Table III). Regarding the lipids in the blood, the serum triglycerides and total cholesterol showed similar trends of changes, and the variance of the resting values became distinctly small after 90 to 100 weeks (Fig. 2). However, it is noteworthy that the performance of treadmill running showed no significant improvement in the three-year training as far as the all-out running time was concerned.

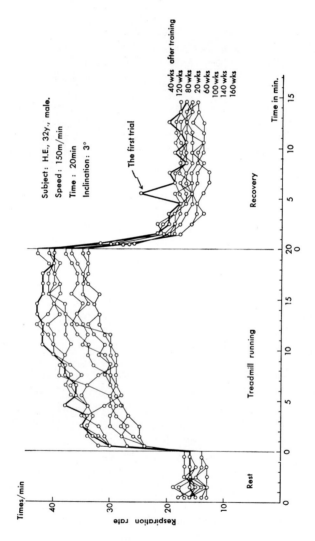

FIG. 6. Effect of long-term physical training on the respiration rate during exercise.

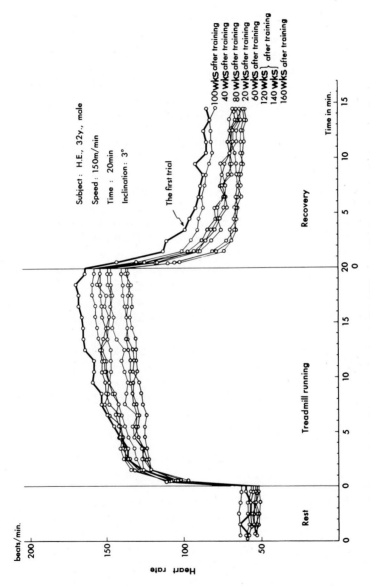

FIG. 7. Effect of long-term physical training on the heart rate during exercise.

Table III. Area of Cardiac Silhouette Before and After Training (cm^2)

Subject	Before Training	85 Weeks After Training	Increase Ratio	Cardiothoracic Ratio B/A
H.E.	128.5	132.0	2.73	26.8/27.4
H.S.	116.0	148.0	27.59	31.4/31.7
Y.G.	121.0	149.0	23.14	31.0/31.3
N.K.	88.0	−	−	29.7/−

Discussion

It has been already pointed out by several scientists that the physical training of the adult can usually cause no marked improvement of physical fitness; in other words, the effect of training is far different from that in the adolescent [1, 2, 6]. In the present experiment, the performance in all the subjects showed no definite trend of change and some of them showed even a decrease in $\dot{V}O_2$ max (Fig. 3). These findings might be related to the physical conditions of each subject [8]. Accordingly, it can be said in general that their physical fitness could not appreciably be improved by the training. As aforementioned, daily regular repetitions of 20-minute exercise of the intensity corresponding to two thirds of the maximal effort could cause in adult men obvious improvement in some physiological functions in the first 20 weeks (Figs. 1 and 2). However, further continuation over three years thereafter resulted in no distinct changes in physiological functions, although a slight improvement was noticed in the circulatory function [4, 7]. Accordingly, the long-term regular physical training in the adult seems to be effective mainly in maintaining the physical fitness level somewhat improved in the early stage of training.

Summary

An experiment was carried out to observe the effect of long-term regular physical training upon the respirocirculatory functions and the blood constituents in adult men, and efforts were made in analyzing the training effect in detail and in following up the time course of appearance of training effect upon physiological functions. The exercise for training was 20-minute running on a treadmill of 3° inclination, and the running speed was regulated so that the exercise intensity corresponded to two-thirds $\dot{V}O_2$ max in each subject. The exercise was one bout a day, five days a week, and continued for about three years. Subjects were five healthy men, ranging in age from 30 to 47.

In the first 5 to 15 weeks, the heart rate at rest showed a decrease of 5 to 6 beats per minute, and increases in the red cell count and oxygen saturation index of the blood were observed in 20 weeks. The decrease in total blood cholesterol became noticeable after 25 to 30 weeks. The hematocrit began to increase after 50 weeks. The radiography disclosed slight increases in the area of heart silhouette and cardiothoracic index after 85 weeks of training. The variance of serum triglyceride became distinctly smaller after 90 to 100 weeks.

Regarding the adaptation to the exercise, the improvement became noticeable in 10 to 15 weeks on the heart rate, ventilatory efficiency, oxygen intake and blood lactate concentration. After 15 to 20 weeks of training, variations of respiration rate became smaller. However, tests could disclose no significant improvement of the performance, such as all-out running time.

In short, it can be said that the training effect in adult men due to regular repetitions of exercise can be noticed in the first 20 weeks, and the further continuous repetitions seem to be effective mainly in maintaining the improved level of physical fitness.

References

1. Astrand, P.O.: Experimental studies of physical working capacity in relation to sex and age. Copenhagen:Ejnar Munksgaard, 1952.
2. Cureton, T.K. and Phillips, E.E.: Physical fitness changes in middle-aged men attributable to equal eight-week periods of training, non-training and retraining. J. Sports Med. 4(2):87-93, 1964.
3. Cureton, T.K.: The Physiological Effects of Exercise Programs on Adults. Springfield, Ill.:Charles C Thomas Publisher, 1972.
4. Ekblom, B., Astrand, P.O., Saltin, B. et al: Effect of training on circulatory response to exercise. J. Appl. Physiol. 24(4):518-528, 1968.
5. Gledhill, N. and Eynon, R.B.: The intensity of training. In Taylor, A.W. (ed.): Training. Scientific Basis and Application. Springfield, Ill.:Charles C Thomas Publisher, 1972, pp. 97-102.
6. Ikai, M. and Kitagawa, K.: Maximum oxygen uptake of Japanese related to sex and age. Med. Sci. Sports 4(3):127-131, 1972.
7. Karlsson, J., Astrand, P.O. and Ekblom, B.: Training of the oxgyen transport system in man. J. Appl. Physiol. 22(6):1061-1065, 1967.
8. Ricci, B.: Physical and Physiological Conditioning for Men. Dubuque, Iowa:Wm. C. Brown Co., 1972.
9. Shephard, R.J.: Intensity, duration and frequency of exercise as determinants of the response to a training regime. Int. Z. Physiol. Einschl. Arbeitsphysiol. 26:272-278, 1968.

10. Shibayama, H. and Ebashi, H.: Effect of 20 minute training of adult men from the viewpoint of respiro-circulatory functions. J. Physiol. Soc. Japan 36(8-9):408, 1974.
11. Shibayama, H. and Ebashi, H.: Effect of long-term physical training of adult men. J. Physiol. Soc. Japan 37(8-9):202-203, 1975.
12. Shibayama, H., Ebashi, H. and Nishijima, Y.: Training effect of adult men from the viewpoint of the heart rate change. J. Phys. Fitness Japan 24(2):72-73, 1975.
13. Shibayama, H. and Ebashi, H.: Administration of physical training of adult men by monitoring the heart rate. J. Physiol. Soc. Japan 38(3-4):199, 1976.

Effects of Physical Training on the Aerobic Power of the Middle and Old Aged

Minoru Itoh, Kazuo Itoh,
Tamotsu Yagi and Kiyoko Maeda

Introduction

The problem of adult physical endurance has been studied by many researchers, among whom the studies of Åstrand et al were especially excellent. However, in Japan, very few studies have been made. In fact, only a few studies of the middle-aged and elderly have to our knowledge been published to date.

The purpose of this paper is to investigate the effects of physical training on middle-aged and elderly Japanese by examination of aerobic power. Taking the maximum oxygen intake ($\dot{V}O_2$ max) as one of the most important functions, we examined the increment of $\dot{V}O_2$ max before and after a certain period of training.

There are several methods for testing $\dot{V}O_2$ max. The treadmill running method and bicycle ergometer method are widely employed. However, for most middle- and older-aged men, continuous running would be somewhat of a strain. For the same reason, the bicycle method did not seem quite appropriate for the elderly either. Therefore, we chose the "inclined treadmill walking" method for the examination of $\dot{V}O_2$ max.

Subjects and Method

Thirty subjects (24 males and six females) were chosen from healthy and sedentary adults of 32 to 65 years of age. The physical characteristics of male subjects are shown in Table I. It also shows the results of their resting ECG and the Master's Double Step Test.

The responses of ECG which were recorded in resting states and the results of the Master's Double Step Test indicated little deviation

Minoru Itoh, Kazuo Itoh and Tamotsu Yagi, Kyoto University, Kyoto, and Kiyoko Maeda, Seian Women's College, Tokyo, Japan.

Table I. Physical Characteristics of the Subjects

No.	Subject	Age	Height (cm)	Weight (kg)	Resting ECG	Master's D. Test
1	E.H.	40	172.4	65.5		
2	U.K.	40	164.0	54.0	S.-ARR.	S.-ARR.
3	K.H.	41	164.8	64.5		
4	T.F.	41	167.0	52.0		
5	T.T.	42	161.7	50.5		
6	M.I.	43	167.0	51.0		
7	K.Y.	45	171.0	65.0		ST–dep.
8	M.K.	45	174.5	70.0		
9	Z.T.	47	162.8	68.0		
10	Y.M.	47	166.1	52.5		
11	O.S.	48	165.7	65.0		
12	S.Hi.	48	165.0	71.8		
13	K.M.	48	172.5	78.0		
14	H.K.	50	171.0	63.0		
15	M.T.	52	172.5	68.0		
16	S.Ho.	52	174.0	55.0		
17	J.E.	52	164.5	48.0		
18	N.Ko.	53	162.0	51.0		
19	R.Y.	57	167.7	56.0	PQ: 0.08 sec (w-p-w)	ST–dep.
20	K.T.	60	165.0	48.0	ST-elev./PQ: 0.24 sec	ST–dep. T–flat
21	M.N.	60	162.0	54.0		
22	T.N.	61	160.8	56.5	L.B.B.–Block/QRS 0.2 sec	ST–dep.
23	N.Ku.	63	170.0	63.5		
24	N.Ku.	65	170.0	65.5		

S.-ARR: sinus arrhythmia
ST–dep: ST–depression
L.B.B.–Block: left bundle branch block

from the norm. After careful consideration, it was agreed that these subjects could join our training.

Table II shows the physical characteristics of female subjects. In this case, with the exception of one person, there were no abnormal responses on the resting ECG and on the Master's Double Step Test.

The treadmill walking method was used for the exhaustive test in order to measure $\dot{V}O_2$ max. This test was modified from the method which was used by Balke et al.

Subjects were required to walk on the treadmill 80 meters/min for men and 70 meters/min for women. Simultaneously, the gradient of slope was increased 2.5% every minute. This was continued until the subjects were exhausted. During the test, the oxygen intake was measured by the Douglas bag method and the maximal heart rate (max H.R.) by either a telemeter or an attached electrocardiogram. The ECG was recorded by the chest bipolar lead.

Table II. Physical Characteristics of Female Subjects

No.	Subject	Age	Height (cm)	Weight (kg) Pre-training	Weight (kg) Post-training	Master's D. Test
1	T.A.	32	154.3	41.0	41.0	
2	T.M.	39	159.0	54.0	53.0	
3	Y.S.	40	144.0	44.0	45.5	
4	K.N.	41	158.0	58.0	57.5	
5	K.M.	42	154.0	51.0	51.0	
6	T.N.	61	152.0	48.0	47.0	ST–dep.

For the purpose of our training, each subject's "load" was calculated to 70% of his $\dot{V}O_2$ max. This "load" also determined the gradient of the inclined treadmill. The training was conducted on the treadmill for five minutes each twice a week for ten weeks.

In order to record the effects of our training, the exhaustive test was given before, during and after training. $\dot{V}O_2$ max, max H.R. and exercised ECG were measured at the exhaustive tests.

Results

Table III shows the $\dot{V}O_2$ max of subjects examined (I) before training; (II) during training; and (III) after training.

Although there were no significant changes caused by training in the age group over 60, in the 40- to 57-year-old bracket, the $\dot{V}O_2$ max increased after the training.

The right-hand side of Table III shows the results of the calculated volume of $\dot{V}O_2$ max per 1 kg of body weight. This table indicates that the younger subjects had a higher value than the older.

Figure 1 is a graph on the variation of $\dot{V}O_2$ max due to training. The "standard" seen at the right end is the mean value of Swedish subjects of the same age as reported by Åstrand.

The absolute $\dot{V}O_2$ max value for Japanese is less than that for Swedes. However, when we calculate this for each by 1 kg, although the value for Japanese before training was a little less than that for Swedes, after training the reverse was true.

Figure 2 shows the change of heart rate in subject K.H. recorded throughout the training. The upper diagram is the result of the 2nd to 8th training sessions and the lower diagram is from the 11th to 19th sessions. The subject tended to decrease his resting heart rate as well as his heart rate at any given time during the successive exercises. Similar results were recorded in other subjects. In this

Table III. Effects of 70% $\dot{V}O_2$ Max Training on $\dot{V}O_2$ Max
and $\dot{V}O_2$ Max per Body Weight (kg)

No.	Subject	B.M. $O_2\,ml$	$\dot{V}O_2\,Max\,(l)$			$\dot{V}O_2\,Max/B.W.\,(ml/kg)$		
			I	II	III	I	II	III
1	E.H.	214	2.84	2.94	3.12	43.4	44.9	47.6
2	U.K.	190	1.97	1.96	2.08	36.5	36.3	38.5
3	K.H.	204	2.42	2.78	2.80	37.5	43.1	43.8
4	T.F.	188	1.89	2.22	2.53	36.4	42.8	48.5
5	T.T.	181	2.19	2.67	2.50	43.3	52.8	51.9
6	M.I.	168	2.17	2.61	2.76	42.0	50.6	54.1
7	K.Y.	211	1.98	2.40	2.13	30.5	36.9	32.8
8	M.K.	226	2.55	2.81	2.95	36.0	39.6	40.9
9	Z.T.	205	2.06	2.27	2.40	30.3	33.4	35.3
10	Y.M.	189	1.76	1.92	2.16	33.5	36.5	41.2
11	O.S.	201	1.90	2.18	2.22	29.2	33.5	34.2
12	S.Hi.	213	1.69	2.21	–	27.2	30.7	–
13	K.M.	226	2.16	2.49	2.69	27.7	31.9	34.4
14	H.Ki.	203	2.02	2.02	2.22	32.1	32.1	35.2
15	M.T.	199	1.96	2.12	2.34	28.8	31.2	34.4
16	S.Ho.	196	1.59	1.64	1.43	28.9	28.8	26.0
17	J.E.	176	1.64	1.67	2.10	33.4	34.1	42.8
18	N.Ko.	181	1.64	2.12	2.27	32.2	41.6	44.5
19	R.Y.	188	2.03	2.24	2.23	36.3	40.0	39.8
20	K.T.	170	1.04	1.05	–	21.7	22.9	–
21	M.N.	177	1.73	1.60	1.71	32.0	29.6	31.7
22	T.N.	179	2.07	–	2.20	36.9	–	38.3
23	N.K.	195	2.13	–	2.25	33.6	–	35.5
24	N.K.	196	1.94	2.03	1.74	29.6	31.0	26.6

B.M.: basal metabolism I: before training II: middle of training III: after training.

figure, the heart rate during the 11th session is higher than that of the eighth due to the increase in the gradient from 12.5% in the first half of training to 15% in the second half.

Next, we examined the max H.R. in the 40- to 60-year age group (Table IV). Very little difference before and after training was found. Most subjects showed increased $\dot{V}O_2$ max throughout the training. Maximal oxygen pulse (max O_2 pulse), therefore, was greater after than before training. The average value increased by 11%.

Figure 3 shows an example of the appearance of an abnormal ECG pattern during the exhaustive test (subject T.N., 60-years-old, male). In exhaustive test I, the arrhythmic symptoms were noticed during a five- to seven-minute exercise and 30 second recovery. A junction type ST depression also appeared in the exercise. In exhaustive test III, however, an arrhythmia was found after only 30 seconds of exercise.

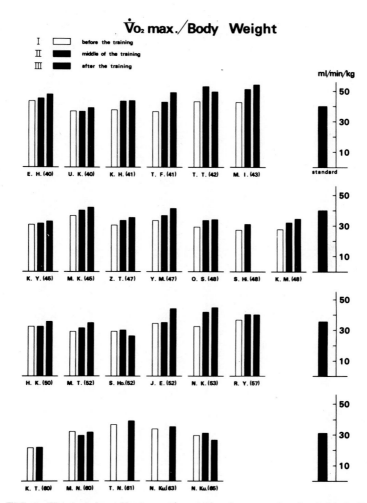

FIG. 1. The training effects on the maximal oxygen intake (ml/min/kg).

Table V shows the abnormal ECG pattern during training. In this table, abnormal patterns which occurred during either the exercise or the recovery periods are shown by symbols.

For the 40 to 49 age group subjects, the abnormal pattern seemed to decrease as the training continued while for the subjects in their sixties, very little difference throughout the training was observed.

The female subjects' $\dot{V}O_2$ max and max H.R. in the exhaustive tests are shown in Table VI (I) before, (II) during, and (III) after

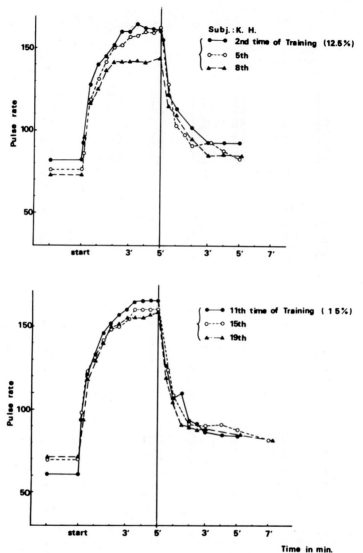

FIG. 2. Pulse rate changes during training and its recovery. (Subject: K.H., 41 years, male.) *Upper*: the before half of the training session. *Lower*: the later half.

training. Every subject showed an increase in $\dot{V}O_2$ max as training progressed, but the max H.R. changed only nominally.

Figure 4 shows the change of $\dot{V}O_2$ max per body weight (kg). It indicates that the $\dot{V}O_2$ max/B W. of all subjects (including the 61-year-old-subject) increased along with the training.

Table IV. Maximal Heart Rate and Maximal
Oxygen Pulse in Exhaustion Tests

Age		Max Heart Rate		Max O_2 Pulse	
		I	III	I	III
	M	186.3	189.5	11.6 ml	13.4 ml
40-49	max	205	205	14.1	15.6
	min	170	175	9.6	10.2
	M	175.2	183.0	10.6 ml	11.8 ml
50-59	max	180	190	12.3	13.1
	min	170	175	8.9	7.7
	M	160.4	164.2	11.1 ml	11.0 ml
60-65	max	180	180	13.1	12.9
	min	111	118	9.4	9.1
Average		178.1	182.6	11.3 ml	12.5 ml

Discussion

The treadmill walking method was devised from the Balke and Pollock method with the gradient of the slope increasing 2.5% per minute. In the beginning, both men and women trained at 80 meters/min.

For male subjects, the value of $\dot{V}O_2$ max from the start was not much lower than with the treadmill running method, but much higher than that with the bicycle method. Many of the female subjects, however, were not able to sustain the exercise at 80 meters/min and reached exhaustion when their heart rates were still low.

For this reason, we decided to turn down the speed of the treadmill to 70 meters/min for all examinations and trainings for females.

The $\dot{V}O_2$ max throughout the training increased from an average of 2.03 liters to 2.31 liters for males, and 1.48 to 1.68 liters for females. Both increased by 14%, which was sufficient value at which to compare the results with those of former researchers.

Concerning the max H.R. during the exhaustive tests, many subjects both male and female did not show any differences before and after training. Therefore, the average max O_2 pulse increased from 11.3 ml to 12.5 ml or 11% for males, and from 8.3 to 9.3 ml or 12% for females.

Figure 5, summarized from Figures 1 and 4, shows the relation between the age and the effects of the training by $\dot{V}O_2$ max increase.

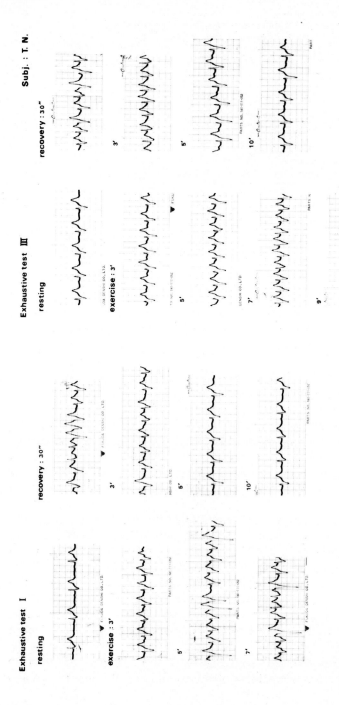

FIG. 3. Changes in the ECG patterns during and after the exercises. Exhaustive test I: prior to the training. Exhaustive test III: after ten weeks training.

Table V. ECG Change in the Training

Age	Subject	Grade	2nd	5th	8th	Grade	12th	15th	18th
	K.H.	12.5%	ST	ST		15 %	ST		
40-44	T.T.	15				17.5	PB		
	M.I.	15	PB			17.5	(PB)		
	Z.T.	12.5%	ST	ST	PB	15 %	ST, T		T
45-49	O.S.	12.5	ST	ST, T	T	15	ST, T	ST	
	K.M.	10		ST	ST	12.5	ST		ARR
	H.K.	15 %	T	ST, T	ST, T	15 %	ST, T	ST, T	T
50-59	J.J.	12.5	ST	ST		12.5	ST	ST	(PB)
	N.Ko.	15	ST	ST	ST	17.5	ST		ST
60-	M.N.	10 %	P	ST	P	10 %	ST	ST	
	N.Ku$_2$	10	ARR	ST,(ARR)	ST, T	10	ST, T	ARR	ST, T

P: Pulmonal P   ARR: Arrhythmia
ST: ST depression   PB: Premature beat
T:T flat or negative

Table VI. Effects of 70% $\dot{V}O_2$ Max Training, on $\dot{V}O_2$ Max and Max Heart Rate

Subject	$\dot{V}O_2$ Max (l)			$\dot{V}O_2$Max/B.W. (ml/kg/min)			Max Heart Rate		
	I	II	III	I	II	III	I	II	III
T.A.	1.37	1.52	1.67	33.4	37.1	40.7	175	165	170
T.M.	1.79	1.85	1.92	33.1	34.3	35.6	185	185	190
Y.S.	1.49	1.58	1.58	33.9	35.9	35.9	185	190	190
K.N.	1.70	1.84	1.91	29.3	31.7	32.9	180	180	185
K.M.	1.29	1.43	1.42	25.3	28.0	27.8	170	170	172
T.N.	1.25	1.33	1.58	26.0	27.7	32.9	170	170	175
Mean	1.48	1.59	1.68	30.2	32.5	34.3	178	177	180
S.D.	0.21	0.20	0.18	3.53	3.65	3.90	6.3	9.0	8.3

From this test it was concluded that the younger subjects showed greater effects of the training than the older ones.

Acknowledgment

We wish to express our sincere thanks to Dr. N. Miyata and the staff of the Research Group of Adult Physical Fitness of Kyoto University. They have given us invaluable help throughout this investigation.

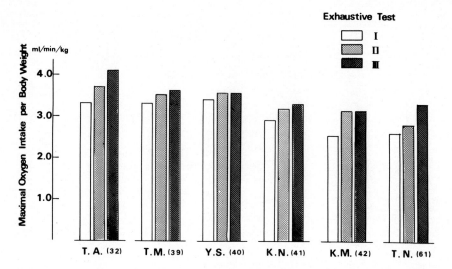

FIG. 4. The training effect on the $\dot{V}O_2$ max (ml/min/kg). I: before training; II: middle of the training; III: after training.

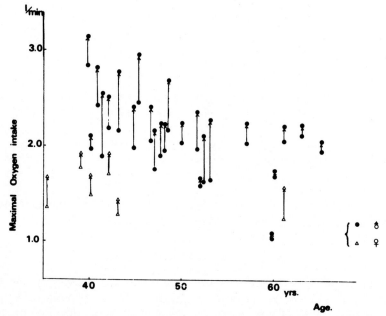

FIG. 5. Correlation between chronological age and maximal oxygen intake.

References

1. Åstrand, I., Åstrand, P.-O., Hallback, I. and Kilbom, A.: Reduction in maximal oxygen uptake with age. J. Appl. Physiol. 35:649-654, 1973.
2. Åstrand, I.: Aerobic work capacity in men and women with special reference to age. Acta Physiol. Scand. 49 Suppl. 169, 1970.
3. Åstrand, P.-O.: Experimental studies of physical work capacity in relation to sex and age. Copenhagen:Ejnar Munksgaard, 1952.
,4. Balke, B. et al: An experimental study of physical fitness of Air Force personnel. U.S. Armed Forces Med. J. 10:675-688, 1959.
5. Itoh, M., Itoh, K., Yagi, T. and Kawahatsu, K.: Training effects of treadmill walking on general endurance in middle and old-aged women. Report of Research Center in Physical Education, vol. 3, 1975 (in Japanese).
6. Itoh, M., Miyata, N., Manni, M. et al: Effect of physical training on general endurance of middle and old age. Report of Research Center in Physical Education, vol. 1:134-143, 1973 (in Japanese).
7. Kato, K., Kaneko, M., Toyooka, J. and Ishii, K.: Effects of training frequency on aerobic work capacity in adult men. Report of Research Center in Physical Education, vol. 1, 1973, pp. 116-124 (in Japanese).
8. Pollock, M.L. et al: Effects of walking on body composition and cardiovascular function of middle aged men. J. Appl. Physiol. 30(1):111-125, 1970.
9. Saltin, B., Hertley, L., Kilbom, A. and Åstrand, I.: Physical training in sedentary middle-aged and older men. II. Scand. J. Clin. Lab. Invest. 24:323-334, 1969.
10. Sandberg, L.: Studies on electrocardiographic changes during exercise test. Acta Med. Scand. 169 Suppl. 365, 1961.

Effects of Long-Term (38 Months) Training on Middle-Aged Sedentary Males: Adherence and Specificity of Training

W. E. Sime, I. T. Whipple, J. Stamler
and D. M. Berkson

Introduction

Considerable evidence is available indicating that habitual exercise may help protect against premature clinical coronary heart disease. Evidence from more than 35 epidemiological studies investigating this hypothesis has been reviewed by Fox, Naughton and Haskell [3] and Froelicher and Oberman [4]. The results of these studies have been inconclusive primarily because there have been no large prospective studies on randomly selected populations with carefully controlled procedures. Conflicting evidence has been reported on the relationship between occupational level of physical activity and coronary heart disease. Stamler et al [17] found that blue collar workers, who presumably were more physically active than white collar workers, exhibited higher rates for the major coronary risk factors than the sedentary white collar workers. On the other hand Brunner et al [2] found that the incidence of coronary heart disease was two to four times higher in sedentary male workers than in nonsedentary workers in an Israeli kibbutz. Investigations in Denmark by Gyntelberg [5] found that the level of physical fitness, as estimated by indirectly measured maximal oxygen uptake, was related to the major coronary risk factors. In addition, the level of physical fitness in these 5249 middle-aged Copenhagen males was related to leisure-time physical activity but not to occupational physical activity. Further efforts to study occupational physical

W. E. Sime, Department of Kinesiology/Health Studies, University of Waterloo, Ontario, Canada; I. T. Whipple, J. Stamler and D. M. Berkson, Department of Community Health and Preventive Medicine, Northwestern University Medical School, Chicago, Illinois, U.S.A.

457

activity levels in relation to coronary heart disease may not be relevant, since the technological developments in industry of Western society have virtually eliminated occupations that require high levels of physical activity. Morris et al [9] have reported encouraging evidence on the role of nonoccupational exercise in the prevention of coronary heart disease. He found that men taking regular, vigorous, leisure-time physical activity had a lower incidence of myocardial infarction. Large-scale and long-term prospective studies are needed to assess this hypothesis. For this purpose, it was first necessary to examine the efficacy and feasibility of leisure-time exercise programs in free-living sedentary males to determine (1) whether cardio-pulmonary fitness levels would be enhanced, (2) whether other coronary risk factors would be affected and (3) whether middle-aged, asymptomatic males would continue to adhere to an exercise program as an integral part of their life-style. The feasibility of a physical training program for middle-aged men up to 18 months' duration has been described by Teraslinna et al [18] and Oja et al [10]. The participation rate varied from 43% to 90% monthly and adherence was 91% for the 18 months of exercise which consisted of bicycle pedaling, bench stepping, swimming, calisthenics, running and volleyball. Adherence rates have also been reported in exercise programs for postinfarct cardiac rehabilitation, wherein patients are presumably highly motivated. However, Bruce et al [1] reported that postcardiac adherence rates had declined to 30% after three years of training. The present study was designed to investigate the physio-logical effects of and the adherence to a long-term (three year) bicycle ergometer training program in middle-aged, asymptomatic, sedentary males. At the end of that period a follow-up program of walking and/or jogging was offered to the participants who remained active to determine whether additional physiological changes could be elicited.

Methodology

Forty-six healthy, sedentary male volunteers were recruited by advertisement for participation in a long-term exercise program at a Chicago Jewish community center. All of the respondents lived or worked near the community center and agreed initially to participate for a minimum of three years. Medical eligibility was established by a complete medical history, physical examination, resting 12 lead ECG, chest X-ray and extensive laboratory tests. Men were excluded when they exhibited ST segment depression equal to or greater than 0.1 mv during or after exercise testing.

Two submaximal exercise tests were performed at one-week intervals on a bicycle ergometer at 300, 600 and 900 kpm/min. One week later, a submaximal treadmill test was administered at 3 mph and 2%, 8% and 14% incline. Reproducibility of heart rate and blood pressure during these procedures has been reported previously. Waistline girth, body weight, vital capacity, skinfold thickness, blood cholesterol, blood triglycerides, heart rate and blood pressure response to exercise were recorded on repeat testing at approximate six-month intervals.

Training facilities were available at the community center four evenings per week from 5:00 to 9:00 p.m. and on Sunday morning from 8:00 to 12:00 a.m. All of the men agreed to participate a minimum of three times per week for training on a bicycle ergometer under supervision of an attendant. Interval training on the ergometer consisted of three work periods of four-minute duration with a three-minute rest between each period. Training sessions were preceded by a warm-up and followed by a brief cooling off period. During the first four weeks of training the workload on the ergometer was adjusted so that training heart rate was approximately 120 beats per minute. After four weeks the workload was gradually increased so that each participant was exercising at an individually prescribed training heart rate of 70% of his age-predicted maximum heart rate. Training pulse rates were recorded at two-minute intervals by the attendant who was experienced in cardiopulmonary resuscitation. Training sessions were individualized with no more than three participants exercising at one time. There was very little opportunity for group interaction during the training sessions; however, several incentive programs were utilized. A social, a team contest and numerous individual awards produced only modest and temporary improvements in adherence. At the end of 36 months of bicycle ergometer training, the participants who remained in the study were switched to a continuous walking and/or jogging program on an outdoor track. Group interaction was encouraged in this follow-up program designed to investigate whether additional physiological changes could be elicited.

Results

Earlier progress reports on this investigation have shown that men who attended more than 50% of the expected exercise sessions had greater reductions in heart rate at 600 kpm/min and blood pressure at 900 kpm/min than those with less than 50% attendance. Small though significant decreases in heart rate and blood pressure were observed on the treadmill test, but only after 18 months of training. Concerning the effect of exercise on other risk factors, only serum triglycerides showed a significant decrease after 21 months. The average attendance at bicycle ergometer training sessions was 2.4 times per week for 22 of the original 46 men who remained in the program after 30 months.

Figure 1 shows the adherence to the bicycle ergometer and to the follow-up jogging exercise program for the 38-month training study. Up to 30 months of training, the adherence rates for this study were comparable with other investigations (54%). Of the 46 men who initially agreed to participate, only 24% remained active at 36 months when the study was scheduled to terminate. During the two-month follow-up jogging program, 17% continued to participate. These results suggest that long-term participation cannot be expected from this type of exercise training program.

Table I shows the heart rate at rest and in response to bicycle ergometer and treadmill exercise in eight men who completed 38 months of training. After 30 months of training significant reductions were observed on the bicycle ergometer test, but not on the treadmill. The results after two months of jogging showed that heart rate was significantly reduced at rest and in response to treadmill

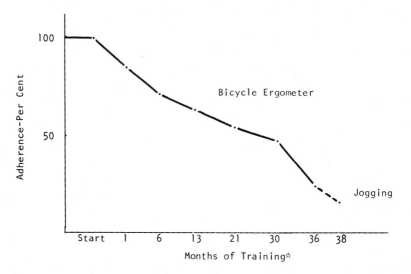

*   Bicycle ergometer training for the first 36 months, jogging from 36 to 38 months.

FIG. 1. Adherence to a bicycle ergometer and a follow-up jogging exercise program — 46 middle-aged, sedentary males for 38 months.

Table I. Heart Rate at Rest and in Response to Bicycle Ergometer
and Treadmill Exercise Test in Eight Men Who Completed
38 Months of Training

| Variable | Months of Training | | | |
	0	30[+]	36	38[++]
Heart Rate (bts/min)				
Resting	64	63	64	57*
Ergometer				
600 kpm/min	131	109*	108	105
Treadmill (3 mph)				
. 14% Grade	140	136	135	132
17% Grade[†]	147	145	147	140*

*$P < 0.05$.

[†]N = 6 men who went on to a higher workload (15%-19%, average = 17%).

[+]Interval training on a bicycle ergometer for the first 36 months of the study.

[++]Continuous walking and/or jogging for the last two months of the study.

testing at 17% inclination. These results strongly suggest that heart rate response to either jogging or ergometer training is specific to the mode of testing. These phenomena, reported previously, were observed in this investigation to occur for jogging even after a long-term bicycle ergometer program.

Table II shows systolic and diastolic blood pressure response to bicycle ergometer and treadmill testing. Significant reductions in systolic blood pressure were noted on the ergometer test after 30 months of training, but not after the jogging program. Diastolic

Table II. Systolic and Diastolic Blood Pressure Response to
Bicycle Ergometer and Treadmill Test in Eight Men
Who Completed 38 Months of Training

| Variable | Months of Training | | | |
	0	30[+]	36	38[++]
Systolic BP[†]				
Ergometer (600 kpm)	189	163*	163	163
Treadmill (3 mph)				
14% Grade	178	175	170	182
Diastolic BP[†]				
Ergometer (600 kpm)	108	88*	92	86*
Treadmill (3 mph)				
14% Grade	91	85*	89	86

*$P < 0.05$.

[†]Systolic and diastolic blood pressure in mm Hg.

[+]Interval training on a bicycle ergometer for the first 36 months of the study.

[++]Continuous walking and/or jogging for the last two months of the study.

blood pressure on the ergometer at 600 kpm was significantly reduced after 30 months of training and after the two-month follow-up jogging program. Results on the treadmill for this parameter showed significant reductions after the bicycle training, but not after the jogging program. The results on systolic and diastolic blood pressure in this study do not support the specificity of training hypothesis.

Table III shows data on eight men for body weight, skinfold thickness, blood cholesterol and attendance. Weight, skinfold and cholesterol were not significantly different after 30 months of bicycle ergometer training. Only skinfold thickness showed a significant reduction after the two-month follow-up jogging program. Attendance during the jogging program was notably higher than during the bicycle ergometer training. These results do not provide any evidence indicating that long-term bicycle ergometer training or jogging training produces significant reductions in other coronary risk factors.

Discussion

The results of this investigation are in agreement with several other studies showing that endurance-type exercise training enhances cardiovascular function in middle-aged sedentary men [6, 16].

The specificity of training effects resulting from programs of bicycle ergometry and walking/running has been studied in great detail by several investigators [12-14]. It was generally concluded that the training effects of bicycle ergometry are more task-specific than those produced by running. The results of the present investigation tend to support that hypothesis, but also suggest that a

Table III. Body Weight, Skinfold Thickness, Blood Cholesterol
and Attendance for Eight Middle-Aged, Sedentary Males
Who Completed 38 Months of Training

| Variable | Months of Training | | | |
	0	30+	36	38++
Weight (kg)	75.5	75.0	75.5	75.9
Skinfold (mm)	50	47	48	43*
Cholesterol (mg%)	221	216	216	209
Attendance (Average/week)	2.4		3.8*	

*P < 0.05.
+Interval training on a bicycle ergometer for the first 36 months of the study.
++Continuous walking and/or jogging for the last two months of the study.

follow-up jogging program after long-term bicycle training elicits additional training effects which are specific to the mode of testing. The adherence rate for the first 30 months in this investigation was comparable to other similar studies [10, 19]. However, the adherence was considerably lower between 30 and 38 months. There are numerous motivational aspects of exercise which have been discussed previously [7, 8, 15]. In general, adherence rates have been much higher for group exercise programs than for individual programs. In light of these results on long-term exercise, it is advisable to utilize group programs or to perhaps consider an unconventional approach described by Pandolf and Goldman [11]. They found that middle-aged sedentary men achieved significant improvements in cardiorespiratory fitness from a six-week program of wearing ankle spats during the waking hours with weights up to 2.25 kg per ankle. It is clear that in order to achieve long-term participation in leisure-time exercise for reducing coronary risk it will be necessary to develop new, highly innovative approaches.

References

1. Bruce, E.H., Frederick, R., Bruce, R.A. and Fisher, L.D.: Comparison of active participants and drop-outs in CAPRI cardiopulmonary rehabilitative programs. Am. J. Cardiol.37:53-60, 1976.
2. Brunner, D., Manelis, G., Modan, M. and Levin, S.: Physical activity at work and the incidence of myocardial infarction, angina pectoris and death due to ischemic heart disease. J. Chronic Dis. 27:217-233, 1974.
3. Fox, S.M., III, Naughton, J.P. and Haskell, W.L.: Physical activity and the prevention of coronary heart disease. Ann. Clin. Res. 3:404-432, 1971.
4. Froelicher, V.F. and Oberman, A.: Analysis of epidemiological studies of physical inactivity as risk factor for coronary artery disease. Progr. Cardiov. Dis. 15:41-65, 1972.
5. Gyntelberg, F.: Physical fitness and coronary heart disease in Copenhagen men aged 40-59. III. Danish Med. Bull. 21:49-56, 1974.
6. Hanson, J.S., Tabakin, B.S., Levy, A.M. and Nedde, W.: Long-term physical training and cardiovascular dynamics in middle-aged men. Circulation 38:783-799, 1968.
7. Heinzelmann, F.: Social and psychological factors that influence the effectiveness of exercise programs. In Naughton, J.P., Hellerstein, H.K. and Mohler, I.C. (eds.): Exercise Testing and Exercise Training in Coronary Heart Disease. New York:Academic Press, 1973.
8. Massie, J.F. and Shephard, R.J.: Physiological and psychological effects of training — A comparison of individual and gymnasium programs, with a characterization of the exercise "drop-out." Med. Sci. Sports 3:110-117, 1971.
9. Morris, J.N., Chave, S.P.W., Adam, C. et al: Vigorous exercise in leisure time and the incidence of coronary heart disease. Lancet 1:333-339, 1973.

10. Oja, P., Teraslinn, P., Partanen, T. and Karava, R.: Feasibility of an 18-months' physical training program for middle-aged men and its effect on physical fitness. Am. J. Public Health 64:459-465, 1974.
11. Pandolf, K.B. and Goldman, R.F.: Physical conditioning of less fit adults by use of leg weight loading. Arch. Phys. Med. Rehab. 56:255-261, 1975.
12. Pechar, G.S., McArdle, W.D., Katch, F.I. et al: Specificity of cardio-respiratory adaptation to bicycle and treadmill training. J. Appl. Physiol 36:753-755, 1974.
13. Pollock, M.L., Dimmick, J., Mi ller, H.S., Jr. et al: Effects of mode of training on cardiovascular function and body composition of adult men. Med. Sci. Sports 7:139-145, 1975.
14. Roberts, J.A. and Alspaugh, J.W.: Specificity of training effects resulting from programs of treadmill running and bicycle ergometer riding. Med. Sci. Sports 4:6-10, 1972.
15. Roth, W.T.: Some motivational aspects of exercise. J. Sports Med. 14:40-47, 1974.
16. Siegel, W., Blomqvist, G. and Mitchell, J.H.: Effects of a quantitated physical training program on middle-aged sedentary men. Circulation 91:19-29, 1970.
17. Stamler, J., Berkson, D.M., Lindberg, H.A. et al: Long-term epidemiological studies on the possible role of physical activity and physical fitness in the prevention of premature clinical coronary heart disease. In Brunner, D. and Jokl, E. (eds.): Physical Activity and Aging. Medicine and Sport, Vol. 4, Basel/New York:Karger, 1970.
18. Teraslinna, P., Partanen, T., Pyorala, K. et al: Feasibility study on physical activity intervention: Report on recruiting design, training program, and three months' experience. Work Environ. Health 6:24-31, 1969.
19. Wilhelmsen, L., Sanne, H., Elmfeldt, D. et al: A controlled trial of physical training after myocardial infarction: Effects on risk factors, nonfatal reinfarction, and death. Prev. Med. 4:491-508, 1975.

Aerobic Work Capacity in
Middle- and Old-Aged Runners

Katsumi Asano, Shinkichi Ogawa
and Yoshinori Furuta

Introduction

Considerable research of aerobic power in young trained and untrained men has been reported. However, little information is available to elucidate the aerobic work capacity of middle- and old-aged athletes [2, 3, 5].

The present study is to research the aerobic work capacity in middle- and old-aged runners who participated in regular running training for a long time.

Subjects and Methods

The subjects were 41 men aged 40 to 81 (Table I) who participated in a training program of running about 10 km for one hr/day four to six days/week for more than two years. The control sedentary group were 11 men aged 40 to 61.

For the maximal aerobic work capacity test, exhaustive running on a treadmill (zero grade) was used. The test included maximal oxygen intake ($\dot{V}O_2$ max), maximal cardiac output ($\dot{Q}$ max) and maximal heart rate (HR max).

$\dot{V}O_2$ max was determined by Douglas bag and Haldane's gas analyzer. $\dot{Q}$ max was measured by the CO_2 rebreathing method using the LB-2 Beckman analyzer.

Heart volume (HV) at rest in standing position was determined by chest radiogram and calculated by the Rohrer-Kahlstorf method.

Results and Consideration

Training Intensity of Running

Three subjects aged 65 to 67 ran for 20 minutes at their own speed.

Katsumi Asano, Shinkichi Ogawa and Yoshinori Furuta, Department of Exercise Physiology, University of Tsukuba, Saiki, Sakura-mura, Niihari-gun, Ibaraki-ken, Japan.

Table I. Physical Characteristics and Blood
Pressure at Rest

Age Groups (yrs)		Height (cm)	Weight (kg)	Blood Pressure (mm Hg)	
				Systolic	Diastolic
40-49	X̄	162.6	58.1	117	70
	SD	±6.98	±4.91	±8.63	±5.12
	N	(9)	(9)	(9)	(9)
50-59	X̄	163.9	58.0	132	79
	SD	±3.39	±6.01	±14.01	±9.85
	N	(13)	(13)	(13)	(13)
60-69	X̄	162.9	52.9	135	82
	SD	±4.29	±6.86	±18.34	±9.98
	N	(14)	(14)	(14)	(14)
70-81	X̄	156.6	51.4	157	78
	SD	±3.92	±5.83	±15.73	±8.00
	N	(5)	(5)	(5)	(5)

X̄:Means; SD:Standard deviation; N:Number of subjects.

Heart rate during running was measured by a telemetric system and $\dot{V}O_2$ was determined during one-minute exercise from the 9th to 10th minute and from the 19th to 20th minute.

These data suggested that daily training intensity of running was approximately 70% to 75% $\dot{V}O_2$ max and 90% to 95% HR max (Fig. 1).

In competition of 25 km running, one 66-year-old runner's heart rate during running was measured by telemetric system.

It appears from these data that running intensity for old-aged runners is approximately 90% to 95% HR max (Fig. 1).

Aerobic Work Capacity of Runners

$\dot{V}O_2$ max was approximately 2.5 l/min (range 2.0 to 2.9 l/min) and $\dot{V}O_2$ max/kg was approximately 45 ml/kg/min (range 39 to 50 ml/kg/min) (Fig. 2; Table II).

This value was 20% to 30% higher than the control group value of 1.8 l/min and 35 ml/kg/min for 50- to 70-year-olds.

In runners over 70 years, $\dot{V}O_2$ max/kg was 40 to 45 ml/kg/min corresponding to 40- to 50-year-olds of the control group. This value was almost the same as Pollock's data of 40 ml/kg/min in trained 75-year-olds [4].

$\dot{Q}$ max was approximately 18 l/min (range 16-22 l/min). This value was 20% higher than the control group of 50- to 55-year-olds.

Respiro -circulatory changes during ground running

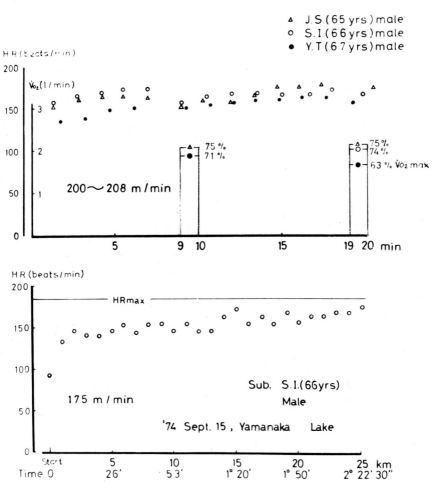

FIG. 1. Changes in oxygen intake and heart rate during usual ground running.

In the 50- to 75-year-olds, $\dot{Q}$ max was almost 15 to 18 l/min corresponding to 40- to 50-year-olds of the control group (Fig. 3).

Maximal stroke volume was approximately 100 ml/beat (range 90 to 120 ml/beat) which was 20% higher than the control group at each age (Fig. 4).

Oxygen pulse max was approximately 15 ml/beat (range 14 to16 ml/beat) in each age group. This value was 30% higher than the control group.

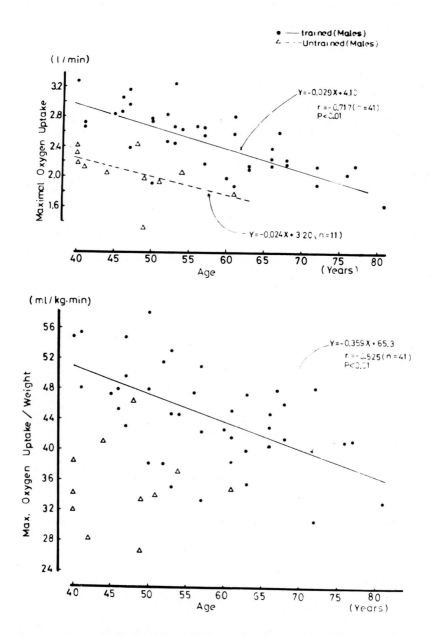

FIG. 2. Individual values for maximal oxygen uptake and maximal oxygen uptake per body weight in relation to ages.

Table II. Maximal Aerobic Power for Middle- and Old-Aged Runners

Age Groups (yrs)		$\dot{V}O_2$ (l/min)	$\dot{V}O_2$ (ml/kg/min)	$\dot{V}_E Max$ (l/min)	$\dot{Q} Max$ (l/min)	HR Max (beats/min)	SV Max (ml/beat)	$A-VO_2D$ (ml/l)
40-49	$\overline{X}$	2.89	49.7	113.2	21.8	183	120	130
	SD	±0.26	±4.21	±11.6	±2.32	±9.38	±8.49	±22.4
	N	(9)	(9)	(9)	(7)	(9)	(7)	(7)
50-59	$\overline{X}$	2.59	45.1	96.4	18.4	176	105	132
	SD	±0.31	±7.13	±16.4	±3.60	±12.9	±21.3	±21.6
	N	(13)	(13)	(13)	(8)	(13)	(8)	(8)
60-69	$\overline{X}$	2.22	42.2	84.7	16.3	168	97	133
	SD	±0.27	±3.86	±9.12	±2.33	±14.8	±12.2	±19.2
	N	(14)	(14)	(14)	(14)	(14)	(14)	(14)
70-81	$\overline{X}$	1.97	38.9	84.2	15.8	168	92	120
	SD	±0.19	±6.25	±8.87	±0.54	±14.7	±8.86	±13.1
	N	(5)	(5)	(5)	(4)	(5)	(4)	(4)

X:Means; SD:Standard deviation; N:Number of subjects.

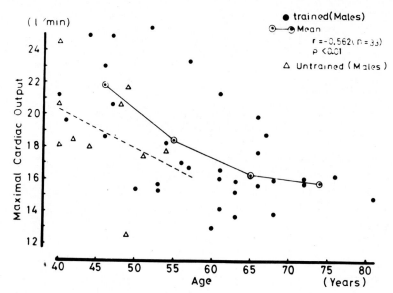

FIG. 3. Individual values for maximal cardiac output in relation to ages.

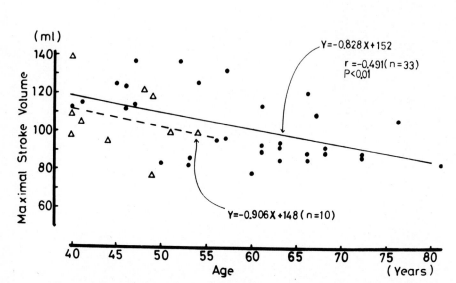

FIG. 4. Individual values for maximal stroke volume in relation to ages.

Heart volume was approximately 15 ml/kg (range 13 to 17 ml/kg) in each age group. This value was 20% to 30% higher than the control group. Benestad's data of 11 ml/kg in HV of 75-year-olds [1] were a little below compared with this present value.

Cardiodynamics of Runners

Systolic pressure at rest in the group over 50 years was significantly lower than that of the Japanese average of the same age group by 8 to 17 mm Hg, but no difference in diastolic pressure was noted. Thirty-three percent of the runners had a heart rate under 60 beats/min in supine position at rest.

Out of the comparatively high occurrence of abnormal resting ECG (II lead) was 35% P lengthening, 20% QT prolongation, 10% QRS widening and 9% PQ prolongation.

Conclusion

It may be concluded that a regular running training program of 70% to 75% $\dot{V}O_2$ max and 90-95% HR max for middle- and old-aged men significantly increased their physical resources and maintained their level of aerobic power 20% to 30% higher than the control group.

It is suggested that regular running training could prevent the development of systolic hypertension with aging in older subjects.

References

1. Benestad, A.M.: Trainability of old men. Acta Med. Scand. 178:321-327, 1961.
2. Grimby, G.N., Nilsson, J. and Saltin, B.: Cardiac output during submaximal and maximal exercise in active-middle aged athletes. J. Appl. Physiol. 21(4):1150-1156, 1966.
3. Grimby, G. and Saltin, B.: Physiological analysis of physically well-trained middle-aged and old athletes. Acta Med. Scand. 179:513-529, 1966.
4. Pollock, M.L.: Physiological characteristics of older champion track athletes. Res. Q. 45:363-373, 1974.
5. Saltin, B. and Grimby, G.: Physiological analysis of middle-aged and old former athletes. Comparison with still active athletes of the same ages. Circulation 38:1104-1115, 1968.

Acute Effects of Exercise on the Circulatory System and on Physical Strength: Results of a Study on the Prevention of Senility

K. Nishimura, I. Hosokawa, K. Kitamura and Y. Nishimura

Introduction

In recent years, the life span of the Japanese has been increasingly extended within the short period of time of 30 years. In turn, this has caused a large increase in the elderly population. The three cardinal diseases — intracranial vascular accidents, cancer and heart attack — constitute about 60% of mortality causes. Therefore, measures to protect the aged from these diseases have been searched for and are in fact regarded as urgent, along with measures to protect humans from pollution caused in the environment.

Despite the well-known fact that humans begin to get senile at about 30 years of age, factors contributory to senility have actually not been satisfactorily clarified as yet. Accordingly, no truly effective medical management of senility has been developed to the present time. Nevertheless, basic and clinical research has made it possible to delay the onset and reduce the factors of senility. For example, it is found that physical exercise is very helpful in preventing senility, exerting a beneficial effect on both prevention and treatment of arteriosclerosis and obesity.

Meanwhile, the development of the transportation systems, especially that of the automobile, has led to drastic decreases in physical activity habits. Lack of physical exercise and overnourishment tend to accelerate senility. It is obviously reasonable and important, in studying the problem of human senility, to pay attention to the relationship between these two factors.

K. Nishimura, Director, Medical Laboratory for Adult Disease and Physical Strength; I. Hosokawa, Osaka College of Physical Education; K. Kitamura, Department of Laboratory Medicine, Kyoto Prefectural University of Medicine; and Y. Nishimura, First Division of Internal Medicine, Kyoto University Hospital, Japan.

Incidentally, a symposium was held for the first time in Kyoto at the time of the 19th Japanese General Congress of Medicine in 1975 on the problem: "The Prevention of Senility and Lack of Physical Exercise Resulting from the Progress of Transportation Systems." In Japan, we have adopted golf since 1967 and marathon running since 1971 for middle- and old-aged persons as a senility-preventive measure or as a positive exercise treatment, periodically checking physical conditions by medical examinations,* performed at the Muromachi Hospital in cooperation with the local Medical Association and Health Center. From our observations, it can be stated that shaping up the middle- and old-aged persons by exercise is basically important in the prevention of senility.

Results

The general health condition and the physical strength of sportsmen were found to be superior to those of non-sportsmen (Tables I and II). Both systolic and diastolic blood pressure were improved after exercise. Their body weight and sugar in urine were found to be decreased, although there was no change observed in the fatigue test. Furthermore, the senility test shows some improvement.

**Table I. General Health and Strength Indices
Before and After One Round of Golf**

	Average Age	Height	Weight	Blood Pressure Systolic	Blood Pressure Diastolic	Physical Strength	Age
Before play			61.4 kg	136.4	87.0	40	44
	48.8	165.8 cm					
After play			60.1 kg	129.5	83.7	35	39

	Sugar in Urine	Abnormality of Electrocardiogram Severe	Abnormality of Electrocardiogram Moderate	Abnormality of Electrocardiogram Slight
Before play	16	1	18	72
After play	6	1	11	60

(The figures are based on the data collected on 493 subjects from September 1970 to September 1974.)

---

*Since 1963 we have been practicing the "Ningen-Dock" (a dock for man) twice a year in Muromachi Hospital and since 1966 we have been examining physical strength together with it. These results were used for control group (non-sportsmen group).

Table II. Apparent Effects of Playing Golf on Health Practices

| | | If One Plays Golf | | | Sports Except Golf | | |
		Improve Health	Increase Appetite	Good Sleep	Daily	Occasion-ally	None
Group I.	15 subjects (~ 40 years)	12 (80%)	11 (73%)	9 (60%)	2 (13%)	4 (27%)	7 (46%)
Group II.	18 subjects (41 ~ 51 years)	16 (88%)	13 (72%)	9 (50%)	0 (0%)	3 (17%)	14 (77%)
Group III.	17 subjects (55 ~ years)	17 (100%)	13 (76%)	12 (71%)	5 (29%)	2 (12%)	9 (52%)
Total	50 Subjects	45 (90%)	37 (74%)	30 (60%)	7 (14%)	9 (18%)	30 (60%)

The electrocardiogram of 174 golfers, 166 men and 8 women with mean age of 49 (Table III), taken immediately before and after one round of golf, revealed that ischemic and other changes were noted in subjects over 40, predominantly in the forties and fifties (Table IV).

Of 46 subjects with abnormal electrocardiograms before the round of golf, 19 showed improvements after play (Table V). It is worth noting that ischemic changes were improved in 12 subjects. The electrocardiogram remained unchanged in 21 subjects. However, six subjects showed some aggravation of the electrocardiogram after play.

Heart rate, blood pressure and the product of heart rate and systolic blood pressure before and after play are tabulated in Table VI. There was a drop in systolic blood pressure in 11 of 12 subjects in whom ischemic changes were improved, and the drop, when

Table III. Age Distribution of Golfers
(Mean : 49)

Age	Number of Examinations
20-29	10
30-39	25
40-49	59
50-59	40
60-69	35
70-79	5
Total	174

Table IV. Electrocardiograms Before a Round of Golf

Age	Normal	Abnormal	
20-29	10	0 (0)	
30-39	24	1 (4.0)	
		Nonspecific ST changes	1
40-49	45	14 (23.8)	
		Ischemic changes	5
		Left axis deviation	4
		Complete RBBB	1
		Incomplete RBBB	1
		Left atrial enlargement	1
		Right atrial enlargement	1
		P–Q prolongation	1
50-59	25	15 (37.5)	
		P–Q prolongation	3
		Old anteroseptal MI	2
		Ischemic changes	2
		Left axis deviation	2
		Complete RBBB Left axis deviation	2
		LVH	2
		Nonspecific axis deviation	2
60-69	26	9 (34.3)	
		Old infarction	2
		Ischemic changes	2
		LVH	2
		Incomplete RBBB − ischemic changes	1
		Nonspecific ST&T changes	1
		P–Q prolongation	1
70-79	4	1 (20.0)	
		P–Q prolongation − ischemic changes	1
Total	134		40
		174	

expressed in percentage, was more pronounced than in those subjects in whom ischemic changes were unchanged or aggravated. Post-exercise changes in heart rate and the product of heart rate and systolic blood pressure were not significantly different in these three groups.

Our "golfer" group was superior to the nonexercise group with regard to all three tests of physical strength: grip strength, side-step, and vertical jump and also vital capacity (Tables I and VII).

In order to investigate the effect of playing golf on physical strength, the latter was measured both before and after one round of

Table V. Electrocardiographic Changes After a Round of Golf

Improved	*19 cases*
1) Ischemic changes normalized or improved	12
2) Left axis deviation normalized	1
3) Incomplete RBBB and ischemic changes normalized	1
4) Nonspecific ST&T changes normalized	5
Unchanged	*21 cases*
1) Ischemic changes	5
2) P–Q prolongation	5
3) Left axis deviation	4
4) Complete RBBB and left axis deviation	2
5) Complete RBBB	1
6) Incomplete RBBB	1
7) Complete LBBB	1
8) Right atrial enlargement	1
9) Left atrial enlargement	1
Aggravated	*6 cases*
1) Ischemic changes appeared	4
2) Left axis deviation appeared	1
3) Occasional ventricular premature beats	1

play. Although there was no remarkable change in the score of grip strength after play, there was a significant improvement of the score side-stepping, especially in three age groups: 25 to 29, 30 to 39 and 45 to 49 years (Table VIII). The result also showed a tendency for the improvement of the score of vertical jumping after play. Playing golf seems to contribute to improved leg strength but has no positive effect on arm strength.

The results of the marathon runner's group tested before and after 5,000 or 10,000 meter runs were similar to those of the golfers' group.

It may be that active participation in sports by the middle aged and the elderly improves their general health, builds up their physical strength, serves to retard senility and helps to alleviate mental stress and strain. In addition, appropriate exercise exerts a beneficial effect on ischemic heart disease. Certain types of sports and exercises are suitable for rehabilitation of selected cases of old myocardial infarction. Physical activities appear useful as a supplement to medical treatment and possibly in the prevention of geriatric diseases. It will become increasingly more important to determine the optimum amount and the most effective method of exercise for those middle-aged and elderly persons who constitute a large portion of our society.

Table VI. Cardiovascular Changes After One Round of Golf

	Case	Heart Rate Before	Heart Rate After	Systolic B.P. Before	Systolic B.P. After	Diastolic B.P. Before	Diastolic B.P. After	Sys. × HR Before	Sys. × HR After
Improved Cases	1	63	94	128	118	78	70	81	111
	2	60	90	140	135	95	85	84	122
	3	78	102	125	130	80	90	98	133
	4	110	126	150	144	95	98	165	181
	5	67	90	160	144	92	90	107	130
	6	66	84	148	134	88	82	98	113
	7	67	62	180	136	78	80	120	84
	8	63	86	144	122	92	86	91	105
	9	73	73	144	118	92	86	105	86
	10	77	70	140	132	102	104	108	92
	11	92	110	126	108	88	76	116	119
	12	80	88	138	130	90	90	110	114
	Mean	74.7	89.6	143.6	129.3	89.2	86.4	106.9	115.8
	± S.D.	±13.8	±16.8	±14.8	±10.4	±7.0	±8.8	±20.9	±24.9
	%		+19.9		−10.0		−3.4		+7.7
Aggravated Cases	1	53	73	160	124	110	86	93	91
	2	95	110	138	144	94	90	131	158
	3	76	82	144	134	88	90	110	110
	4	67	88	134	134	78	72	90	100
	Mean	72.8	88.3	144.0	134.0	92.5	84.5	106.0	114.8
	± S.D.	±15.4	±13.6	± 9.9	± 7.1	±11.6	±7.4	±16.3	±25.9
	%		+10.8		−6.9		−8.7		+8.3
Unchanged Cases	1	70	96	140	128	80	80	98	123
	2	110	126	150	144	95	98	165	181
	3	59	83	148	136	90	82	87	113
	4	73	88	121	138	82	86	88	121
	5	78	73	138	132	94	94	108	96
	Mean	78.0	93.2	139.4	135.6	88.2	88.0	109.2	126.8
	± S.D.	±17.1	±18.0	±10.3	± 5.4	±6.1	±6.9	±28.9	±28.7
	%		+19.5		−2.7		−0.3		+15.2

Table VII. Vital Capacity in Japanese Nonathletes, Golfers and Marathon Runners

Age	Nonathletes Cases	Nonathletes Vit. Cap.	Golfers Cases	Golfers Vit. Cap.	Marathon Runners Cases	Marathon Runners Vit. Cap.
30-39	298	2421-2361	138	3857		
40-49	197	2311-2187	78	3396		
50-59	84	2198-2051	54	2956		
60-	77	1849-1510	78	2370	52	2597
Method	Spirometer			Spirometer		

Table VIII. Motor Fitness Scores Before and After One Round of Golf

Age	N	Before Play Grip Strength		Vertical Jump		Side Step		After Play Grip Strength		Vertical Jump		Side Step	
		M	SD	M	SD	M	SD	M	SD	M	SD	M	SD
20-24	3	55.83	4.093	59.66	4.505	42.33	3.775	52.33	3.663	61.00	3.265	46.66	4.035
25-29	10	49.35	5.617	49.80	6.108	38.50	5.277	48.50	5.970	54.95	5.672	42.40	3.583
30-34	19	51.81	5.509	48.81	7.631	37.26	3.042	52.68	6.219	52.23	6.901	41.15	2.733
35-39	14	48.42	5.369	44.25	3.839	37.00	5.818	47.39	5.380	46.60	3.446	41.42	4.811
40-44	37	51.91	8.290	45.48	7.399	36.21	7.231	51.98	7.969	48.61	6.642	39.02	7.152
45-49	28	46.46	6.284	39.26	6.065	34.57	4.341	47.42	6.796	39.51	8.160	37.28	5.261
50-54	14	45.89	6.783	35.28	5.991	33.35	3.559	45.82	7.804	39.78	6.516	34.64	3.703
55-59	35	46.45	6.399	33.01	7.704	30.71	5.280	46.83	7.024	35.61	6.402	33.14	5.472
60-64	21	44.09	6.205	32.21	3.998	29.52	7.225	45.73	5.358	33.19	3.740	30.95	5.949
65-69	13	40.98	3.822	31.34	4.286	29.30	3.433	40.01	4.599	32.76	5.309	30.61	3.588
70-	2	29.75	1.250	21.00	1.000	18.50	0.500	23.25	1.280	23.00	4.080	22.00	4.000

Analysis of Cardiac Function of Well-Trained Men During Prolonged Exercise in Hot Air Temperature

Yoji Suzuki, Yoshio Kuroda,
Katsumi Tuskakoshi, Teruya Amemiya
and Shizuo Ito

Introduction

In temperatures as high as 40 C, despite an increase of skin blood flow, the cardiac output ($\dot{Q}$) during prolonged exercise decreases successively from a high level during the initial period. Shortly after the start of this decrease, $\dot{V}O_2$ starts to decrease as well. On the other hand, the heart rate (HR) does not reach the maximum level when $\dot{V}O_2$ max is determined. This fact suggests the distribution of $\dot{Q}$ must be altered to facilitate heat dissipation [2]. The change in these cardiovascular functions during exercise in hot temperatures must affect the mechanical ventricular systole and the heart's hemodynamics.

In this study, cardiac function, during a prolonged period of exercise at various air temperatures, was investigated in well-trained men by means of mechanocardiography (MCG) and by measuring $\dot{Q}$.

Methods

The subjects were four well-trained men (20 to 21 years old) who had been distance running since their school days. Table I lists their physical characteristics along with $\dot{V}O_2$ max and their individual best time in 5,000 meter running. The temperature conditions set up in an artificial climate chamber, at atmospheric pressure, were as follows: 0 C-80% relative humidity, 10 C-80%, 20 C-60%, 30 C-60%, and 40 C-60%. The clothing worn was minimal, only running shorts and shoes.

Yoji Suzuki, Yoshio Kuroda, Katsumi Tuskakoshi, Teruya Amemiya and Shizuo Ito, The Institute for Sports Science and Medicine of the Amateur Sports Association of Japan.

Table I. Characteristics of Subjects

Subjects	Age yr	Height cm	Weight kg	Best Results 5,000 meter Running min, sec	$\dot{V}E$ (BTPS) l/min	Maximum Oxygen Uptake			
						$\dot{V}O_2$ l/min	$\dot{V}O_2$/Wt ml/kg/min	HR beats/min	RF cycles/min
A.M.	20	163.0	54.08	16'27"2	141.65	3.79	70.04	190.0	68.0
B.S.	20	164.0	52.76	15'33"0	154.69	3.90	73.90	192.0	67.0
C.W.	21	159.7	53.11	16'08"0	127.63	3.77	70.95	187.0	56.0
D.K.	21	175.5	62.55	15'34"0	155.59	4.16	66.54	181.0	63.0

After a rest time of 30 minutes while sitting in a 25 ± 1 C room, the subject entered the climate chamber and the rest period was continued for 15 minutes. Exercise was performed on a bicycle ergometer with a workload of 1,080 kpm/min. This corresponded to about 65% $\dot{V}O_2$ max at 20 C while in a sitting posture until exhaustion. Exercise was stopped for 10 to 20 seconds every ten minutes so as to record MCG. The intervals for each measurement were as follows: every minute for rectal and skin temp., HR and respiratory frequency (RF), every ten minutes for the collection of expired air and every five minutes for blood pressure (BP) measurement. $\dot{Q}$ was measured after 10 minutes, and then at 30 minute-intervals, and just before exhaustion. All measurements were continued for 15 minutes after the end of the exercise period.

Expired air for oxygen uptake ($\dot{V}O_2$) determination was collected and measured in a Douglas bag. The expired air was analyzed with a Scholander microgas analyzer within accuracy to ± 0.05 vol%. HR was calculated from the ECG and RF was found by using a thermistor connected to a pen-writing oscillograph. The skin temperature was measured at four sites: the forehead(Ts-fh), calf(Ts-c), thigh(Ts-t) and chest(Ts-ch) by thermistors. Rectal temperature(Tre) was measured with a thermistor inserted to a depth of 8 cm. The thermistors were calibrated in a thermoregulated water-bath just before and after each experiment against a mercury thermometer standardized by the Meteorological Institute of Japan. Measurement of BP was made using a Riva-Rocci mercury manometer. The cuff was attached to the arm about 2 cm above the antecubital space. During measurement, the point of first appearance of an audible pulse beat was recorded as the systolic pressure(MaBP), and then the sound was noted to become quite suddenly muffled(IVP) and shortly to disappear(VP). IVP was used as diastolic pressure(MiBP) [3]. Mean blood pressure(MeBP) and pulse pressure(PP) were determined as follows: MeBP = (MaBP + MiBP)/2, PP = MaBP – MiBP. $\dot{Q}$ was measured by a CO_2 rebreathing method. Each expired gas sample during rebreathing was analyzed for CO_2 content with the Scholander microgas analyzer. CO_2 content in the rebreathing gas was 5% mixed with 95% O_2. The gas volume in the bag was determined to equal the subject's tidal volume. End-tidal PCO_2 was measured by the end-normal-expiratory method. Breathing rate was regulated by using a metronome set at 15 cycles/min at rest and 40 cycles/min during exercise. From the arteriovenous CO_2 difference and the CO_2 output, $\dot{Q}$ was calculated according to Fick's principle [5]. Also, other cardiovascular parameters were calculated: oxygen pulse

$(O_2$ pul) = $\dot{V}O_2/HR$(ml/beat), stroke volume(SV) = $\dot{Q}/HR$(ml) and arteriovenous oxygen difference $(A\text{-}VO_2D)$ = $\dot{V}O_2/\dot{Q}$(ml/liter). The duration of time for left ventricular systole was measured from simultaneous recording of the electrocardiogram (ECG), the phonocardiogram (PCG) and the carotid arterial pulse (CAP) tracing employing a pen-writing oscillograph (described as MCG). ECG was a vectocardiogram with the Frank's lead. The PCG was recorded using a microphone with an air conducting tube placed on fifth intercostal space of left midclavicular line (KA5) to pick up the initial high frequency vibrations of the first cardio (IA) and the second cardio (IIA) sounds. The onset of IA was determined at the beginning of the first main vibration (40-150) and the onset of IIA at the first vibration of high vibration for a short time indicated on a space between the end of the T wave of the ECG and just before the dicrotic notch (DN) of CAP. The CAP was picked up by a semiconductor-strain-gauge with a metal tubing (length = 5 cm, internal diameter = 10 mm) [4, 8]. As shown in Figure 1, the total electromechanical systolic interval (Q-IIA), the left ventricular

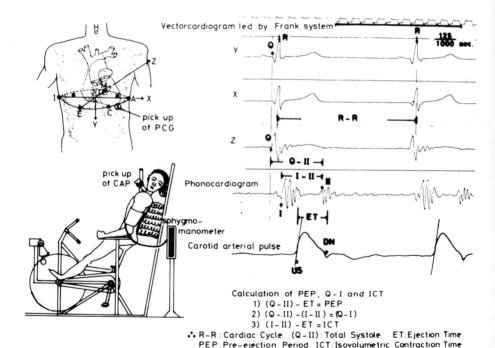

FIG. 1. A record of mechanocardiograph and a method of measurement.

ejection time (ET) and the interval between IA and IIA were measured directly from MCG. From these measurements, other intervals were calculated as shown in Figure 1. All interval times (mm sec) were determined as the mean of measurements made on six consecutive beats. Q-IIA, ET and PEP were corrected with Weisseler's equation and ICT with MiBP. Hemodynamic index (HDMi) was derived from the relation of PEP to ET [9-11], that is, Q-IIi = 2.1 $\times$ HR + Q-II, ETi = 1.7 $\times$ HR + ET, PEPi = 0.4 $\times$ HR + PEP, ICTi = ICT/MiBP, HDMi = PEP/ET. Then, the cardiac work (CaW) and CaW/min (CaW/M) were calculated as follows: CaW = MeBP $\times$ SV = 0.0013 gr/cm^2 $\times$ xmm Hg $\times$ ycm^3 (cc), CaW/M = CaW $\times$ HR/min.

Results

The mean of the maximum exercise time(ExT) was greatest at 10 C, even though two subjects had their longest ExT at 20 C. However, ExT of all subjects decreased in the two highest temperatures: 30 C and 40 C. At 40 C, the decrease in ExT varied from 11.5% to 26.7% of the maximum value. The rate of increase in Tre during exercise was greater as environmental temperature increased; however, highest Tre was about the same. $\dot{V}O_2$ was highest at 10 C and significantly lower at 40 C even though the work rate was the same. HR increased to higher values as temperatures were raised and, conversely, O_2 pul dropped gradually with the rising temperature. Ts-t rose progressively with each temperature condition, till 37.8 C at 30 C and 39 C at 40 C. Q-II became shorter at higher temperatures than at lower and, in higher temperatures, shortened gradually with the continuing exercise. ICT in high temperature was a little shorter than in lower. PEP and ET also shortened in higher temperatures. MaBP at 40 C fell only on approaching exhaustion. MeBP indicated about the same value in the initial period of exercise, but as the exercise continued, it fell notably in higher temperatures. $\dot{Q}$ was about the same at every condition in the initial period of exercise, but at exhaustion it decreased. This decrease was greater at 40 C probably because of SV variation (Fig. 2).

All of the values measured at exhaustion are shown in Figure 3, the values being the mean and range of four subjects. MeBP and CaW fell, and SV and $\dot{Q}$ decreased in higher temperatures. These changing ratios became larger with increasing temperatures. A-VO$_2$D became higher at 40 C; O_2 pulse fell accordingly as the temperature became higher. Q-IIi was a little higher at 40 C, but a significant difference from the values at other temperatures was not shown. ETi became

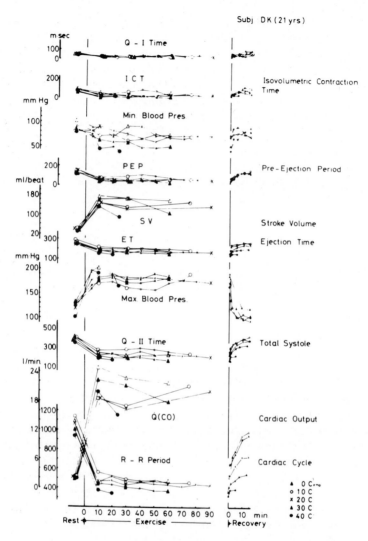

FIG. 2. The effect of external temperature on the variation of cardiac function during prolonged exercise.

higher with the rising temperature and, conversely, PEPi fell. ICTi shortened notably in conditions above 20 C as compared to conditons below 10 C. HDMi was almost the same for every condition. The relation of the indices of the cardiac muscle contractile strength and HDMi to SV during rest and exercise is shown in Figure 4. Even when the cardiac muscle contraction was

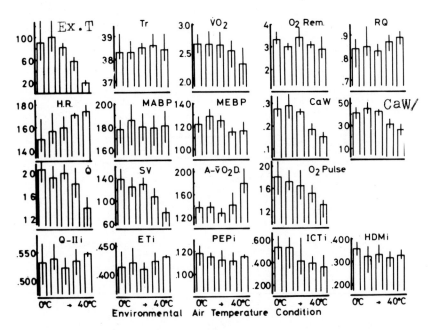

FIG. 3. The effect of external temperature on the respiratory and cardiovascular function at the exhaustion point of submaximum exercise and the exercise time.

strengthened as exercise continued at 30 C and 40 C, SV decreased. HDMi became lower at higher temperatures despite the decrease in SV. Average variation of $\dot{V}O_2$ and several parameters of cardiac function during exercise are shown in Figure 5. HR was increased along with the rising temperature and also as exercise continued, but it never attained the maximum value determined $\dot{V}O_2$ max. ICTi decreased to a lower level with the rising temperature, but did not show a time-to-time variation during exercise. Whereas SV decreased with both raised temperature and continuing exercise. CaW also decreased due to decrease in SV.

Discussion

A criterion for the strength of cardiomuscular contraction is given by ICTi and ETi; also a hemodynamic state is observed by HDMi. That is, ICTi is in inverse proportion to the strength of cardiomuscular contraction. A negative correlation is shown in the relation between the cardiomuscular strength and PEPi. Also, ETi is in inverse proportion to HR and in proportion to SV. The extension of ETi indicates the high $\dot{Q}$ state, and the shortening, the low state. If

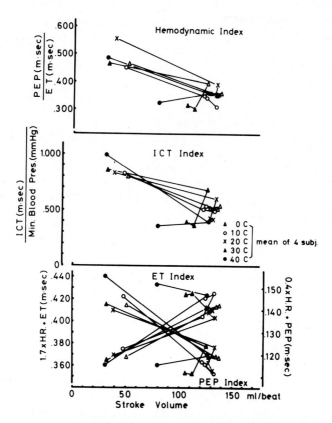

FIG. 4. The effect of external temperature on relation of PEPi, ETi, ICTi, and HDMi to stroke volume during rest and prolonged exercise.

the inotropic action is accelerated, despite the shortening of PEP, the extension of ET is not shown and Q-II is shortened. In this case, the increase of SV resulted from the elevation of ejection rate, as HDMi becomes smaller [6, 7, 9-12].

In high temperature, the cardiomuscular contraction was strengthened because ICTi was shortened, but SV decreased gradually with the continuing exercise. On the other hand, ETi did not shorten in high temperature despite the decrease of SV, and HDMi became smaller. This fact suggests an acceleration of inotropic action due to the decline in heart filling at high temperature. In this case, because of the decreased SV, even if the strength of contraction of the heart muscle was increased, the reason for the extended ETi cannot be explained because of the decrease in blood quantity

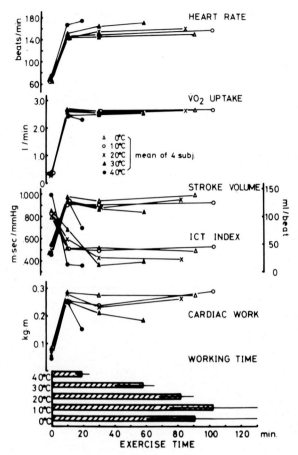

FIG. 5. The effect of external temperature on the variation of HR, $\dot{V}O_2$, SV, ICTi and CaW during prolonged exercise.

ejected into the aorta. The reason why HDMi becomes smaller in high temperature results from the decline in the heart filling.

Despite the same exercise Tre. at each temperature, greater A-VO$_2$D at higher temperatures indicates oxygen intake ratio in active muscle rises. However, the decrease of $\dot{V}O_2$ suggests the change in this ratio has a limit and oxygen intake in the muscle is determined by the muscle blood flow (BF). On the other hand, a fall of MiBP at higher temperatures may suggest an output of systolic reserve is increased because the aortic valve must be shut when the left intraventricular pressure becomes lower than the aortic pressure. However, SV in high temperature decreases. These facts mean that the increase of skin capillary blood in high temperature makes the distribution of $\dot{Q}$ change and BF in the muscles decreases.

A fall of CaW at high temperature due to a decrease in SV, despite the strengthened contraction of the heart muscle, suggests a fall in efficiency of the heart's action. This does not mean the heart is itself fatigued because the HR at exhaustion was not the maximum HR, as was attained during $\dot{V}O_2$ max determination. Cardiac function is almost the same at initial period during exercise in every condition, then SV and CaW both decrease with the continuation of exercise in high temperature, and muscular contraction of the heart strengthens. Also, these changes suggest the cardiac function is affected by the length of time in high temperature. From the above consideration, when exercise is prolonged in high temperature, the distribution of $\dot{Q}$ is altered to increase skin BF, without reference to muscle activity, for the purpose of thermoregulation. An increase in skin BF means a decrease in venous return and this causes the filling of the heart to decrease, but aortic pressure is maintained by growing peripheral resistance and increasing amount of skin blood flow. The contractile strength of the heart muscle and the HR increase to cause an increase in $\dot{Q}$, despite the decrease in venous return. The contraction strength is probably regulated by the length of heart muscle depending upon a certain level of the diastolic reserve volume. So, even if HR increase at higher temperatures, if the venous return decreases, the increase of $\dot{Q}$ dependent upon HR may be limited to maintain the muscle length, because despite the decrease of SV, Q-IIi was extended in high temperature and CaW became lower. Overall, it would be concluded that the increase of skin BF becomes fundamentally and directly a causative factor of the decrease in venous return which makes the filling of the heart decline and $\dot{Q}$ decrease.

Summary

Performing a prolonged exercise with about 65% $\dot{V}O_2$ max load until exhaustion by four well-trained men, the cardiac function was measured by means of MCG, $\dot{Q}$, SV, BP and $\dot{V}O_2$ in five temperature conditions of 0 C to 40 C. High temperature made $\dot{V}O_2$, $\dot{Q}$, and SV drop, but HR increased. A-VO_2D became greater in high than in lower temperature. MeBP fell, ICTi shortened and CaW dropped in high temperature, but HDMi was almost the same or a little shortened in comparison with it at lower temperatures despite the extension of Q-IIi. These results suggest the decline of cardiac function, but cannot be considered the fatigue of the heart muscle itself. The decrease of venous return because of altering the distribution of Q̇ makes the heart filling decline and this affects the cardiac function during exercise in high temperature. So, in high temperature, because the increase of skin BF due to the thermoregulation makes the venous return decrease, the cardiac function during exercise is limited by the increasing degree of skin BF.

References

1. Blumberger, K. and Meiners, S.: Studies of cardiac dynamics. *In* Luisada, A.A. (ed.): Cardiology and Encyclopedia of the Cardiovascular System, Vol. II, Part 4. New York:McGraw-Hill, 1957, 372 pp.
2. Kuroda, Y., Suzuki, Y., Tuskagoshi, K. et al: Temperature and Endurance Exercise. IV. The effect of temperature on circulatory function in sub-maximum exercise (in Japanese). The 1972 Reports of Sports Science Committee of the Japanese Amateur Sports Association, Vol. VII, 1974.
3. Kuroda, Y., Tamura, M., Toyoda, H. et al: Comparison of Direct Method and Auscultatory Method Measuring of Arterial Blood Pressure during Exercise. Proceedings of the Dept. of Physical Ed., College of General Ed., University of Tokyo, No. 4, Aug. 1967.
4. Luisada, A.A., MacCannon, D.M., Kumar, S. and Feiger, L.P.: Change views on the mechanism of the first and second heart sounds. Am. Heart J. 88(4):503, 1974.
5. Magel, J.R. and Anderson, K.: Cardiac output in muscular exercise measured by CO_2 rebreathing procedure. *In* Ergometry in Cardiology. 1967, 147pp.
6. Metzger, C.C., Chough, C.D., Krootz, F.W. and Leonard, J.J.: True isovolumic contraction time. Its correlation with two external indexes of ventricular performance. Am. J. Cardiol. 25:434, 1970.
7. Reeves, T.J., Hefner, L.L., Jones, W.B. et al: Hemodynamic determinants of the rate of change in pressure in left ventricle during isometric contraction. Am. Heart J. 60:745, 1960.
8. Sakamoto, J., Kaito, G. and Ueda, H.: Electrocardiographic and phonocardiographic studies in hypertension. II. Phonocardiographic study with special reference to the atrial sound and "Q-I" interval. Jap. Heart J. 1:213, 1960.
9. Wallance, A.G., Mitchell, J.H., Skinner, H.S. and Sarnoff, S.J.: Duration of the phase of left ventricular systole. Cire. Rev. 12:611, 1962.
10. Weissler, A.M., Perler, R.G. and Rochill, W.H., Jr.: Relationship between left ventricular ejection time, stroke volume, and heart rate in normal individuals and patients with cardiovascular disease. Am. Heart J. 62:367, 1961.
11. Weissler, A.M., Harris, L.C. and White, G.D.: Left ventricular ejection time index in man. J. Appl. Physiol. 18(5):919, 1963.
12. William, B.J. and Foster, G.L.: Determinants of duration of left ventricular ejection in normal young men. J. Appl. Physiol. 19(2):279, 1964.

Sympathoadrenal Changes in Athletes and Nonathletes During Graded Exercise in a Cold Environment

A. K. Chin, N. Gledhill and I. Fedchun

Introduction

The sympathoadrenal system plays an important role in maintaining homeostatic functions during exercise and cold stress [4, 6]. The increased secretion of epinephrine (E) from the adrenal medulla and of norepinephrine (NE), mainly from the adrenergic vasomotor system, elicited by homeostatic reflexes, serves to increase the availability of fuel or to prevent disturbances in the cardiovascular system [8]. Since many of the physiological systems are influenced by E and NE, it is possible that the enhanced physical performance by trained athletes may be related in part to an adaptation of the sympathoadrenal function. This study was designed to examine the plasma E and NE responses in untrained men and in highly trained athletes during graded exercise in a cold environment.

Materials and Methods

The subjects in this study were 14 healthy male university students ranging in age from 20 to 26 years. Seven of the subjects were highly trained athletes who competed in track at the provincial and/or national level. The other seven subjects were the untrained group. Special efforts were made to minimize the emotional factors involved in the study. The subjects visited the laboratory several times prior to the experimental day and were familiarized with the entire testing protocol, including several trial runs on the treadmill. All subjects had participated in at least one to three previous studies

A. K. Chin, N. Gledhill and I. Fedchun, Human Performance Laboratory, York University, Toronto, Ontario, Canada; and Biosciences Division, Defence and Civil Institute of Environmental Medicine, Toronto, Ontario, Canada.

The research for this paper was supported by the Defence Research Board of Canada Grant # 9310-147 and the York University Faculty of Science.

which had involved catheterization during exhaustive treadmill testing. A 21-gauge thin-wall vein needle was introduced into one of the superficial dorsal hand veins near the dorsal venous arch [9]. Clotting was prevented by repeated flushing with heparinized saline solutions. Two 10-ml control blood samples were taken, one at least 30 minutes after catheterization and one immediately prior to the start of exercise. During the treadmill test at 4±1 C, the work intensity was increased progressively every two minutes from an initial 4 mph at a 0% grade to a maximum of 8 mph at a 10% grade. Ten milliliters of blood was sampled serially in cooled heparinized syringes during the second minute of each new workload. The catecholamine levels were assayed in duplicate by a modification of the trihydroxyindole method of Anton and Sayre [1] using a Turner spectrofluorometer (model 430). A Student t analysis with appropriate corrections for multiple comparisons was used to analyze the data [22].

Results

An inspection of Figure 1 reveals that when the plasma NE concentrations are compared at various work intensities expressed as O_2 uptake in ml/kg/min, the athletes showed lower NE levels at moderate and higher intensities of exercise at 4 C than the untrained men. Figure 2 shows that when the E values are compared at the same absolute workloads, the athletes had lower E levels at higher intensities of exercise than the untrained subjects. As shown in Figure 3, when the NE levels are compared at various work intensities expressed as a percentage of maximal O_2 uptake ($M\dot{V}O_2$), the NE concentrations increased slowly up to approximately 50% to 65% $M\dot{V}O_2$ of the untrained group and 75% to 85% $M\dot{V}O_2$ of the athletes; thereafter the NE levels increased rapidly. Figure 4 reveals that the plasma E levels increased slowly up to about 65% to 75% $M\dot{V}O_2$ of the untrained men and 80% to 90% $M\dot{V}O_2$ of the athletes; whereafter the E concentrations increased markedly.

Discussion

The plasma NE and E responses during graded exercise at 4 C were similar to the findings we reported previously at 25 C [5], but the catecholamine levels were slightly higher in the cold environment. The results of the present investigation are in agreement with the findings of several studies at ambient temperatures which showed that muscular activity caused an increase in plasma catechol-

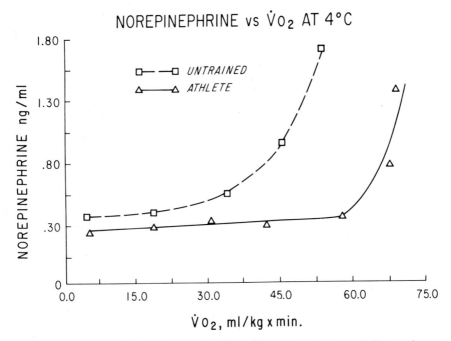

FIG. 1. Plasma norepinephrine responses to graded exercise at 4 C. Comparisons between untrained men (□) and highly trained athletes (△) are made at various work intensities expressed as O_2 uptake in ml/kg/min.

amines [2, 10, 11, 14-17, 24]. When the NE levels are compared at the same absolute workloads (Fig. 1), the athletes showed lower NE concentrations at moderate and higher intensities of exercise than the untrained subjects. These findings are in accord with the results of several authors [11, 14, 16] who reported that plasma NE levels were lower in trained than in untrained men at the same workloads. In contrast to these findings, Vendsalu [24] reported that there were no significant differences in the NE concentrations between trained and untrained subjects working at comparable loads.

When the E concentrations are compared at the same absolute workloads (Fig. 2), the athletes showed lower E levels at higher intensities of exercise than the untrained men. Several authors [2, 16, 17, 24] have reported a gradual increase in plasma E levels during prolonged heavy exercise. These findings are at variance with the results of Haggendal et al [11] who indicated that the plasma E values were unaltered during heavy work. Hartley et al [14, 15] reported that the plasma E levels were elevated significantly above resting values only at exhaustion. He also found that the E response

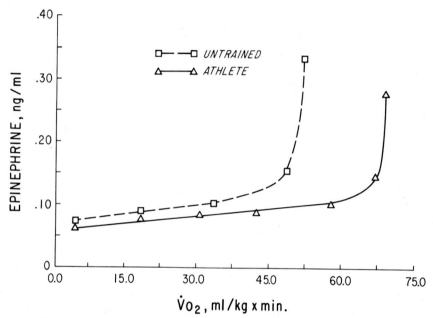

FIG. 2. Plasma epinephrine responses to graded exercise at 4 C. Comparisons between untrained men (□) and highly trained athletes (△) are made at various work intensities expressed as O_2 uptake in ml/kg × min.

to exercise was unchanged by physical training. Johnson et al [16] reported lower plasma E and NE levels in racing cyclists as compared to untrained subjects at the end of heavy exercise. Ostman et al [20] found lower E and NE excretion in urine in trained rats as compared to untrained rats after two hours of swimming.

When the plasma NE and E concentrations are compared at various work intensities expressed as a % $M\dot{V}O_2$, the onset of the increased NE and E secretions occurred at lower intensities of exercise for the untrained men and at higher intensities of work for the athletes (Figs. 3 and 4). Hartley [13] reported that after a seven-week program of endurance training, the NE levels were lower at any absolute value of O_2 uptake, but the NE concentrations at each relative work intensity (% $M\dot{V}O_2$) were not affected. Haggendal et al [11] reported that the plasma NE levels increased slowly, up to about 75% $M\dot{V}O_2$; thereafter, the NE concentrations increased rapidly. It should be noted that in the latter study only one of the subjects was involved in regular endurance training.

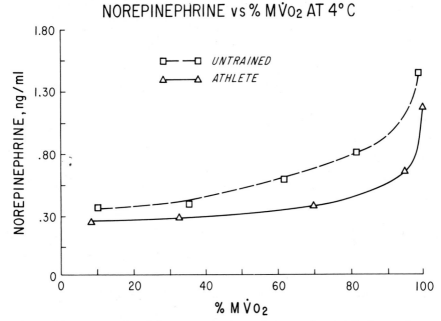

FIG. 3. Plasma norepinephrine responses to graded exercise at 4 C. Comparisons between untrained men (□) and highly trained athletes (△) are made at various work intensities expressed as a percent of maximal O_2 uptake.

An organism must be capable of secreting sufficient amounts of biologically active amines in order to maintain metabolic balance in a cold environment [18]. NE represents the first line of defense in the cold because of its heat production role. Hannon et al [12] reported that the calorigenic action of NE is achieved largely through a stimulation of lipid metabolism. Radomski [21] found an increased lipid mobilization with an enhanced utilization of free fatty acids as a fuel substrate for heat production during cold stress. Leduc [18] reported that in the cold, E acts as a second line of defense which supplements the readily limited synthesis and/or secretion of NE.

The increased secretion of catecholamines and corticosteroids is necessary to mobilize lipids, proteins, and glycolytic substrates to facilitate the increased energy demands of exercising in a cold environment [25]. Corticosteroids potentiate E action in glucose oxidation [23], fat mobilization [19] and catabolic production of keto acids for oxidation [23]. Bergstrom and Hultman [3] found that muscular fatigue was associated with the depletion of muscle glycogen. NE and E influence the rate of depletion of muscle glycogen through the activation of phosphorylase [7]. The lower

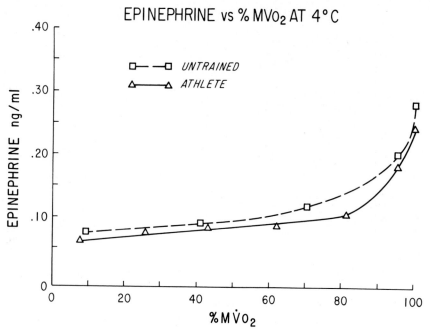

FIG. 4. Plasma epinephrine responses to graded exercise at 4 C. Comparisons between untrained men (□) and highly trained athletes (△) are made at various work intensities expressed as a percent of maximal O_2 uptake.

concentrations of NE and E in the athletes may have decreased the rate of utilization and thus may have delayed the breakdown of muscle glycogen. This lower rate of glycogen depletion would lead to an increase in endurance performance and a decrease in blood lactate levels [15] which the athletes showed. The athletes were capable of running two to four minutes longer than the untrained group at 8 mph at a 8% to 10% grade. This enhanced physical performance by the athletes may be related in part to a modification of the sympathoadrenal function. In summary, the lower sympathoadrenal response by the highly trained athletes suggests an improvement in the mechanisms of adaptation to the increased demands of exercising in a cold environment.

References

1. Anton, A.H. and Sayre, D.F.: J. Pharmacol. Exp. Ther. 138:360-375, 1962.
2. Banister, E.W. and Griffiths, J.: J. Appl. Physiol. 33:674-676, 1972.
3. Bergstrom, J. and Hultman, E.: Scand. J. Clin. Lab. Invest. 19:218-228, 1967.

4. Chin, A.K.: *In* Taylor, A.W. (ed.): Application of Science and Medicine to Sport. Springfield, Ill:Thomas Publishing Co., 1975, pp. 127-136.
5. Chin, A.K., Gledhill, N. and Fedchun, I.: Fed. Proc. 35:528, 1976.
6. Chin, A.K., Seaman, R. and Kapileshwarker, M.: J. Appl. Physiol. 34:409-412, 1973.
7. Ellis, S.E.: Physiol. Pharmacol. 4:179-226, 1967.
8. Euler, U.S.V.: Med. Sci. Sports. 6:165-173, 1974.
9. Forster, H.V., Dempsey, J.A., Thomson, J. et al: J. Appl. Physiol. 32:134-137, 1972.
10. Galbo, H., Holst, J.J. and Christensen, N.J.: J. Appl. Physiol. 38:70-76, 1975.
11. Haggendal, J., Hartley, L.H. and Saltin, B.: Scand. J. Clin. Lab. Invest. 26:337-342, 1970.
12. Hannon, J.P., Evonuk, E. and Larson, A.M.: Fed. Proc. 22:783-788, 1963.
13. Hartley, L.H.: Med. Sci. Sports 7:34-36, 1975.
14. Hartley, L.H., Mason, J.W., Hogan, R.P. et al: J. Appl. Physiol. 33:602-606, 1972.
15. Hartley, L.H., Mason, J.W., Hogan, R.P. et al: J. Appl. Physiol. 33:607-610, 1972.
16. Johnson, R.H., Park, D.M., Reunie, M.J. and Sulaiman, W.R.: Proc. Physiol. Soc. 23P-25P, April 1974.
17. Kotchen, T.A., Hartley, L.H., Rice, T.W. et al: J. Appl. Physiol. 31:178-184, 1971.
18. Leduc, J.: Acta Physiol. Scand. Suppl. 183:1-101, 1961.
19. Masoro, E.J.: Physiol. Rev. 46:67-101, 1966.
20. Ostman, I., Sjostrand, N.O. and Swedin, G.: Acta Physiol. Scand. 86:299-308, 1972.
21. Radomski, M.W.: Can. J. Physiol. Pharmacol. 44:711-719, 1966.
22. Ryan, T.: Psychopharmacol. Bull. 56:26-47, 1959.
23. Smith, R.E. and Hoijer, D.J.: Physiol. Rev. 42:60-142, 1962.
24. Vendsalu, A.: Acta Physiol. Scand. 49: Suppl. 173, 1960.
25. Wilson, O., Hedner, P., Laurell, S. et al: J. Appl. Physiol. 28:543-548, 1970.

Physical Responses to Various Ambient Temperatures During Treadmill Walking at Various Speeds and During Recovery

Introduction

Performance of exercise is affected by ambient temperature; generally, the effect is dominant under hot environment. Moreover, these effects from ambient temperature may be affected according to the degree of exercise. In this sense, there have been few systematic reports, especially with light-loaded performances. In this study, the physiological responses during walking at various speeds under various ambient temperatures were measured and discussed with reference to thermoregulation and performance.

Method

The exercise consisted of walking on a treadmill at the speeds of 3, 4, 5 and 5.5 km/hr in an artificial climate room at ambient temperatures (Ta) of 25, 30, 33 and 36 ± 0.5 C, humidity 60 ± 10% and wind velocity below 30 cm/sec. Experiments were conducted in July on three healthy males aged 20 to 23 years. They were required to rest on a chair for 40 minutes; then they were asked to walk for 40 minutes (at each speed) followed by a recovery period of 40 minutes (while sitting on a chair). This protocol was repeated for each ambient temperature with subjects wearing working clothes. Heat production, body temperatures, heat flow, heart rate, blood pressure, reaction time, etc., were recorded.

Measurement Techniques: Heat Production (Hp)

Five-minute expired air samples were taken every ten minutes by the Douglas bag method. *Rectal temperature* (TR) was measured by

Masatoshi Tanaka, Centre de recherche en sciences de la santé Université du Québec à Trois-Rivières, Québec, Canada.

501

a thermistor inserted to a depth of 10 cm. *Skin temperature* was also measured with a thermistor. Measurements were taken at eight places: forehead (7.4), neck (2.4), upper arm (8.2), lower arm (11.4), abdomen (16.6), back (16.2), thigh (17.2) and leg (20.6); mean skin temperature ($\overline{Ts}$) was calculated from these values, numbers representing weighting coefficient for calculating $\overline{Ts}$. Mean body temperatures ($\overline{TB}$) were calculated as follows: $\overline{TB} = 0.2\ \overline{Ts} + 0.8\ TR$. *Heat flow* values were measured at the thigh, abdomen, leg and upper arm by heat flow meter. *Reaction time* was the time elapsed between initiation and cessation of three kinds of light (red, blue and yellow); measures were taken at rest, after walking and after 40 minutes of recuperation.

Results

Thermal Responses

In Figure 1, TR and $\overline{TB}$ are shown at each Ta at two walking speeds (rest, exercise and recovery). TR increased at rest for 40 minutes in Ta 36 C, but tended rather to decrease in this period in another Ta. During walking, TR increased to above 38 C in high Ta and at heavy exercise loads. There were smaller differences of TR in higher exercise loads than that in lower exercise loads. At 25 C Ta, increase of TR was rather greater than at other Ta, although the absolute value of TR was lower than that at other Ta. At recovery, decrease of TR at lower exercise load was smaller than at higher load in high Ta. The difference of TR between low and high exercise load in high Ta was smaller than at low Ta. The differences of $\overline{TB}$ in each exercise load during exercise were clear, but at recovery the difference was smaller. Heat flow showed higher value at lower Ta under all conditions. But heat flow at the abdomen was smaller than at the peripheral part and the change due to Ta was smaller at higher Ta. With walking, these values increased especially in the peripheral parts; lower Ta and higher exercise load showed the highest heat flow values.

Cardiac Responses

HR in high Ta was higher than HR observed at Ta at each exercise load. The difference of HR at high load in elevated Ta was smaller than at low Ta. HR at recovery was higher at high Ta and high exercise load. HR at Ta 25 C was the smallest in each case. Blood pressure and pulse pressure (= systolic pressure − diastolic pressure) due to exercise load was obvious, but the difference due to

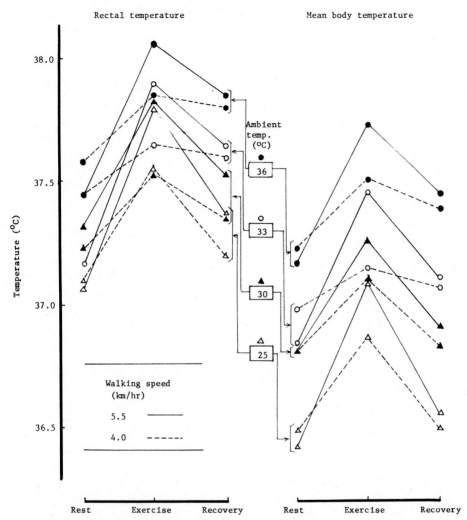

FIG. 1. Change in rectal temperature and in mean body temperature at various ambient temperatures and walking speeds.

Ta was not so obvious. Although systolic pressure at 25 Ta was low, systolic and diastolic pressure at higher Ta and exercise load did not demonstrate a discernible pattern (Fig. 2).

Reaction time with foot was slower than that with hands in all conditions. Reaction time at rest in 25 C Ta tended to be faster than in other Ta, but after exercise it did not demonstrate a discernible pattern at each walking speed and Ta. At recovery, reaction time at

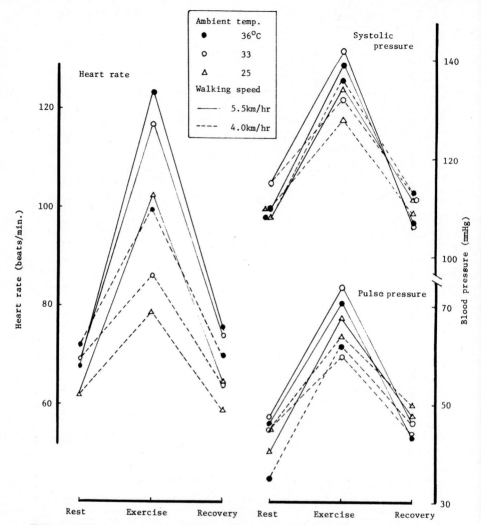

FIG. 2. Change in heart beats and in blood pressure (systolic blood pressure and pulse pressure) at various ambient temperatures and walking speeds.

high Ta and high exercise load tended to be slower in average. The numbers of times mistaken were maximal at speed 5.5 km/hr after exercise, which had no relation with Ta (Fig. 3).

Relationship Between Thermal and Cardiac Responses

In Figure 4, the relationship between TR and HR was shown at exercise 40 minutes in all cases for each individual. No interrelation-

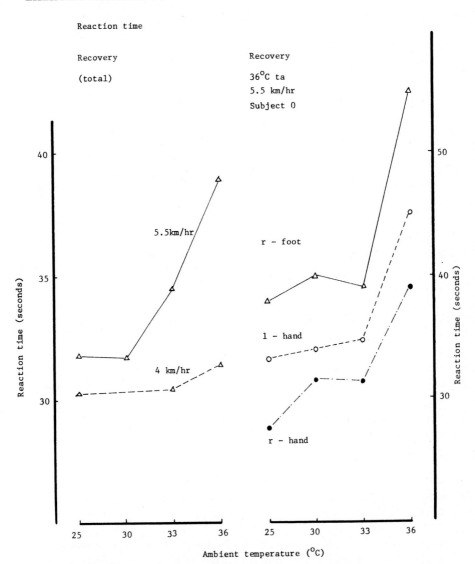

FIG. 3. Reaction times at recovery period (40 min), the difference due to hands and foot; the relations between speeds and ambient temperatures.

ship with Ta seemed to exist. The regression line fitted equation: HR = 39.96 TR − 1402.19 (beats/min., °C), coefficient correlation (r) = 0.46 HR against metabolic heat production (Me), the regression line fits equation HR = 0.28 Me + 56.37 (beats/min, Cal/m^{2}h), r = 0.37, but at 36 C Ta, the regression line, HR = 0.34 Me + 51.79, r = 0.56

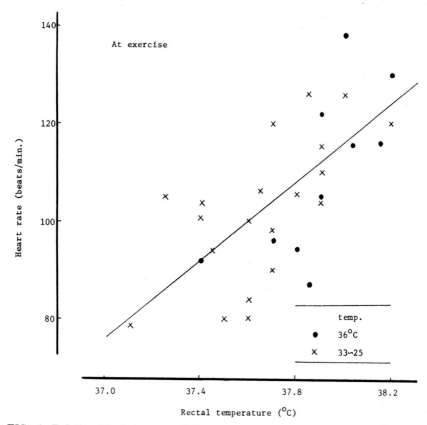

FIG. 4. Relationship between rectal temperature and heart beats at exercise in various ambient temperatures.

and Ta 25 C, HR = 0.27 Me + 45.52, r = 0.50. The effect due to Ta seems to appear in this relation. In the same way, the regression line against Me fits equation, TR = 0.0046 Me + 36.94 ($^\circ$C, Cal/m^{2}h) r = 0.39, and at Ta 36 C, TR = 0.0048 Me + 37.05, r = 0.68, in the case of higher Ta, TR appeared high level. Figure 5 showed the relationship between $\overline{\text{TB}}$ and Me. This relation appears to be affected by Ta, especially at Ta 36 C. Therefore on the whole, correlative coefficient was low, (r = 0.28). But, at Ta 36 C, $\overline{\text{TB}}$ = 0.0049 Me + 36.71 ($^\circ$C, Cal/m^{2}h), r = 0.72, at 33 $\sim$ 25 C Ta, $\overline{\text{TB}}$ = 0.0055 Me + 36.17, r = 0.46.

Cardiac and Thermal Efficiency

Figure 6 showed the relation between cardiac efficiency and thermal index. Cardiac efficiency is introduced as follows:

$$\frac{W \cdot D}{\Sigma \triangle \ HR} \left((Kg - m) \middle/ beat \right)$$

Where

W = body weight

D = total walking distance

$\triangle$HR = number of heart beats (exercise and recovery period) above the testing level.

Thermal index is introduced from the formula of Body Storage Index:

$$\frac{0.83 \cdot W}{A} \cdot \triangle\overline{T}B$$

Where

0.83 = body specific heat

A = body surface area

$\triangle\overline{T}B$ = increase of $\overline{T}B$ due to exercise above the resting level at Ta 25 C.

These indices were introduced for a cost comparison in various environments and exercise loads. At 5.5 km/hr, cardiac efficiency was low above Ta 30 C although thermal index increased. At 4.0 km/hr, according to decreasing thermal index, cardiac efficiency increased remarkably. When thermal index became high, cardiac efficiency tended to decrease to a certain level, then the difference due to individuals and in various conditions tended to become smaller.

Discussion and Conclusion

At all ambient temperatures remarkable changes in thermal responses were observed during exercise and recovery. The heart rate increased progressively as the ambient temperature passed from 25 to 36 C. It was reported that there is no difference in cardiac output for light-load exercise between neutral and hot ambient temperatures and that stroke volume decreases under hot temperatures [2]. This relationship is complex. The heart rate at exercise changes with the dynamic relationship due to cardiac output, stroke volume, A-V difference which are affected by ambient temperatures and work

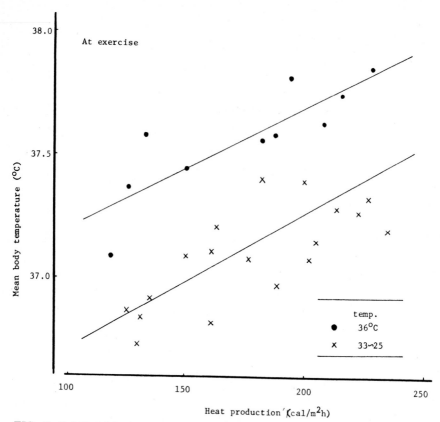

FIG. 5. Relationship between heat production and mean body temperature at exercise in various ambient temperatures.

intensities. The increase in skin thermal responses indicates an increase in vasodilatation, a reduced peripheral resistance and a drop in stroke volume, which is compensated by an increase in heart rate as the cardiac output is constant. HR or TR when plotted against heat production showed higher coefficient correlation at each Ta, in which tended to show higher value against the same heat production in higher Ta. The relation between HR and TR was not interrelated with Ta, but TR against HR was lower than that reported by Kamon et al [1]. This fact may be caused with the difference of Ta. $\overline{T}B$ against heat production was related with Ta, in which the difference between 36 C and other Ta was greater at lower heat production, and as shown in reaction time at recovery, the time became late and numbers mistaken was great in 36 C Ta and 5 km/hr walking speed.

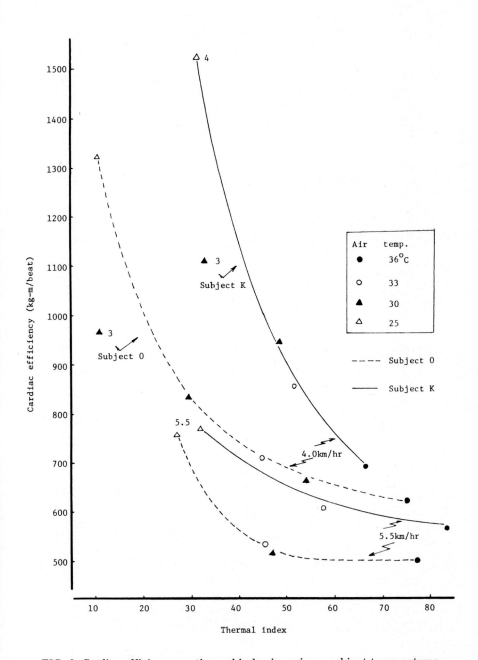

FIG. 6. Cardiac efficiency vs. thermal index in various ambient temperatures.

Therefore, the effect of the ambient temperature in physiological response and performance cannot be neglected at low exercise load.

There were some differences in the individual thermal and cardiac responses and performance. Cardiac efficiency reached limitation at a certain Ta, which did not relate to thermal index, and in the case of low exercise load, the change of thermal index was greatly affected when plotted against cardiac efficiency.

References

1. Kamon, E. and Belding, H.S.: Heart rate and rectal temperature relationships during work in hot humid environments. J. Appl. Physiol. 31 (3):472-477, 1971.
2. Rowell, L.B. et al: Reductions in cardiac output, central blood volume, and stroke volume with thermal stress in normal men during exercise. J. Clin. Invest. 45 (11):1801-1816, 1966.

Relationship Between Muscle Temperature and O_2 Debt

E. Saar and Y. Cassuto

Introduction

According to the hypothesis of Hill [8], later modified by Margaria et al [12], elevated O_2 uptake after exercise (O_2 debt) represents the extra O_2 required for reconversion of lactate to glycogen, restoration of O_2 stores, and re-esterification of high energy phosphate compounds. This hypothesis has recently been challenged by showing that the O_2 debt exceeds the O_2 deficit (O_2 discrepancy). Part of the O_2 discrepancy was attributed to the exponential decrease in the heart rate and the work of breathing at cessation of work [13, 17]. Brooks et al [1-3] suggested that O_2 debt is partly due to the increased temperature of muscle and other tissues during exercise. The increased temperature impairs the efficiency of the oxidative phosphorylating system [1, 3, 4] causing a need for higher volume of O_2 for re-esterification of high energy phosphate bonds. These arguments gain relevance when conflicting reports about the existence and magnitude of O_2 deficit encountered at the onset of eccentric (ecc.) work are considered [6, 9].

It was found that temperature of working muscles during ecc. work is higher than during concentric (con.) work of similar $\dot{V}O_2$ [14]. In light of this fact and that a linear relationship exists between O_2 debt and steady state $\dot{V}O_2$ following light to moderate exercise [10, 17], it was decided to test the hypothesis of Brooks et al [1-3] about the connection between higher muscle temperature and O_2 debt in humans.

This work attempts to correlate the values of O_2 debts measured after prolonged periods of con. and ecc. work at similar $\dot{V}O_2$, with the muscle temperature at the termination of exercise. Also presented are data which support the result of Knuttgen and Klausen [10] who did not find any O_2 deficit at the onset of ecc. work.

E. Saar and Y. Cassuto, Department of Biology, Ben-Gurion University of the Negev, Beer Sheva, Israel.

Methods

Five healthy adult males (mean values of 24 years, 63 kg and 173 cm for age, weight and height, respectively) were subjects of this study.

Resting O_2 consumption ($\dot{V}O_2$) was measured following 20 minutes of rest while the subjects were standing on a treadmill. Thereafter, the subjects walked on the treadmill for 60 minutes, either on a positive slope of 9° (con. work), at a speed of 2 km/hr, or on a negative slope of 9° (ecc. work), at a speed of 6.5 km/hr, a condition which yielded a similar steady state $\dot{V}O_2$. Ambient temperature and relative humidity were 22 C and 53%, respectively. Expired air samples were collected into meteorological balloons connected to a low resistance breathing valve. Frequent samples were taken during the first six minutes of the work and during the first ten minutes of recovery period. Additional samples were taken between the 30 to 32 and 58 to 60 minutes of work; O_2 and CO_2 concentrations were measured with Beckman E_2/O_2 analyzer and Godart Capnograph, respectively. Both instruments were calibrated, using a Haldane apparatus as reference. Heart rates (HR) were measured from a continuous recording of the electrocardiogram.

Rectal temperatures were recorded using thermistor probes (yellow spring). Muscle temperatures were measured immediately after the end of the work period, using a thermistor needle (yellow spring) inserted 3 cm into the vastus lateralis.

Spirometric measurements were conducted using a Godart Pulmotest. Muscle temperatures and the spirometric measurements were performed in replicative experiments at the same conditions and at the same steady state $\dot{V}O_2$ on three and two subjects, respectively.

Results

Figure 1 demonstrates the rate of O_2 consumption at the onset, steady state and at recovery of con. and ecc. works. Similar values of steady state $\dot{V}O_2$ (l/min) 0.92 ± 0.02 and 0.88 ± 0.01 for con. and ecc. work, respectively, were recorded. The O_2 deficit during con. work is significantly larger than that during ecc. work (P < 0.05). Average values for the five subjects were −36 ± 73 ml during ecc. work and 241 ± 82 during con. work. The O_2 debts accumulated during the work periods were also significantly different (P < 0.01). A value of 552 ± 21 ml O_2 was obtained for ecc. work and 425 ± 26 ml O_2 for con. work.

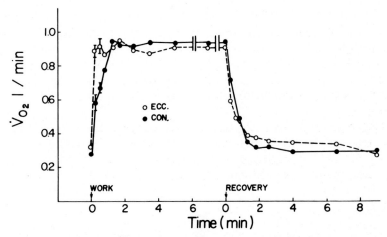

FIG. 1. Mean values of $\dot{V}O_2$ (STPD) during onset, steady state and recovery periods of con. and ecc. work. Values given in $1O_2$/min. Standard errors are given only where the differences are statistically significant (n = 5).

Figure 2 depicts the values of the minute ventilation ($\dot{V}_E$) during periods of work and recovery. Although the steady state values were the same for con. and ecc. work, a significant difference was found during the onset of work. A steep increase of $\dot{V}_E$ at the onset of ecc. work was recorded compared with moderate elevation of $\dot{V}_E$ while performing con. work.

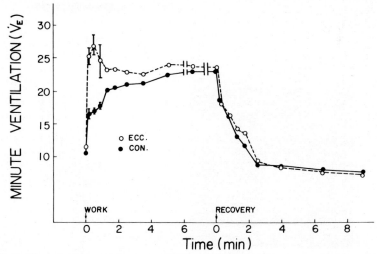

FIG. 2. Mean values of minute ventilation (STPD) during onset, steady state and recovery periods of con. and ecc. work. Values given in liters per minute. Standard errors as in Figure 1 (n = 5).

Figure 3 shows a detailed study of the ventilatory pattern during the onset of work as recorded by a spirometer on the subject E.S. The experiments represented in Figure 3A and 3B were conducted at the same $\dot{V}O_2$ as those represented in Figures 1 and 2. Figure 3C depicts the respiratory pattern of the subject walking on a positive slope at the same speed (6.5 km/hr) as in the ecc. work ($\dot{V}O_2$ = 2.35 l/min).

Table I summarizes the spirometric data of the subjects E.S. and M.A. It can be seen that ecc. work initiates markedly decreased values of Functional Residual Capacity (FRC) and rapid ventilatory response, mainly due to increased tidal volume.

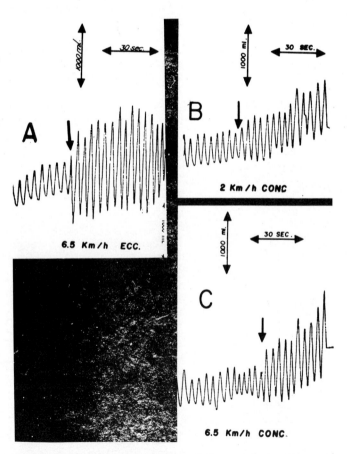

FIG. 3. Spirometric recordings at the onset of con. and ecc. work. Arrow indicates the onset of work.

Table I. Spirometric Measurements of Subjects M.A. and E.S. (BTPS)
During First 20 Seconds of Con. and Ecc. Work

Subjects	Type of Work and Speed	Respiratory Frequency min⁻¹	Tidal Volume ml	Increase in Minute Ventilation l/min	Decrease FRC at the Onset of Work ml
M.A.	con. (+9°) 2.0 km/hr	15 [14]	760 [530]	3.98	100
M.A.	ecc. (−9°) 6.5 km/hr	14 [12]	1560 [660]	13.92	660
M.A.	con. (+9°) 6.5 km/hr	15 [14]	1150 [660]	8.00	270
E.S.	con. (+9°) 2.0 km/hr	15 [16]	660 [500]	1.90	60
E.S.	ecc. (−9°) 6.5 km/hr	16 [14]	1500 [480]	17.28	510
E.S.	con. (+9°) 6.5 km/hr		1000 [500]	8.50	90

[ ] values recorded while standing before the onset of work.

Con. work, either at the same steady state $\dot{V}O_2$ or at the same walking speed ($\dot{V}O_2$ = 2.35 l/min), had much less effect on the FRC and ventilation.

The patterns of the respiratory quotient (RQ) during onset, steady state and recovery periods from con. and ecc. work are seen in Figure 4. There were no significant differences between the two types of work during the onset and steady periods. However, the

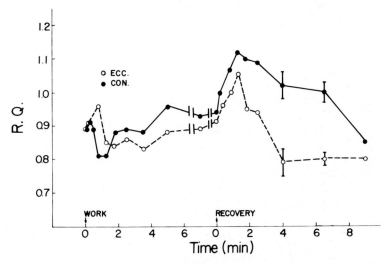

FIG. 4. Mean values of RQ during onset, steady state and recovery periods of con. and ecc. work. Standard errors as in Figure 1 (n = 5).

return of RQ values to the resting levels was markedly faster during recovery from ecc. work.

The average steady state values of HR were similar in ecc. and con. work (103 ± 3 and 101 ± 4, respectively). However, the kinetics of the HR response during the onset of the work were different.

Figure 5 shows kinetics of the HR response during the first three minutes of work in the subject M.A. It can be seen that in this period the heart rate overshoots while performing ecc. work. Average values of the five subjects showed the same trend, but due to individual variabilities the differences between average values of con. and ecc. works were not statistically significant.

The temperatures of the vastus lateralis were measured in three subjects upon termination of the work period. Data given in Table II show that the average muscle temperature (Tm) after performing ecc. work was 1.1 C higher (P < 0.02) than after con. work, whereas rectal temperatures were not significantly different: 37.65 ± 0.19 C for ecc. work and 37.40 ± 0.11 C for con. work (P > 0.1).

Discussion

The concept that muscle temperature plays a role in determining the extent of "O_2 discrepancy" was supported by experiments on rats exercising to exhaustion [2]. Since the same phenomenon is shown in human subjects performing low and moderate exercise [9],

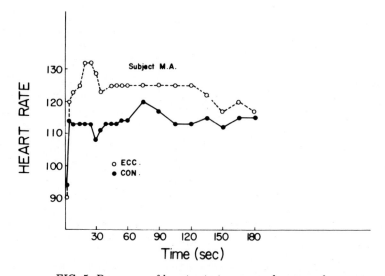

FIG. 5. Response of heart rate to con. and ecc. work.

Table II. Muscle Temperatures (Vastus Lateralis) at
Termination of 60 Minutes of Ecc. and Con. Work

Subject	Eccentric	Concentric
E.S.	38.70°C	37.30°C
A.M.	38.10°C	37.00°C
I.N.	38.30°C	37.60°C
Mean ± S.E.	38.4 ± 0.17	37.3 ± 0.17*

* P < 0.02

it was of relevance to find whether under such circumstances muscle temperatures affect the extent of "O_2 discrepancy."

Preliminary studies, where attempts to control the muscle temperatures by performing work at a water pool at different temperatures or while working an ergometer wearing a cooling suit in which cold or warm water was circulated, proved unsuccessful in achieving different muscle temperatures at constant workloads. Therefore, it was decided to compare the O_2 debts accumulated after ecc. and con. work at the same steady state of O_2 consumption.

The data shown in Figure 1 demonstrates that pertaining to O_2 debt a significant (P < 0.01) difference was obtained between the two experiments. O_2 debts of 425 ± 26 ml O_2 and 552 ± 21 ml O_2 were measured after con. and ecc. work of similar steady state O_2, respectively.

As expected, Table II demonstrates that muscle temperatures measured after identical experiments were also higher after ecc. than those recorded after con. work. The extent of the increased muscle temperatures from the resting level of 35 C [16] to the recorded values of 38.4 C in our study, and the difference between the muscle temperatures at con. and ecc. work (1.1 C P < 0.02), can be considered as a cause of reducing the oxidative phosphorylation mechanism of the muscle mitochondria as suggested by Brooks et al [1] and Cassuto, [4]. Thus it can be concluded that the results presented seem to support the hypothesis that muscle temperatures have a role in regulating O_2 uptake.

Contrary to the increased O_2 debt, no O_2 deficit was accumulated at the onset of ecc. work. The abruptly increased O_2 consumption seen in Figure 1 can be partially explained by changes in FRC (Table I). Figure 3 demonstrates that about 500 ml were expired from the lungs at the onset of ecc. exercise compared to only 60 ml during con. work. If one assumes that the P_{O_2} of the alveolar gas is 100 mm Hg, then an increased $\dot{V}O_2$ of about 25 ml could be due to the technique used, a value which cannot account for the difference in O_2 deficit measured: -36 ml O_2 and 241 ml O_2 for ecc. and con. work, respectively. An additional factor which could decrease the O_2 deficit could be a faster gas exchange between the working tissues and the lungs, namely, increased cardiac output with concomitant elevation of minute ventilation. Figure 2 shows that $\dot{V}_E$ was indeed greatly accelerated during the first minute of ecc. work. This was not a hyperventilation response, but a true O_2 utilization, as can be judged by equivalent respiratory exchange ratios shown in Figure 4. Although no direct measurements of cardiac output were performed on the subjects, abruptly increased heart rate at the beginning of ecc. work, shown in Figure 5, can be taken as a sign of an equivalent change of cardiac output.

The fast ventilatory response to ecc. work is probably not due to chemical stimuli. Figure 3C demonstrates that con. work of over twice the magnitude of ecc. work did not stimulate a similar effect. Moreover it shows that the rate at which the muscles contract does not have a significant role. It can be suggested that the ventilation was stimulated via a mechanoreceptor reflex caused by lung deflation (Fig. 3A) [5, 15, 18]. We cannot see a direct connection between performing ecc. work and lung deflation and can only suggest that a change in body position due to walking on the negative slope of the treadmill causes this deflation.

Glick et al [7] found in dogs a relationship between the activation of pulmonary stretch receptors in the lung and inhibition of the sympathetic tone of the heart. It seems possible that decreased discharge from these receptors due to the deflation of the lungs accelerates the sympathetic tone with a consequent increase of the heart rate. Recently, Linnarson [11] showed in human subjects a correlation between the decreased FRC and increased HR at the onset of the work.

The comparison between the magnitude of the O_2 deficit and the O_2 debt is of prime relevance. Subjects performing con. work have shown both a deficit and a debt, suggesting that O_2 debt restored the O_2 deficit. The values recorded during ecc. work are puzzling. On the one hand no O_2 deficits were accumulated, as was shown also by Knuttgen and Klausen [10] and on the other hand, the O_2 debts were even greater than those obtained after con. work of comparable steady state $\dot{V}O_2$. If so, what does the O_2 debt after ecc. work cover? Can the differences between muscle temperatures during con. and ecc. work account for these differences? At present, no conclusive answer can be given.

References

1. Brooks, G.A., Hittelman, D.J., Faulkner, S.A.: Temperature, skeletal muscle mitochondrial functions, and oxygen debt. Am. J. Physiol. 220:1053-1059, 1971.
2. Brooks, G.A., Hittelman, D.J., Faulkner, J.A. and Beyer, R.E.: Tissue temperature and whole animal oxygen consumption after exercise. Am. J. Physiol. 221:427-431, 1971.
3. Brooks, G.A., Hittelman, K.J., Faulkner, J.A. and Beyer, R.E.: Temperature, liver mitochondrial respiratory functions, and oxygen debt. Med. Sci. Sports 3:72-74, 1971.
4. Cassuto, Y.: Oxidative activities of liver mitochondria from mammals, birds, reptiles and amphibia as a function of temperature. Comp. Biochem. Physiol. 39B:919-923, 1971.
5. Culver, G.A. and Rahn, H.: Reflex respiratory stimulation by chest compression in the dog. Am. J. Physiol. 169:686-693, 1952.
6. Flemming, B.P., Knuttgen, H.G. and Heriksson, S.: Muscle metabolism during exercise with concentric and eccentric contractions. J. Appl. Physiol. 33:792-795, 1972.
7. Glick, G., Wechsler, A.S. and Epestein, S.E.: Reflex cardiovascular depression produced by stimulation of pulmonary stretch receptors in the dog. J. Clin. Invest. 48:467-473, 1969.
8. Hill, A.V. and Lupton, H.: Muscular exercise, lactic acid, and the supply and utilization of oxygen. Q. J. Med. 16:135-171, 1923.
9. Knuttgen, H.G.: Oxygen debt after submaximal physical exercise. J. Appl. Physiol. 20:651-657, 1970.
10. Knuttgen, H.G. and Klausen, K.: Oxygen debt in short-term exercise with concentric and eccentric muscle contraction. J. Appl. Physiol. 30:632-635, 1971.
11. Linnarson, D.: Dynamics of pulmonary gas exchange and heart rate changes at start and end of exercise. Acta Physiol. Scand. Suppl. 415, 1974.
12. Margaria, R., Edwards, H.T. and Dill, D.B.: Possible mechanisms of contracting and paying oxygen debt and the role of lactic acid in muscular contraction. Am. J. Physiol. 106:689-715, 1933.
13. Martin, T.P.: Oxygen deficit, oxygen debt relationship at submaximal exercise. J. Sports Med. 14:152-258, 1974.
14. Nielsen, B.: Thermoregulation in rest and exercise. Acta Physiol. Scand. Suppl. 323, 1969.
15. Reed, E.A. and Scott, S.: Effect of position upon the respiratory rate of anesthetized dogs. Fed. Proc. 8:130, 1949.
16. Saltin, B., Gagge, A.P. and Stolwijk, J.A.: Muscle temperature during submaximal exercise in man. J. Appl. Physiol. 25:679-688, 1968.
17. Welch, H.G., Faulkner, J.A., Barclay, J.K. and Brooks, G.A.: Ventilatory response during recovery from muscular work and its relation with O_2 debt. Med. Sci. Sports 2:15-19, 1970.
18. Widdicombe, G.J.: Respiratory reflexes. In Fenn, O.W. and Rahn, H. (eds.): Respiration, Sec. 3, Vol. I, Handbook of Physiology, 1964.

Prediction of Heat Tolerance and $\dot{V}O_2$ Max From Heart Rate and Rectal Temperature

E. Shvartz, A. Meroz,
A. Magazanik and Y. Shapiro

Introduction

When men are assigned to work in hot environments, or when athletic events are performed in hot conditions, it is important to know who is going to show poor tolerance to heat or inability to acclimatize. While some attempts to predict performance in heat were made [3] and factors which contribute to heat tolerance or heat intolerance such as age [7], weight [8] and $\dot{V}O_2$ max [7] were identified, when these three factors were combined they accounted for only 63% of the cases [2]. Preliminary data collected by the present author [4] showed that submax heart rate and rectal temperature in a temperate environment were highly correlated with the same responses in heat. The relationship between heat tolerance and physical fitness was also considered. $\dot{V}O_2$ max was shown to have a moderate relationship to heat tolerance [2, 9] and physical training resulted in decreases in submax rectal temperature [5, 6]. Despite the linear relationship which exists between submax heart rate and oxygen consumption, predicting $\dot{V}O_2$ max from submax heart rate includes a substantial error for reasons such as large individual variations in $\dot{V}O_2$-heart rate relationship at high workloads, the decline of max heart rate with age and high, but not perfect, correlations between $\dot{V}O_2$ and cardiac output [1]. Therefore, it was interesting to determine if the prediction of $\dot{V}O_2$ max could be improved by combining both, submax heart rate and rectal temperature, instead of heart rate alone. Thus, the purpose of this study was to develop a test for the prediction of heat tolerance and $\dot{V}O_2$ max from submax heart rate and rectal temperature.

E. Shvartz, A. Meroz, A. Magazanik and Y. Shapiro, Heller Institute of Medical Research, Sheba Medical Center, Israel.

Methods

Forty healthy young men participated in the experiment. The subjects' age ranged from 18 to 24 years and their physical characteristics are listed: (means±SD): 175±6.6 cm; 68±9.5 kg; and 1.83±0.15 m^2. Ten subjects were untrained (mean $\dot{V}O_2$ max of 41.8 ml/kg/min), 20 subjects were trained (mean $\dot{V}O_2$ max of 55.9 ml/kg/min), and the other 10 subjects were untrained but in good physical condition (mean $\dot{V}O_2$ max of 51.9 ml/kg/min). There were minor and insignificant differences in physical characteristics between these groups. Ten additional subjects were also tested but their data were not considered because of errors in rectal temperature measurements. The experiments were conducted during late fall and winter when the subjects were unacclimatized to heat.

Procedure

All subjects were first tested at room temperature (23 C DB, 16 C WB). The subjects performed bench stepping, on a bench 30 cm high, at a rate of 12 steps/min for 60 minutes. This constituted moderate work with the average workload equal to 40 w. No more than 60 minutes of exercise were necessary since at this workload rectal temperature levels off after about 40 minutes. Heart rate and rectal temperature were recorded every 15 minutes and sweat rate was recorded for the entire hour. After at least two hours of rest, $\dot{V}O_2$ max was determined on a treadmill by grade running at a constant speed of 10 km/hr. The grade was elevated every two minutes until the subjects were exhausted after seven or eight minutes. Oxygen consumption was determined during the last minute of exercise. On the following day, the subjects attempted to perform the same workload for three hours in heat (40 C DB, 30 C WB), and the same measurements were made as on the first day.

Following these tests, the ten untrained subjects underwent three weeks of a moderate training program (daily, one hour exercise, at 70% of $\dot{V}O_2$ max), and the other ten untrained subjects underwent eight days of heat acclimation (three hours of daily exposure to the same conditions as during testing in heat). These two groups were retested in the temperate and hot environments following training and acclimation.

Results

Table I shows that the trained subjects (group B) had lower heart rates and rectal temperatures than the untrained subjects (groups A,

Table I. Responses to Exercise of Different Groups of Subjects in Temperate and Hot Environments

Group		Responses at 23C			Responses in Heat			
		Heart Rate beats/min	Rectal Temp. C	Sweat Rate ml/hr	Heart Rate beats/min	Rectal Temp. C	Sweat Rate ml/hr	$\dot{V}O_2$ Max ml/kg/min
A	Before training	117 ±13.2	38.1 ±0.34	240 ±60	152 ±22.0	38.9 ±0.49	560 ±90	41.8 ±8.7
	After training	106 ± 9.1	37.9 ±0.21	235 ±58	145 ±19.0	38.7 ±0.42	557 ±143	47.0 ±8.6
	(N = 10)							
B	Trained	102 ± 9.6	37.9 ±0.31	262 ±95	135 ±15.3	38.5 ±0.39	610 ±138	55.9 ±4.4
	(N = 20)							
C	Before acclim.	111 ± 5.5	38.0 ±0.18	251 ±87	150 ±11.2	38.8 ±0.40	575 ±167	51.9 ±6.4
	After acclim.	101 ± 7.5	37.6 ±0.17	180 ±92	125 ± 9.0	38.2 ±0.28	644 ±180	57.1 ±5.3
	(N = 10)							

Data are means ± SD after 30 minutes of exercise at 23C and after three hours of exercise in heat.

C before training and acclimation) in all conditions. Training in group A resulted in decreases in heart rate and rectal temperature responses at 23 C but in small changes in heat. Heat acclimation in group C resulted in large improvements in responses at 23 C and in heat. The trained subjects in group B showed partial heat acclimation. Training in group A resulted in 12% increase in $\dot{V}O_2$ max while heat acclimation in group C resulted in a corresponding increase of 10%. Table II shows the relationships among physiological responses in the different conditions. It is noted that the various parameters are only moderately interrelated. Table III shows the distribution of heart rate and rectal temperature data at 23 C and in heat, and the corresponding $\dot{V}O_2$ max data. Thirty minute values at 23 C were considered instead of 60 minute values, because there were no heart rate differences between responses after 30 and 60 minutes and rectal temperature after 30 minutes was by only 0.1 C lower than that after 60 minutes. The scores at the right column are arbitrary ones. A score of 1 indicates poor responses and a score of 9 indicates very good responses. The correlation coefficients shown in Figures 1 and 2 were computed according to this Table. Figure 1 shows the

Table II. Correlation Coefficients Among Responses at 23C, in Heat and $\dot{V}O_2$ Max

Condition		r
23C	T_{re} vs. T_{re} at rest	0.85
	vs. T_{re} in heat	0.80
	vs. HR at 23C	0.68
	vs. HR in heat	0.62
	vs. $\dot{V}O_2$ max	-0.66
23C	HR vs. HR in heat	0.77
	vs. T_{re} in heat	0.63
	vs. $\dot{V}O_2$ max	-0.85
	SR vs. SR in heat	0.81
Heat	T_{re} vs. T_{re} at rest	0.62
	vs. HR in heat	0.73
	vs. $\dot{V}O_2$ max	-0.60
	HR vs. $\dot{V}O_2$ max	-0.65

T_{re} = rectal temperature; HR = heart rate; and SR = sweat rate. The correlation coefficients for heart rate and rectal temperature are between values recorded at rest, after 30 minutes of exercise at 23C and after three hours of exercise in heat. Sweat rate for one hour at 23C was correlated with average sweat rate values for three hours in heat.

Table III. Scores for Heart Rate and Rectal Temperature Responses
at 23C, in Heat and for $\dot{V}O_2$ Max

| 23C | | Heat | | | |
Heart Rate beats/min	Rectal Temp. C	Heart Rate beats/min	Rectal Temp. C	$\dot{V}O_2$ Max ml/kg/min	Score
130	38.4	170	39.5	38	1
124	38.2	160	39.2	42	2
117	38.1	153	38.9	46	3
112	38.0	146	38.7	49	4
107	37.9	140	38.6	51	5
102	37.8	134	38.5	53	6
97	37.7	127	38.3	56	7
92	37.6	120	38.1	59	8
85	37.4	110	37.8	62	9

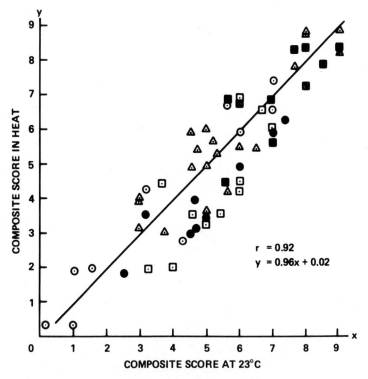

FIG. 1. Correlation coefficient between the composite scores at 23 C and in heat. ○ = Group A before training, and ● = after training; △ = Group B, and □ = Group C before acclimation and ■ = after acclimation.

relationship between heart rate and rectal temperature responses at 23 C and in heat. These two parameters are expressed in terms of composite scores according to Table III. Each individual's composite score at 23 C or in heat was calculated according to the equation:

$$CS = T_{re} \cdot 0.7 + HR \cdot 0.3$$

in which CS is the composite score at 23 C or in heat; T_{re} = rectal temperature score shown in Table III and HR = heart rate score in Table III. More weighting was given to rectal temperature than to heart rate because rectal temperature, indicating susceptibility to develop heat stroke, was considered to be of more importance than heart rate, indicating susceptibility to develop heat syncope [6], in the assessment of heat tolerance. Figure 2 shows the relationship

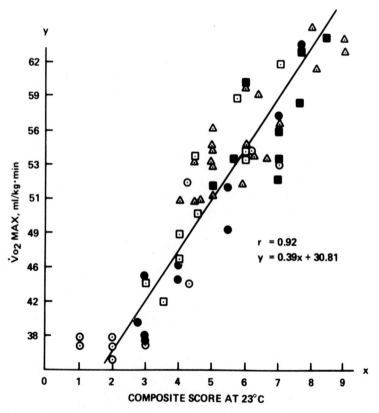

FIG. 2. Correlation coefficient between composite scores at 23 C and VO$_2$ max. Symbols are the same as in Figure 1.

between the composite scores at 23 C and $\dot{V}O_2$ max. In this case, the composite scores at 23 C were computed according to the equation:

$$CS = T_{re} \cdot 0.3 + HR \cdot 0.7$$

in which CS is the composite score at 23 C; T_{re} = rectal temperature score shown in Table III and HR = heart rate score in Table III. More weighting was given to heart rate than to rectal temperature in this case because heart rate, reflecting cardiovascular responses, was considered to be of more importance than rectal temperature, indicating thermoregulatory responses, in the prediction of aerobic capacity.

Discussion

This study has presented a simple test for the prediction of heat tolerance and $\dot{V}O_2$ max which requires the measurement of heart rate and rectal temperature after 30 minutes of bench stepping at a moderate workload. Like any other test of this nature, it is important to make sure that the subjects have not participated in physical activity for several hours before testing. At this stage, it is not expected that this test would provide a quantitative assessment of heat tolerance and $\dot{V}O_2$ max before more data are available. Obviously, the main purpose of this test would be to predict heat tolerance and information about $\dot{V}O_2$ max would be helpful because the two capacities are related anyhow. At present, this test could certainly provide qualitative information in separating heat-tolerant and fit individuals (composite scores above 7.0) from heat-intolerant and unfit individuals (composite scores below 3.0).

References

1. Astrand, P.-O. and Todahl, K.: Textbook of Work Physiology. New York:McGraw-Hill, 1970, pp. 352-360.
2. Kok, R., Wyndham, C.H., Strydom, N.B. and Rogers, G.G.: A comparison of certain physiological and anthropometrical characteristics of heat-intolerant and heat tolerant Bantu from climatic room acclimatization. Chamber of Mines Research Report, No. 14/72, Johannesburg, South Africa, 1972.
3. Lavenne, L. and Belayew, D.: Exercise tolerance test at room temperature for the purpose of selecting rescue teams for training in a hot climate. Rev. Inst. Hyg. Mines 21:48-58, 1966.
4. Shvartz, E: Physical performance of heat adapted individuals. Proc. of the XXVI Inter. Congress Physiol. Sci., New Delhi, India, Vol. X, pp. 264-265, 1974.
5. Shvartz, E., Magazanik, A. and Glick, Z.: Thermal responses during training in a temperate climate. J. Appl. Physiol. 36:572-577, 1974.

6. Shvartz, E., Strydom, N.B. and Kotze, H.: Orthostatism and heat acclimation. J. Appl. Physiol. 39:590-595, 1975.
7. Strydom, N.B.: Age as a casual factor in heat stroke. J. S.A. Inst. Min. Metall. 72:112-114, 1971.
8. Strydom, N.B., Wyndham, C.H. and Benade, A.J.S.: The responses of men weighing less than 50 kg. to the standard climatic room acclimatization procedure. J. S.A. Inst. Min. Metall. 72:101-104, 1971.
9. Wyndham, C.H., Strydom, N.B., Benade, A.J.S. et al: Heat stroke risks in unacclimatized and acclimatized men of different maximum oxygen intakes working under hot and humid conditions. Chamber of Mines Research Report, No. 12/72, Johannesburg, South Africa, 1972.

Effects of Residual Tobacco Smoke on Nonsmokers

J. R. White

Introduction

There is increasing evidence that more smokers than nonsmokers die prematurely from coronary disease. But nonsmokers who involuntarily inhale residual tobacco smoke (any and all smoke from tobacco, whether from the cigarette, cigar or pipe or from the exhalation of the smoker) experience nasal congestion, eye irritation, headache, nausea and gastric upset, and the smoke can be particularly harmful to nonsmokers with cardiorespiratory and allergy problems, a sizable group of between 8 and 34 million Americans (Zussman, *Journal of Asthma Research*, June 1974, and Banzhaf, *Today's Health*, April 1972).

Definitive evidence that inhaling residual smoke constitutes a health hazard to otherwise healthy nonsmokers has not as yet appeared in the literature. However, a reasonable hypothesis is that when a nonsmoker is exposed to residual smoke, he will experience adverse physiological responses.

This paper presents an analysis of cardiac, pulmonary and neural changes caused by inhalation of residual tobacco smoke. These changes are simultaneously reflected in each of the following parameters:

1. Minute volume ($\dot{V}_E$)
2. Oxygen consumption ($\dot{V}O_2$)
3. Oxygen consumption/kg
4. Carbon dioxide production ($\dot{V}CO_2$)
5. R.Q.
6. Respiratory rate
7. Perspiration production
8. Heart rate
9. Systolic blood pressure

J. R. White, Department of Physical Education, University of California, San Diego, La Jolla, Calif., U.S.A.

10. Diastolic blood pressure
11. Pulse pressure
12. Hand steadiness

Method

Fifty subjects, aged 11 to 65 years, were used in this study. Each was exposed to the residual smoke from a smoker seated 4½ feet away in a well-ventilated room (five to six air changes per hour in a 20' × 30' research laboratory) for approximately three minutes. The subject was seated in a comfortable chair, blindfolded, wore a noseclip and breathed directly into a low-resistance Beckman Metabolic Measurement Cart (MMC). The entire process of collecting data, calculating the physiological variables and printing them on a strip recorder was under the control of the processor. Complete data could be collected as often as every 30 seconds. Each subject was tested on two separate occasions. On the first occasion, after 20 minutes of stabilization a cigarette smoker was seated 4½ feet away from the subject. He smoked a popular low-tar, low-nicotine filtered cigarette. The smoker was not allowed to exhale smoke directly toward the subject and the subject inhaled the tobacco smoke only by chance. At no time were the subjects aware that tobacco smoke had been introduced into their environment.

On the second occasion, an identical procedure was followed except that in place of the cigarette a plastic toy cigarette was used to simulate the smoking movement.

Stabilization data were collected for 20 minutes (one recording each minute), 30-second recordings were made for the next 5 minutes (during which the smoking or simulated smoking took place) and one-minute postsmoke exposure recordings were taken for the next 30 minutes.

Results

The results indicate that the inhalation of residual tobacco smoke causes significant physiological changes (Table I).

Discussion

The results support the hypothesis that involuntarily inhaling residual smoke will cause physiological changes to occur in otherwise healthy nonsmokers. In this study, the overall effect of inhaling tobacco smoke appeared to be remarkably consistent, i.e., inhaling tobacco smoke caused a significant increase in total ventilation, total

Table I. Physical Response to Inhalation of Tobacco Smoke on Nonsmokers

Parameter	Material	20 Min. Stabiliz.	S.D.	Two Minutes After Lighting Material	S.D.	15 Minutes After Exting. Material	S.D.	30 Minutes After Exting. Material	S.D.
$\dot{V}_E$ ml/min (BTPS)	Tobacco	5,105	1116	8,379	977	6,684	1010	6,183	987
	Placebo	5,271	1261	5,255	1184	5,329	1250	5,258	1200
$\dot{V}O_2$ ml/min (STPD)	Tobacco	200	61	391	104	233	88	224	80
	Placebo	210	69	207	75	215	69	211	71
$\dot{V}O_2$ ml/min/kg (STPD)	Tobacco	3.5	0.3	7.14	1.25	4.38	2.10	4.05	2.20
	Placebo	3.6	0.3	3.50	0.30	3.60	0.03	3.50	0.03
$\dot{V}CO_2$ ml/min (STPD)	Tobacco	167	80	229	96	144	73	131	76
	Placebo	169	72	171	74	170	72	172	73
R.Q.	Tobacco	0.57	.13	0.67	.18	0.62	.17	0.59	.13
	Placebo	0.59	.11	0.59	.10	0.58	.11	0.59	.10
Resp. rate (beats/min)	Tobacco	12.3	2.1	13.98	3.9	13.5	3.9	12.9	3.4
	Placebo	12.1	2.3	12.00	2.3	12.2	2.2	12.1	2.3
Perspiration (gm/min)	Tobacco	0.01	.003	.06	.008	.04	.007	.03	.005
	Placebo	0.01	.003	.01	.003	.01	.003	.01	.003
Heart rate (beats/min)	Tobacco	72.4	13.8	78.7	12.7	78.1	11.6	74.7	10.6
	Placebo	72.2	14.3	72.0	14.2	72.1	14.0	72.0	13.6
Systolic BP (mm Hg)	Tobacco	124	9.7	129.8	11.6	126.9	12.2	126.1	11.1
	Placebo	124	9.8	123.1	9.7	122.8	9.6	122.1	9.7
Diastolic BP (mm Hg)	Tobacco	80	7.2	84.4	8.8	84.2	8.5	82.6	7.9
	Placebo	79	7.4	80.1	7.5	79.6	7.4	79.3	7.4
Pulse pressure	Tobacco	44	8.7	45.4	9.1	42.7	9.0	43.5	9.0
	Placebo	43	8.7	43.0	8.9	43.2	9.0	42.8	8.9
Hand steadiness	Tobacco	35	4.6	160	102.0	140	80.0	112	52.0
	Placebo	37	4.3	40	4.4	38	4.2	35	4.3

oxygen consumption and total carbon dioxide production and an increase in R.Q., respiratory rate, perspiration production, heart rate and both systolic and diastolic blood pressure, as well as a reduction in pulse pressure. The effects on hand steadiness suggest that some neural changes occur; many children and teenagers displayed hand tremor that would usually be expected only in 60- to 70-year-old adults.

Summary

Inhaling residual tobacco smoke from a smoker seated 4½ feet away caused statistically significant increases in ventilation, oxygen consumption, carbon dioxide production, R.Q., respiratory rate, perspiration production, heart rate and systolic and diastolic blood pressure and decreases in hand steadiness and pulse pressure.

The degree of change in these parameters caused by inhaling residual smoke varied somewhat from subject to subject; however, this may have been because the exact amount of inhaled smoke could not be determined, since the smoke being emitted by the smoker circulated within the room in a random manner.

Although data collected in this study show that residual smoke does significantly alter physiological responses in humans, at this time it is impossible to determine the total harm that residual smoke has on the nonsmoker. It is true, however, that inhaling residual smoke increases the number and severity of coronary disease risk factors in nonsmokers. One must consider that the smoker has a choice regarding the adding of smoking to his own health risk factors — it is his own personal choice. The nonsmoker should also have a choice. The convenience to a smoker of being able to smoke wherever he pleases is far less important than the health risk to his nonsmoking neighbor.

The Influence of Polycythemia, Induced by Four-Week Sojourn at 4300 Meters, on Sea Level Work Capacity

D. Horstman, R. Weiskopf, R. Jackson
and J. Severinghaus

Introduction

There has been increased participation recently in physical training at high altitude, with the hope of improving subsequent athletic performance at sea level. However, there is little scientific evidence recommending this procedure. For example, if one examines maximal oxygen consumption ($\dot{V}O_2$ max), perhaps the best physiological indicator of potential for performance in endurance-related events, the literature is equivocal as to any beneficial effects of high altitude training. Several studies utilizing trained athletes have indicated no change or decreases of $\dot{V}O_2$ max measured at sea level following training at high altitude [3, 7, 16]. Other studies, utilizing both athletes and trained individuals who were not athletes, have demonstrated increases in sea level $\dot{V}O_2$ max subsequent to training at high altitude [2, 6, 13].

Further attesting to this fact was the joint meeting of the British Association of Sport and Medicine with the British Olympic Association held in November 1973. This meeting brought together an international group of physicians, exercise physiologists and coaches to review the available knowledge of altitude training and its effects on both physiological indices of performance and on performance per se at sea level. The consensus from this meeting was that it is uncertain whether performance at sea level is improved after training at altitude [15]. One factor, which was common to all of these previous studies, was the use of training in conjunction with high altitude sojourn. With exposure to altitude, the potential for

D. Horstman, R. Weiskopf, R. Jackson and J. Severinghaus, U.S. Army Research Institute of Environmental Medicine, Natick, Massachusetts, U.S.A.

detraining in previously trained individuals is high due to disruption of training schedules resulting from decreased physiological capacity, gastrointestinal infection, acute mountain sickness and/or psychological disturbances. Perhaps, a more logical first step would be to evaluate the effects of high altitude sojourn, independent of training, on $\dot{V}O_2$ max and endurance performance, measured subsequently at sea level.

Maximal oxygen consumption is a function of maximal systemic oxygen transport [10, 11], the product of maximal cardiac output and arterial oxygen content. Prolonged sojourn at high altitude results in increased hematocrit with a resultant increase in arterial oxygen content [9, 17]. Therefore, one might expect a concomitant improvement in $\dot{V}O_2$ max, as suggested by Ekblom et al [4, 5] in studies in which hematocrit was elevated by the infusion of packed red cells, resulting in an increase of $\dot{V}O_2$ max. However, the situation is not quite this simple. It has also been suggested that prolonged exposure to hypoxia depresses myocardial function, thereby diminishing maximal cardiac output and in turn maximal systemic oxygen transport [1]. In addition to increasing arterial oxygen content, increased hematocrit also results in increased blood viscosity [10, 12]. It is possible that within the normal range of hematocrit, hematocrit-induced increases of arterial oxygen content will not improve maximal systemic oxygen transport, since maximal cardiac output may be reduced because of increased peripheral resistance and reduced venous return resulting from an increase in blood viscosity [8, 11]. Chronic hypoxia has been reported to reduce maximal cardiac output [17, 18].

The primary purpose of this study was to determine the effects of a four-week sojourn at 4300 meters without physical training, on sea level work capacity and related factors. A secondary purpose was to evaluate the specific role of high altitude-induced polycythemia relative to any observed improvements in sea level work capacity and related factors.

Procedures

Nine healthy male volunteers served as subjects for this study. Each volunteer was informed of the procedures to be used and signed a statement of informed consent. Potential subjects were excluded from the study if they were born at an altitude in excess of 1000 meters or had resided for over one month at an altitude in excess of 1000 meters within three years prior to the study. Further basis for exclusion included evidence of any hemoglobinopathy or other illness which would contraindicate sojourn at high altitude.

Table I illustrates the experimental protocol followed during the course of the study. As can be seen, on day 1 and at seven-day intervals throughout the study, $\dot{V}O_2$ max was determined for all subjects. On day 2 and at seven-day intervals throughout the study, endurance time to exhaustion at a work intensity ranging between 75% and 90% $\dot{V}O_2$ max was determined for all subjects.

For purposes of this study, we will compare results obtained during the third week of testing at sea level prior to high altitude sojourn (SL_1) to those obtained at sea level immediately following high altitude sojourn (SL_2), i.e., the days indicated by asterisks in Table I. Maximal oxygen consumption and endurance time to

Table I. Experimental Protocol

Location	Day	Procedure
	1	$\dot{V}O_2$ max
	2	Endurance run (30 min)
	8	$\dot{V}O_2$ max
Sea level	9	Endurance run (90 min or to exhaustion)
	*15	$\dot{V}O_2$ max
	*16	Endurance run (to exhaustion)
	22	$\dot{V}O_2$ max
	23	Endurance run (to exhaustion)
	28	Travel to high altitude
	29	$\dot{V}O_2$ max
	30	Endurance run (to exhaustion)
	36	$\dot{V}O_2$ max
	37	Endurance run (to exhaustion)
High altitude	43	$\dot{V}O_2$ max
	44	Endurance run (to exhaustion)
	49	Phlebotomy
	50	$\dot{V}O_2$ max
	51	Endurance run (to exhaustion)
	56	Travel to sea level
Sea level	*57	$\dot{V}O_2$ max
	*58	Endurance run (to exhaustion)

exhaustion measured during the third week did not differ from that measured during the fourth week prior to high altitude sojourn.

All exercise testing was performed in the running mode on a motor-driven treadmill. For each subject running speed was constant; variation in work intensity was produced by varying the grade of incline of the treadmill. Maximal oxygen consumption was determined with an interrupted procedure similar to that described by Mitchell et al [14].

The criterion for $\dot{V}O_2$ max was a plateauing of $\dot{V}O_2$ concomitant with an increase in work intensity. Endurance time to exhaustion was performed at a work intensity corresponding to 85% of $\dot{V}O_2$ max as determined on day 15 of the study; thereafter, the treadmill speed and grade remained constant for each subject. Endurance tests were interrupted in nature; the initial work/rest cycle was 18 minutes work/3 minutes rest. Failure to complete 18 minutes of running was followed by a work/rest cycle of 12 minutes work/2 minutes rest. Failure to complete 12 minutes of running was followed by a work/rest cycle of 6 minutes work/1 minute rest. Finally, failure to complete the six minutes of running resulted in termination of the test.

In addition to $\dot{V}O_2$ max, resting hematocrit (Hct) and maximal values of minute ventilation ($\dot{V}_E$ max), cardiac output ($\dot{Q}$ max), heart rate (HR max) and stroke volume (SV max) were also obtained. Oxygen consumption was also measured during the endurance run. Minute ventilation was measured using timed collections of expired gas into Douglas bags. Expired gas fractions (O_2 and CO_2) were ascertained by mass spectroscopy. Oxygen consumption was calculated by the Haldane formula. Heart rate was determined from EKG tracings, since EKG was monitored continuously throughout all tests. Cardiac output was measured by a single breath method utilizing a vital capacity inspiration of a gas mixture containing 1% acetylene, 1% dimethyl ether, 10% helium, 21% oxygen, balance nitrogen. With this method, two simultaneous estimations of cardiac output were obtained from the rate of disappearance of both acetylene and dimethyl ether from alveolar air. The mean of these two estimations was used as the final value of cardiac output. Stroke volume was calculated as $\dot{Q}$/HR.

On day 49 of the study, one week prior to return to sea level, 450 ml of whole blood was removed from five of the subjects (BLED). The remaining four subjects (SHAM) underwent venipuncture without blood removal. Volume was replaced with lactated Ringer's solution. Phlebotomies and fluid replacement were performed by trained personnel under the supervision of the physician serving as medical monitor for the study. A double-blind design was utilized with all subjects following identical procedures, with the exception of blood removal. Following venipuncture the subject's arm was screened from his view and knowledge of which subjects had actually been bled was withheld from both the subjects and all members of the research team, with the exception of the medical monitor.

Statistically, we compared the differences between results obtained before high altitude sojourn and those obtained after with a t-test for differences using the 10% level of significance.

Results

In Table II, we can see that SL_2 Hct for BLED was not different from that of SL_1. While for SHAM, SL_2 Hct was 10% greater than that of SL_1. For BLED there were no differences between SL_1 and SL_2 $\dot{V}O_2$ max while for SHAM, SL_2 $\dot{V}O_2$ max was 6% greater than that of SL_1. Maximal minute ventilation increased significantly in both groups.

Table III indicates that there were no differences for BLED· between SL_1 and SL_2 measures of $\dot{Q}$ max, HR max and SV max. However SHAM demonstrated a 5% decrease of $\dot{Q}$ max and SV max, with no change in HR max.

As seen in Table IV, SL_1 and SL_2 endurance times were not different for BLED while for SHAM, SL_2 endurance time was 25% greater than that of SL_1. As $\dot{V}O_2$ max did not change for BLED, both SL_1 and SL_2 endurance tests were performed at a work intensity corresponding to 86% $\dot{V}O_2$ max. SHAM's SL_1 endurance

Table II. Mean ±SE Resting Hct, Maximal $\dot{V}O_2$ and $\dot{V}_E$
for SHAM and BLED, Measured at Sea Level Before (SL_1)
and After (SL_2) High Altitude Sojourn

		SL_1	SL_2	P
Hct	SHAM	45.8 ± 1.9	50.2 ± 2.1	<0.01
(%)	BLED	46.0 ± 1.6	45.4 ± 1.7	n.s.
$\dot{V}O_2$ max	SHAM	50.8 ± 0.5	53.8 ± 0.4	<0.01
(ml/kg/min)	BLED	50.4 ± 1.9	49.7 ± 1.8	n.s.
$\dot{V}_E$ max	SHAM	2289 ± 184	2454 ± 194	<0.01
(ml/kg/min)	BLED	2424 ± 121	2751 ± 90	<0.01

Table III. Mean ±SE Maximal $\dot{Q}$, HR, and SV for SHAM and BLED,
Measured at Sea Level Before (SL_1) and After (SL_2)
High Altitude Sojourn

		SL_1	SL_2	P
$\dot{Q}$ max	SHAM	272 ± 9	258 ± 8	<0.10
(ml/kg/min)	BLED	273 ± 15	274 ± 15	n.s.
HR max	SHAM	192 ± 2	194 ± 3	n.s.
(bpm)	BLED	188 ± 2	190 ± 2	n.s.
SV max	SHAM	1.42 ± .06	1.36 ± .04	<0.10
(ml/kg/beat)	BLED	1.45 ± .08	1.44 ± .09	n.s.

Table IV. Mean ±SE Endurance Values for SHAM
(6.1 mph, 4.5% grade) and BLED (6.3 mph, 4.7% grade)
Measured at Sea Level Before (SL_1) and After (SL_2)
High Altitude Sojourn

		SL_1	SL_2	P
$\dot{V}O_2$	SHAM	42.5 ± 0.8	42.6 ± 0.9	n.s.
(ml/kg/min)	BLED	43.2 ± 1.8	43.0 ± 1.9	n.s.
% $\dot{V}O_2$ max	SHAM	84 ± 1	79 ± 1	<0.01
	BLED	86 ± 1	86 ± 1	n.s.
End Time	SHAM	58.0 ± 6.8	71.5 ± 7.4	<0.05
(min)	BLED	57.2 ± 8.4	52.2 ± 6.0	n.s.

test was performed at a work intensity corresponding to 84% max, but since SL_2 $\dot{V}O_2$ max increased, SHAM's SL_2 endurance test was performed at a work intensity corresponding to 79% $\dot{V}O_2$ max.

Conclusions

We conclude that when excluding the complications of physical training, extended sojourn at high altitude improves subsequent sea level work capacity. It is likely that increased sea level work capacity resulted from the increased systemic oxygen transport afforded by high altitude-induced polycythemia. This supports the work of Ekblom et al [4, 5] who found increases in $\dot{V}O_2$ max and endurance time resulting from increased hematocrit following the infusion of packed red cells. However, it should be noted that the 6% increase in $\dot{V}O_2$ max was not to the same extent as the expected 10% increase in arterial oxygen content. Maximal cardiac output was reduced and $\dot{V}O_2$ max was strictly related to systemic oxygen transport.

References

1. Alexander, J.K., Hartley, L.H., Modelski, M. and Grover, R.F.: Reduction of stroke volume during exercise in man following ascent to 3100 m. altitude. J. Appl. Physiol. 23:849-858, 1967.
2. Balke, B., Faulkner, J.A., and Daniels, J.T.: Maximum performance capacity at sea-level and at moderate altitude before and after training at altitude. Schweiz. Z. Sportmed. 14:106-116, 1967.
3. Buskirk, E.R., Kollias, J., Akers, R.F. et al: Maximal performance at altitude and on return from altitude in conditioned runners. J. Appl. Physiol. 23:259-266, 1967.
4. Ekblom, B., Goldberg, A.N. and Gullbring, B.: Response to exercise after blood loss and reinfusion. J. Appl. Physiol. 33:175-180, 1972.
5. Ekblom, B., Wilson, G. and Astrand, P.-O.: Central circulation during exercise after venesection and reinfusion of red blood cells. J. Appl. Physiol. 40:379-383, 1976.
6. Faulkner, J.A.: Training for maximum performance at altitude. In Goddard, R.F. (ed.): The Effects of Altitude on Physical Performance. Athletic Institute, 1967, pp. 88-90.
7. Grover, R.F.: Exercise performance of athletes at sea level and 3100 meters altitude. In Goddard, R.F. (ed.): The Effects of Altitude on Physical Performance. Athletic Institute, 1967, pp. 80-87.
8. Guyton, A.C. and Richardson, T.Q.: Effect of hematocrit on venous return. Circ. Res. 9:157-164, 1961.
9. Hansen, J.E., Vogel, J.A., Stelter, G.P. and Consolazio, C.F.: Oxygen uptake in man during exhaustive work at sea level and high altitude. J. Appl. Physiol. 23:511-522, 1967.
10. Horstman, D.H., Gleser, M. and Delehunt, J.: Effects of altering O_2 delivery on $\dot{V}O_2$ of isolated, working muscle. Am. J. Physiol. 230:327-334, 1976.
11. Horstman, D.H., Gleser, M.A., Wolfe, D. et al: Effects of hemoglobin reduction on $\dot{V}O_2$ max and related hemodynamics in exercising dogs. J. Appl. Physiol. 37:97-102, 1974.
12. Levy, M.N. and Share, L.: The influence of erythrocyte concentration upon the pressure-flow relationships in the dog's hind limb. Circ. Res. 1:247-255, 1953.
13. Mellerowicz, H., Meller, W., Woweries, J. et al: Vergleichend untersuchungen über wirkung von hohën training auf die dauerleistung in meereshöhe. Sportarzt Sportmed. 21:207-215, 1970.
14. Mitchell, J., Sproule, B. and Chapman, C.: The physiological meaning of the maximal oxygen intake test. J. Clin. Invest. 37:538-546, 1958.
15. Richardson, R.G. (ed.): Altitude training. Br. J. Sports Med. 8:1-65, 1974.
16. Saltin, B.: Aerobic and anaerobic work capacity at an altitude of 2,250 meters. In Goddard, R.F. (ed.): The Effects of Altitude on Physical Performance. Athletic Institute, 1967, pp. 97-102.
17. Saltin, B., Grover, R.F., Blomquist, C.G. et al: Maximal oxygen uptake and cardiac output after 2 weeks at 4300 m. J. Appl. Physiol. 25:400-409, 1968.
18. Vogel, J.A., Hansen, J.E. and Harris, C.W.: Cardiovascular responses in man during exhaustive work at sea level and high altitude. J. Appl. Physiol. 23:531-539, 1967.

Physiological Studies on Cardiorespiratory Response to Exercise and Validity of Endurance Tests in Ten-Year-Old Boys

T. Yoshida and T. Ishiko

Introduction

Studies on cardiorespiratory responses of boys to exercise are rather few in cases where cardiac output is included in the measurements [1, 4, 5, 10]. The authors, therefore, measured cardiac output and related parameters of the boys by administering a maximal bicycling exercise in order to clarify the characteristics of their cardiorespiratory functions and to examine the validity of endurance tests in boys.

Method

Twenty-five 10-year-old school boys and 19 21-year-old healthy adults served as subjects. None of them had been undertaking regular high stress physical training. Their physical characteristics are shown in Table I.

Experiments were performed at the laboratory in the afternoon at least two hours after meals. Following rest in a sitting position, the

Table I. Physical Characteristics of Subjects

Subjects	N	Age yr	Weight kg	Height cm
Boys	25	10.2 ±0.3	32.2 ±7.4	135.8 ±6.4
Adult men	19	21.6 ±1.8	64.3 ±7.8	170.8 ±5.4

T. Yoshida, School of Dental Medicine, Tsurumi University, Japan and T. Ishiko, School of Health and Physical Education, Juntendo University, Japan.

subjects exercised on a mechanical bicycle ergometer. They were given three workloads progressively increased every four minutes in such a way that their heart rate reached about 120, 140 and 160 beats/min. The workload was further increased every minute by 75 kg/min for boys and 150 kg/min for adults until exhaustion.

Oxygen intake was determined by means of the Douglas bag method. The volume of expired air was measured by a wet gas meter and samples of the air were analyzed by polarographic O_2 analyzer (Beckman OM-11) for oxygen and rapid infrared CO_2 analyzer (Beckman LB-1) for carbon dioxide. These apparatus were calibrated by modified Haldane gas analyzer. Heart rate was determined by continuously recorded ECG. Using CO_2 rebreathing method [3, 8], mixed venous CO_2 pressure was calculated graphically and arterial CO_2 pressure was determined by end tidal method. Fick's equation was applied for calculating the cardiac output and arteriovenous oxygen difference. Stroke volume was obtained as cardiac output per heart beat.

At another opportunity, 800-meter distance run and step test were administered to the boys. Step test was a modified Harvard test especially devised for boys as 35 cm bench height, 30 mounts/min, three minutes' duration; it was evaluated as fitness index from recovery heart rate according to the original [2].

Results

The data obtained during maximal exercise are shown in Table II. Maximal oxygen intake was significantly lower in boys than in adults ($p < 0.001$). But this difference disappeared when expressed in milliliter per minute per kilogram of body weight. $Paco_2$ did not

Table II. Cardiorespiratory Functions During Maximal
Bicycling Exercise in Boys and Adult Men

		Boys	Adult Men
$\dot{V}O_2$ max	l/min	1.33 ± 0.21	2.79 ± 0.41‡
	ml/kg/min	41.8 ± 4.9	43.4 ± 4.7
$Paco_2$	mm Hg	33.2 ± 3.3	34.4 ± 4.4
$P\bar{v}co_2$	mm Hg	66.6 ± 5.3	80.6 ± 8.4‡
$\dot{Q}$ max	l/min	10.0 ± 1.3	18.7 ± 2.9‡
HR max	beats/min	195 ± 10	188 ± 7*
SV max	ml	51.6 ± 8.0	99.0 ± 15.8‡
	ml/kg	1.64 ± 0.25	1.53 ± 0.19
(a-v) O_2	diff vol %	13.3 ± 1.7	15.2 ± 1.7†

* $p < 0.05$, † $p < 0.01$, ‡ $p < 0.001$.

show significant difference between boys and adults. On the contrary, $Pvco_2$ in adults was higher compared with boys.

Maximal cardiac output in boys was significantly lower than that in adults ($p < 0.001$), while maximal heart rate was slightly higher in boys than in adults ($p < 0.05$). Maximal stroke volume in boys was only a half of that in adults, but significant difference between the two groups was not detected when expressed in milliliter per kilogram of body weight. Arteriovenous O_2 difference was more remarkable in adults than in boys ($p < 0.01$).

As the measures of endurance tests in boys, the following were considered: fitness index of the step test, 800-meter running performance and PWC_{170}. The validity of these three measures was examined by computing correlation matrix as shown in Figure 1. As a result, step test index was not significantly correlated to any cardiorespiratory functions. Running performance had significant correlation to $\dot{V}O_2$ max (ml/kg/min). PWC_{170} was significantly correlated to $\dot{V}O_2$ max (l/min), $\dot{Q}$ max, SV max and fitness score.

Discussion

Maximal oxygen intake of the subjects was 41.8 ml/kg/min in boys and 43.4 ml/kg/min in adults. These values were almost the same as the values reported previously [6, 7, 9]. Therefore, the subjects of the present study were considered to have ordinary aerobic capacity.

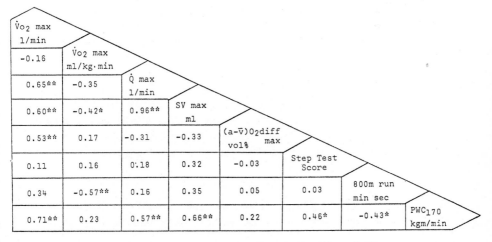

* $p < 0.05$ ** $p < 0.01$ *** $p < 0.001$

FIG. 1. Correlation matrix among the parameters obtained in boys.

According to Fick's principle, oxygen intake is the function of three independent variables: heart rate, stroke volume and arterio-venous oxygen difference. Since maximal oxygen intake (ml/kg/min) and maximal stroke volume (ml/kg) were almost the same between boys and adults, maximal heart rate and arteriovenous oxygen difference should take reverse response mutually, the former and the latter being dominant in boys and in adults, respectively. The fact that arteriovenous oxygen difference was marked in adults would partly be derived from high concentration of hemoglobin in adults, since arteriovenous oxygen difference is known to be dependent of hemoglobin concentration [5].

From the fact that mixed venous CO_2 pressure at maximal exercise was lower in boys, lactacid anaerobic capacity in boys is considered lower compared with adults. This may partly explain the reason why work performance of adults is superior to boys despite equal aerobic capacity (ml/kg/min) between them.

Since the most valid physiological measure of endurance is considered to be $\dot{V}O_2$ max (ml/kg/min), 800 meters was appropriate for evaluating endurance fitness for boys. On the contrary, step test is not valid as shown in correlation matrix and, therefore, is not appropriate insofar as the test is applied to boys.

Conclusion

Cardiorespiratory functions at maximal exercise were studied in boys (10.2 years) and adults (21.6 years). Both groups had almost the same maximal oxygen intake (ml/kg/min) and maximal stroke volume (ml/kg). However, the former had higher maximal heart rate and the latter had higher arteriovenous oxygen difference. Therefore, contribution of these two variables to maximal oxygen intake is different between boys and adults. Moreover, lower mixed venous pressure of CO_2 observed in boys may postulate lower lactacid anerobic capacity in boys. The 800-meter run as a field test was valid for the evaluation of endurance fitness in boys. On the contrary, the step test for boys was not valid as applied in modified form.

References

1. Bar-Or, O., Shephard, R.J. and Allen, C.L.: Cardiac output of 10- to 13-year-old boys and girls during submaximal exercise. J. Appl. Physiol. 30:219-223, 1971.
2. Brouha, L., Graybiel, A. and Heath, C.W.: The step test. A simple method of measuring physical fitness for hard muscular work in adult man. Rev. Can. Biol. 2:86-91, 1943.

3. Defares, J.G., Wise, M.E. and Duyff, J.W.: New indirect Fick procedure for the determination of cardiac output. Nature 192:760-761, 1961.

4. Eriksson, B.O.: Physical training, oxygen supply and muscle metabolism in 11- to 13-year-old boys. Acta Physiol. Scand. Suppl. 384, 1972.

5. Eriksson, B.O., Grimby, G. and Saltin, B.: Cardiac output and arterial blood gases during exercise in pubertal boys. J. Appl. Physiol. 31:348-352, 1972.

6. Ikai, M. and Kitagawa, K.: Maximum oxygen uptake of Japanese related to sex and age. Med. Sci. Sports 4:127-131, 1972 (Japanese).

7. Ishiko, T., Katamoto, S. and Yoshida, T.: Validity of evaluating endurance capacity in young boys and girls from cardiac response to the step test. Rep. Res. Cent. Phys. Ed. 2:42-51, 1974.

8. Klausen, K.: Comparison of CO_2 rebreathing and acetylene methods for cardiac output. J. Appl. Physiol. 20:763-766, 1965.

9. Miyamura, M. and Honda, Y.: Maximum cardiac output related to sex and age. Jap. J. Physiol. 23:645-656, 1973.

10. Rode, A., Bar-Or, O. and Shephard, R.J.: Cardiac output and oxygen conductance. A comparison of Canadian Eskimo and city dwellers. Proceedings of the 4th International Symposium on Pediatric Work Physiology. Wingate Institute, Israel, 1972.

Methode pour une estimation integrale de l'état de vigueur chez les jeunes

L'étude des indices de force chez l'homme a suscité l'intérêt des gens dès les temps les plus anciens. Parallèlement au perfectionnement des méthodes d'investigation scientifique, ce problème ne cesse, de nos jours aussi, de préoccuper les scientifiques et les practiciens.

Nombre de recherches et l'expérience pratique acquise montrent que, tant dans la vie que dans les sports, l'un des facteurs primordiaux dont dépendent les actes moteurs efficaces de l'homme est l'état de vigueur de l'individu (Boïtchev Kl., Barzakov P., 1970; Verkhochanskij Ju., 1970; Zatsiorskij V., 1966; Plotkin B., 1966; Fidelus K., 1970, etc.).

Notre tâche dans cette recherche menée sur une vaste échelle était d'étudier objectivement l'état de vigueur chez des jeunes à l'âge de 18 à 20 ans. Plus précisément, nous nous sommes proposés comme but de fonder une nouvelle méthode d'estimation intégrale de la condition de vigueur.

La fraction représentative fut déterminée par échantillonnage aléatoire, suivant la méthode de loterie, sur 1000 personnes examinées. A chacune de ces personnes, on avait mesuré 9 indices de base et 48 indices dérivés caractérisant leur possibilités de force. Pour plus de brièveté et de netteté dans cette communication, nous nous arrêterons plus en détail sur 24 tests pour chaque individu soumis à l'expérience, dont 8 tests de base et 16 dérivés, comme suit:

No. 1 — Force maximale des muscles extenseurs du tronc ($F_{max.1}$ en kg).

No. 2 — Force maximale des muscles fléchisseurs de la plante du pied ($F_{max.2}$ en kg).

No. 3 — Force maximale des muscles extenseurs des articulations iliaques ($F_{max.3}$ en kg).

No. 4 — Force maximale des muscles extenseurs de l'épaule ($F_{max.4}$).

No. 5 — Force maximale des muscles extenseurs de l'avant-bras ($F_{max.5}$).

N. Hadjiev, Chargé de cours, agrégé en pédagogie, Sofia, Bulgarie.

No. 6 — Force maximale des muscles fléchisseurs des articulations iliaques ($F_{max.6}$).

No. 7 — Force maximale des muscles fléchisseurs de l'avant-bras ($F_{max.7}$).

No. 8 — Force maximale des muscles extenseurs du genou ($F_{max.8}$).

Du No. 9 au No. 16 compris, ce sont les gradients maxima des huit indices de base ou Gr_{max} 1,2 .... 8 en kg/sec.

Du No. 17 au No. 24 compris, ce sont les forces de départ des huit indices de base ou F_{st} 1,2 ...... en keg.

Le mesurage des tests susmentionnés fut réalisé à l'aide d'un banc d'expérimentation spécialement construit assurant une immobilisation maximale des articulations voisines, comme on peut le voir à la Figure 1.

L'enregistrement des paramètres de force fut réalisé par le système tensiométrique "Hettinger".

Pour la lecture des résultats, nous avons utilisé un capteur tensiométrique à induction type standard, fabriqué par la même firme. Sa haute sensibilité et son pouvoir séparateur permettent de procéder aux analyses des paramètres de force à une précision de ± 1 kg. Le capteur tensiométrique ne se laisse pas influencer par les perturbations venant de l'extérieur. Les signaux reçus étaient amplifiés à l'aide d'un amplificateur tensiométrique monocanal KW/T5. A titre d'enregistreur, nous nous servions d'un électrocardio-

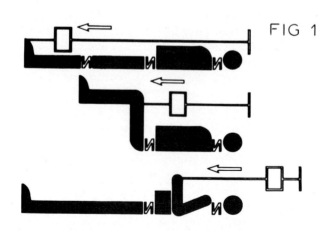

FIG 1

TECHNIQUE DE MESURAGE DES INDICES DE FORCE

FIGURE 1.

graphe monocanal portatif à transistors VEK 3. Lors des enregistrements, nous utilisions sa vitesse maximale de 50 mm/sec. et sa largeur
utile maximale, elle aussi de 50 mm.

Le traitement des enregistrements et l'extraction des caractéristiques numériques des indices étudiés étaient réalisés d'une manière
standard telle qu'indiquée à la Figure 2, notamment:

a) force maximale
b) gradient maximal
c) force de départ.

Tout sujet examiné faisait 3 essais pour chaque indice. Pour les
calculs, nous prenions le meilleur résultat dans chaque test. Avant de
commencer le travail à l'aide de l'ensemble d'appareils tensio-
métriques, on procédait à un étalonnage de l'amplificateur et du
dispositif d'enregistrement. Cela assurait des conditions indentiques
pour l'enregistrement des indices chez tous les examinés.

Les 24 indices fixés pour les personnes soumises aux tests sont
présentés au Tableau I. Y figurent également certains paramètres
statistiques de variabilité, comme m_x, σ et V%. L'analyse de ces
données permet de pénétrer plus en détail dans le problème étudié.
Ainsi, par exemple, une comparaison des valeurs moyennes pour la
force maximale dégage les différences quantitatives entre les groupes
musculaires étudiés. Comme on peut le voir au tableau, en première
place pour l'indice de force maximale viennent les fléchisseurs de la
plante du pied — 161.9 kg (No. 2), en deuxième et troisième places
se trouvent les extenseurs du tronc et les extenseurs des articulations
iliaques avec, respectivement, 138.4 kg (No. 1) et 120.6 kg (No. 3).

Les paramètres statistiques de variabilité font voir un tableau un
peu différent. La plus grande variance des cas individuels est mise en

FIG 2

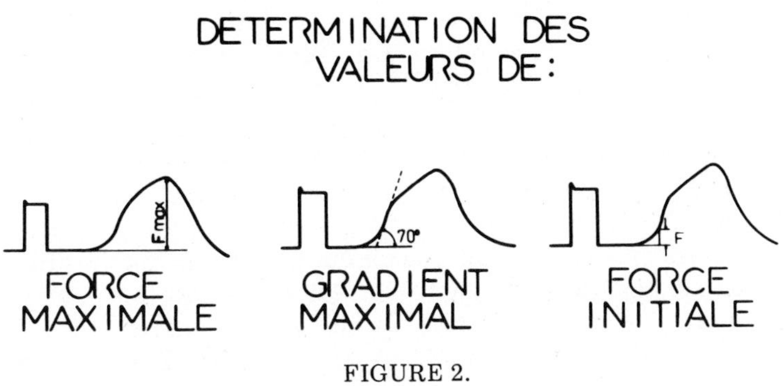

DETERMINATION DES
VALEURS DE:

FORCE   GRADIENT   FORCE
MAXIMALE   MAXIMAL   INITIALE

FIGURE 2.

Tableau I.

TABLEAU DES VARIATIONS DES INDICES CARACTERISANT LA TOPOGRAPHIE DE LA FORCE MUSCULAIRE

		X	m_r		V		R
1	8	138,4	0,724	224,0	16,6	55,0	230,0
2	15	161,9	1,266	40,04	24,7	35,0	300,0
3	22	120,6	0,829	26,22	21,7	35,0	250,0
4	24	53,6	0,561	17,72	27,9	25,0	140,0
5	36	48,0	0,433	23,69	28,6	15,0	105,0
6	43	71,5	0,504	15,92	22,3	30,0	140,0
7	50	52,7	0,284	8,98	17,1	20,0	100,0
8	57	102,8	0,766	24,22	23,6	45,0	245,0
9	10	1041,4	12,569	397,46	38,2	235,0	4758,0
10	17	799,3	8,650	273,53	34,2	189,0	2836,0
11	24	995,5	14,430	456,32	45,8	210,0	4057,0
12	31	469,9	6,572	207,84	44,2	106,0	2029,0
13	38	314,5	4,371	138,29	44,0	91,0	933,0
14	45	558,3	6,025	190,51	34,1	99,0	1422,0
15	52	378,2	4,821	152,47	40,3	101,0	1286,0
16	59	659,8	8,010	253,30	38,4	202,0	2029,0
17	12	49,1	0,514	16,26	33,1	10,0	110,0
18	19	55,0	0,637	20,15	36,7	8,0	160,0
19	26	53,3	0,546	17,28	42,4	7,0	150,0
20	33	28,8	0,423	13,39	46,5	5,0	100,0
21	40	21,8	0,324	10,20	46,9	5,0	85,0
22	47	32,8	0,333	10,57	32,1	10,0	85,0
23	57	21,3	0,224	7,07	33,1	5,0	80,0
24	61	32,4	0,364	11,51	35,5	5,0	95,0

évidence pour les extenseurs de l'avant-bras (No. 5) et de l'épaule (No. 4), respectivement 28.6 et 27.9 kg, ce qui montre que ces indices sont porteurs d'une information relativement indépendante.

Fort intéressantes sont les valeurs du gradient maximal et de la force de départ. En ce qui concerne le gradient, on voit que l'accroissement maximal de la force par unité de temps est plus prononcé pour les groupes musculaires plus puissants (extenseurs du tronc (No. 9) — 1041.4 kg/sec. et extenseurs des articulations iliaques (No. 5) — 995.5 kg/sec.).

Un moment essentiel lors de l'estimation intégrale des indices de force représentent la valeur informatrice des tests choisis et leur autonomie relative. A cet effet, ils ont été soumis à une analyse par corrélation suivant le système chacun contre chacun. Les résultats du traitement de ces données ont revélé que la plupart des coefficients de corrélation sont insignifiants, ce qui montre nettement que les tests choisis sont porteurs d'une information indépendante et

peuvent servir de base lors de la formulation d'une estimation
intégrale. Il n'y a que quelques coefficients avec des valeurs
numériques près de 0.70.

Ce qui, relativement, présente le plus d'intérêt est la tentative de
constituer des indices intégraux d'estimation. A cette fin, les résultats
effectifs furent traités par les méthodes de l'analyse matricielle. Pour
ce faire, ils furent préalablement normalisés, après quoi fut extrait
l'indice de premier ordre (M_I). L'ensemble du traitement mathématique et statistique fut accompli à l'aide d'une calculatrice
électronique IBM-40/30.

L'analyse matricielle et, plus précisément, l'indice de premier
ordre qu'on avait extrait donne la possibilité d'une estimation
objective de l'état de vigueur, ce qui permet d'établir une caractéristique quantitative relativement précise des possibilités de force d'un
individu donné.

Disposant des valeurs normalisées des tests étudiés, nous con-
struisîmes un nomogramme sur lequel on peut déterminer et
procéder à l'estimation du dénommé "polygone des indices de force"
de tout individu. A titre d'exemple, sur la Figure 3 sont indiqués
trois cas sous les Nos. 721, 723 et 727 (numéro de la personne
examinée dans la fraction représentative étudiée). Comme on peut
s'assurer du nomogramme, l'estimation de l'état intégral de vigueur

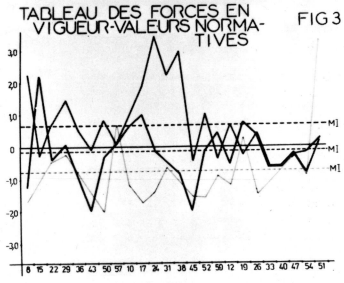

FIGURE 3.

(suivant M_I), tout aussi bien que des maillons faibles et forts dans les indices de force de chaque individu, peut se faire d'une manière très facile, commode et rapide.

Nous sommes convaincus que la méthode décrite par nous est commode et applicable en pratique dans tous les cas où il est nécessaire de procéder à une estimation quantitative, objective et intégrale de l'état de vigueur de l'individu vivant.

Maximal Oxygen Uptake, Body Composition and Running Performance in Japanese Young Adults of Both Sexes

Kaoru Kitagawa, Keizo Yamamoto
and Mitsumasa Miyashita

Introduction

The purposes of the present study are (1) to determine whether there are sex differences in $\dot{V}O_2$ max per lean body mass (LBM) (concerning this question, Döbeln [6] reported no difference between both sexes, while McNab et al [11] and Dill et al [5] showed significant difference); (2) to determine the correlation between $\dot{V}O_2$ max versus body weight and LBM (in the case of men, many studies have shown statistically higher correlations between $\dot{V}O_2$ max and LBM than that between $\dot{V}O_2$ max and body weight [3, 5, 6, 10, 15], but in women, these correlations have not been fully studied); and (3) to examine the best index among aerobic powers ($\dot{V}O_2$ max, $\dot{V}O_2$ max per body weight, $\dot{V}O_2$ max per LBM) to predict endurance-running capacity.

Methods

Thirty-nine healthy young Japanese men and 33 women volunteered as subjects. All of them were university students who did not engage in regular physical conditioning. Their body dimensions are listed in Table I.

$\dot{V}O_2$ max was determined by an exhaustive running test on a motor-driven treadmill. A three-minute warm-up of running at 160 meter/min was given to men and 130 meter/min to women with a

Kaoru Kitagawa and Mitsumasa Miyashita, Laboratory of Exercise Physiology and Biomechanics, Faculty of Education, University of Tokyo and Keizo Yamamoto, Department of Health and Physical Education, College of General Education, University of Tokyo, Japan.

Table I. Body Dimensions and 2400-Meter Running Time

		Age (yrs)	Height (cm)	Weight (kg)	VR (ml)	DB (g/ml)	% Fat (%)	ATM (kg)	LBM (kg)	2400-Meter Run (min, sec)
Men	$\overline{X}$	19.3	172.1	62.03	1360	1.0696	13.1	8.21	53.86	10' 16"
	SD	0.8	5.0	6.69	263	0.0106	4.3	3.00	5.75	1' 28"
Women	$\overline{X}$	18.7	157.0	53.21	992	1.0487	21.6	11.61	41.59	12' 16"
	SD	0.3	4.5	5.07	242	0.0109	4.5	3.16	3.17	48"

VR: residual lung volume; DB: body density; ATM: adipose tissue mass.
Sex differences in all items except age were significant ($p < 0.01$) by t-test.

constant slope of 2 degrees. After a ten-minute rest, the subjects ran at the same speed with a zero degree grade for the first three minutes. Thereafter the grade was increased by 2 degrees every minute until exhaustion. Most running times for all subjects ranged from six to eight minutes. After four minutes of running, expired air was collected every minute into a Douglas bag through a rubber tube of 33 mm diameter and its volume was measured in a dry gasometer. Fraction of O_2 and CO_2 of expired air sample was analyzed by Expired Gas Analyzer (model 1 HO2-2, San-ei Instruments, Inc., Tokyo, Japan), which was calibrated with the Scholander microgas analyzer. The results showed that the oxygen uptake reached almost a steady level despite increasing grade near exhaustion. Therefore, in the present study, the highest value among two or three values of oxygen uptakes was determined as $\dot{V}O_2$ max. Heart rate was monitored on an electrocardiograph during the exhaustive running test.

Body density was determined by the underwater-weighing method [2]. Water temperature was approximately 36 C. Body weight in water was measured using a force electric transducer, of which minimum sensitivity was adjusted to 20 g and calibrated with a known weight. LBM and adipose tissue mass (ATM) were computed from body density (DB), employing the revised formula of Brozek et al [1]; % fat = (4.570/body density − 4.142) × 100. Residual lung volume (VR) was measured just after underwater weighing by use of the oxygen dilution method of Rahn et al [14].

The time required to run 2400 meters by best effort was measured as an index of endurance-running capacity on 25 men and 15 women on a 400-meter outdoor track.

Results

Men showed significantly ($p < 0.01$) higher values in height, body weight, residual lung volume, body density and LBM than women, while lower values in % fat, adipose tissue mass and 2400-meter running time (Table I). Sex difference was also statistically clear in aerobic powers, even in $\dot{V}O_2$ max per LBM (men > women, Table II). Correlations between aerobic powers versus body weight, LBM and 2400-meter running time are listed in Table III. In men, $\dot{V}O_2$ max correlated with LBM higher than with body weight, but vice versa in women. Among indices of aerobic powers, $\dot{V}O_2$ max per LBM shows the lowest correlation with 2400-meter running time in both sexes.

Table II. Aerobic Powers

		$\dot{V}O_2 Max$ (l/min)	$\dot{V}O_2 Max/Wt$ (ml/kg/min)	$\dot{V}O_2 Max/LBM$ (ml/kg/min)
Men	$\overline{X}$	3.22	51.8	59.7
	SD	0.56	6.6	6.9
Women	$\overline{X}$	2.08	39.2	50.0
	SD	0.21	3.0	3.9

Sex differences were significant ($p < 0.01$) by t-test.

Table III. Correlations Between Aerobic Powers Versus
Body Weight, LBM and 2400-Meter Running Time

	Sex	Weight	LBM	2400-Meter Run
$\dot{V}O_2 max$	M	0.702[†]	0.814[†]	−0.633[†]
	W	0.701[†]	0.655[†]	−0.416
$\dot{V}O_2 max/wt$	M			−0.627[†]
	W			−0.461
$\dot{V}O_2 max/LBM$	M			−0.562*
	W			−0.314

M: Men; W: Women; *$p < 0.01$; [†]$p < 0.001$.

Discussion

There have been some studies of body composition and aerobic power in sedentary young Japanese adults. Nagamine and Suzuki [13] presented 13.1% fat in men aged 18 to 27 and 22.2% fat in women aged 18 to 23. Kitagawa et al [10] showed that 17 men (aged 19 to 21) had 12.1% fat on an average. These two studies employed the same formula of Brozek et al as was used in the present study. The mean values obtained in the present study were in agreement with these previous studies. The values of aerobic power were reported by Ikai et al [8] and Matsui et al [12] by an exhaustive running test on a treadmill. The former showed $\dot{V}O_2$ max per body weight of 49.1 ml for men aged 19 to 25 and 36.6 ml for women aged 20 to 21. The latter also presented the similar values which were 50.02 ml for men and 39.62 ml for women at the same age of 18. Based on these comparisons, it can be said that the present subjects were considered to be typical sedentary Japanese.

Sex Difference in $\dot{V}O_2$ Max per LBM

The results obtained in the present study agreed well with the general concept that the absolute $\dot{V}O_2$ max of sedentary women is less than that of the sedentary men.

But as for this sex difference, no definite conclusion has been presented. $\dot{V}O_2$ max depends mainly upon two factors such as the circulorespiratory function and the amount of muscles activated in exhaustive work, assuming that the amount of muscles activated is in proportion to LBM, and moreover, if there is the difference in $\dot{V}O_2$ max per LBM, the circulorespiratory factors might play the main role in determining the difference in $\dot{V}O_2$ max per LBM.

A few studies have been performed about the sex difference in $\dot{V}O_2$ max based on LBM. Döbeln [6] showed that $\dot{V}O_2$ max per kg of $(Wt - Fat/0.62)2/3$ presented statistically nonsignificant sex differences. But, MacNab et al [11], Dill et al [5] and the present study indicated a significant difference in $\dot{V}O_2$ max per LBM (Table IV). The values calculated from Döbeln's data listed in a supplement showed that there were still nonsignificant differences ($p > 0.05$). That is to say, sex differences in $\dot{V}O_2$ max of Döbeln's study were found to be fairly less than that of other studies. Döbeln's subjects were classified to be "well-trained" subjects, while the subjects of MacNab et al [11], Dill et al [5] and the present study were volunteers or randomly selected students. In conclusion, therefore, sex differences of $\dot{V}O_2$ max might mainly be due to the ability of circulorespiratory systems in the case of sedentary subjects.

Correlations Between Absolute $\dot{V}O_2$ Max
Versus Body Weight and LBM

Correlations between $\dot{V}O_2$ max versus body weight and LBM of men in the present study agreed with previous studies as shown in Table V. All studies showed that the correlation of men was higher between $\dot{V}O_2$ max and LBM than between $\dot{V}O_2$ max and body weight. On the contrary, correlation between $\dot{V}O_2$ max and body weight was higher than that between $\dot{V}O_2$ max and LBM in women of the present study. This reverse trend agreed with the study of Dill et al, but didn't with the results by Döbeln [6] and Katch et al [9].

One of the reasons is the metabolism of adipose tissue. Gitin et al [7] pointed out the increase of metabolic level of adipose tissue during exercise in the case of most obese subjects (103 kg with 35% fat). That is to say, "The increase in oxygen consumption of adipose tissue alone would account for 8% to 10% of his maximal

Table IV. Comparison of Aerobic Power and Percent Fat

Reporters	Sex	N	Age (yrs)	Method#	% Fat## (%)	V̇O₂max (l/min)	W/M### (%)	V̇O₂max/wt (ml/kg/min)	W/M (%)	V̇O₂max/LBM (ml/kg/min)	W/M (%)
v. Döbeln [6]	M	35	19-40	B°°	12.1	3.90		56.5		63.3	
	W	34	19-36		22.7	3.04**	(78)	48.7**	(86)	60.6	(96)
MacNab et al [11]	M	24	18-22	T	12.7	3.92		51.7		59.4	
	W	24	18-20		23.4	2.32**	(59)	39.1**	(76)	50.4**	(85)
	M	24	18-22	B	12.7	3.52		46.5		53.3	
	W	24	18-20		23.4	2.12**	(60)	35.7**	(77)	46.9**	(89)
Dill et al [5]	M	11	16-20	B	14.5	3.30		45.2		52.9	
	W	10	16-19		21.7	1.93**	(59)	35.9**	(79)	46.0**	(87)
Present study	M	39	18-21	T	13.1	3.22		51.8		59.7	
	W	33	18-21		21.6	2.08**	(65)	39.2**	(76)	50.0**	(84)

B: bicycle ergometer; T: treadmill; ## calculated by Brozek et al eq. (1963); ### W/M: ratio of women's value to men's; °° indirect measure;
**statistically significant sex difference by t-test (p < 0.01).

Table V. Correlations Between Absolute $\dot{V}O_2$ Max Versus
Body Weight and LBM in Young Adults

Reporters	Sex	N	Body Weight	LBM
v. Döbeln[#] [6]	M	35	0.563‡	0.726‡
	W	34	0.326	0.362*
Buskirk and Taylor [3]	M	54	0.63‡	0.85‡
Welch et al [15]	M	28	0.59‡	0.65‡
Dill et al[#] [5]	M	11	0.708*	0.810‡
	W	10	0.860†	0.706*
Katch et al [9]	W	17	0.66†	0.76‡
Kitagawa et al [10]	M	17	0.736‡	0.821‡
Present study	M	39	0.702‡	0.814‡
	W	33	0.701‡	0.655‡

*p < 0.05; †p < 0.01; ‡ p < 0.001.
[#]Correlations were calculated from their listed data.

consumption." The present study showed 8.21 kg of adipose tissue mass corresponding to 13.1% of body weight for men and 11.61 kg to 21.6% for women on an average, respectively. Absolute and relative values of adipose tissue mass for women were significantly higher than those for men. Consequently, it might be said that the metabolism in adipose tissue must be taken into consideration to evaluate $\dot{V}O_2$ max, especially in women.

Relations Between Aerobic Powers and 2400 Meter-Running Time

The 2400-meter running time is thought to be one of the best endurance running tests. In the present study, men covered 2400 meters in 10 minutes and 16 seconds, and women in 12 minutes and 16 seconds on an average, respectively. Although each aerobic power of men significantly correlated with 2400-meter running time, there was no significant correlation in women. Our result in women was similar to the study of Katch et al [9]. One of the reasons for sex differences might be due to sex difference in running experience or in running skill.

Cooper [4] preferred $\dot{V}O_2$ max per LBM among three aerobic powers as a best index of the 12-minute performance test. From the results of the present study, however, $\dot{V}O_2$ max per LBM showed the lowest correlation with 12-minute running time on both sexes and might not be a good index.

Conclusion

The results obtained in the present study to determine the relations between aerobic powers, body composition and 2400-meter running performance in Japanese young adults of both sexes were as follows:

1. $\dot{V}O_2$ max per LBM was significantly higher in men than in women.

2. $\dot{V}O_2$ max of men correlated with LBM higher (r = 0.814) than with body weight (r = 0.702).

$\dot{V}O_2$ max of women correlated with body weight higher (r = 0.701) than with LBM (r = 0.655).

3. $\dot{V}O_2$ max per LBM showed the lowest correlation with 2400-meter running test among aerobic powers in both sexes.

References

1. Brozek, J., Grande, F., Anderson, J.T. and Keys, A.: Densitometric analysis of body composition: Review of some quantitative assumptions. Ann. N.Y. Acad. Sci. 110:113-140, 1963.

2. Buskirk, E.R.: Underwater weighing and body density: A review of procedures. *In* Brozek, J. and Henschel, A. (eds.): Techniques for Measuring Body Composition. Washington, D.C.:National Academy of Sciences National Research Council, 1961.

3. Buskirk, E. and Taylor, H.L.: Maximal oxygen intake and its relation to body composition, with special reference to chronic physical activity and obesity. J. Appl. Physiol. 11:72-78, 1957.

4. Cooper, K.H.: A means of assessing maximal oxygen intake. JAMA 203:201-204, 1968.

5. Dill, D.B., Myhre, L.G., Greer, S.M. et al: Body composition and aerobic capacity of youth of both sexes. Med. Sci. Sports 4:198-204, 1972.

6. v.Döbeln, W.: Human standard and maximal metabolic rate in relation to fat free mass. Acta Physiol. Scand. 37. suppl. 126, 1956.

7. Gitin, E.L., Olerud, J.E. and Carroll, H.W.: Maximal oxygen uptake based on lean body mass: A meaningful measure of physical fitness? J. Appl. Physiol. 36:757-760, 1974.

8. Ikai, M., Shindo, M. and Miyamura, M.: Aerobic work capacity of Japanese people. Res. J. Phys. Educ. 14:135-140, 1970.

9. Katch, F.I., McArdle, W.D., Czula, R. and Pechar, G.S.: Maximal oxygen intake, endurance running performance, and body composition in college women. Res. Q. 44:301-312, 1973.

10. Kitagawa, K., Ikuta, K., Hirota, K. and Hara, Y.: Investigation of lean body mass as a limiting factor of maximum oxygen uptake. J. Phys. Fitness Japan 23:96-100, 1974.

11. McNab, R.B.J., Conger, P.R. and Taylor, P.S.: Differences in maximal and submaximal work capacity in men and women. J. Appl. Physiol. 27:644-648, 1969.

12. Matsui, H., Miyashita, M., Miura, M. et al: Maximal oxygen intake and its relationship to body weight of Japanese adolescents. Med. Sci. Sports 4:29-32, 1972.
13. Nagamine, S. and Suzuki, S.: Anthrometry and body composition of Japanese young men and women. Hum. Biol. 36:8-15, 1964.
14. Rahn, H., Fenn, W.O. and Otis, A.B.: Daily variations of vital capacity, residual air, expiratory reserve including a study of the residual air method. J. Appl. Physiol. 1:725-736, 1949.
15. Welch, B.E., Riendeau, R.P., Crisp, C.E. and Isenstein, R.S.: Relationship of maximal oxygen consumption to various components of body composition. J. Appl. Physiol. 12:395-398, 1958.

A Comparative Study on Physical Fitness Between Canadian and Japanese Rugby Players Over Forty

T. Hatakeyama, T. Higashitani, K. Koga, T. Meshizuka,
M. Nakamura and M. Tanaka

Introduction

It is reported that there is a rapid decrease of physical strength in middle-aged people over 40 years of age. Many investigators have tried to research their physical strength internationally. In 1975, the Tokyo Fuwaku Rugby Club, which is composed of players over 40, went on an expedition to British Colombia, Canada. This provided the opportunity to investigate the physical strength, physical fitness and health condition of rugby players in order to compare the differences between the athletes of both countries.

Methods

Subjects

Twenty-six Canadians 40 to 63 years of age and 80 Japanese 40 to 72 years were the subjects in this study.

Tests and Measurements

Physical characteristics of height, weight, chest girth, blood pressure, skin fold and arterial pulse rate were measured.

Performance tests included the 50-meter dash, standing long jump, grip strength, side-step test, closed eyes one foot balance and bar gripping reaction time.

Results

We found that age varied from 40 to 72. Among the Canadians, there was only one player over 60, so he was included in the

T. Hatakeyama, Seikei University; T. Higashitani, Chiba Institute of Technology; K. Koga, Musashi Institute of Technology; T. Meshizuka, M. Nakamura and M. Tanaka, Tokyo Metropolitan University, Tokyo, Japan.

50-year-old group. It was easy to measure Japanese players because
we tested them when they were in Japan, but it was quite difficult to
measure the Canadians because of lack of time and equipment.
Tables I and II show the average physical check and performance test
scores of each nation and each age group. Tables III and IV show the
difference between scores of 40- to 50-year-olds of both countries.
"$\overline{X}1$" and "$\overline{X}2$" equal average scores of Japanese and Canadians.

   Rugby is influenced by physical characteristics such as height,
weight and chest girth. According to Table V there are great
differences between Japanese players and the Canadians in physique.
In comparing Japan with Canada, Canadians are taller by 11.9 cm,
heaver by 12.5 kg and broader by 11.9 cm in chest girth than the
Japanese. This means that Japanese players have large handicaps in
physique besides rugby skill. The results become obvious when we
analyze the results of nine games in Canada. The difference of the
average weight between the two countries is 12.5 kg. The average
weight of the forward players (eight persons) is 100 kg. So Japanese
players had to spend their physical power to support the scrimmage,

Table I. Average Scores of Canada and Japan
Physical Check

		Age year	Height cm.	Weight kg.	Chest Girth cm.	Blood Pressure		Pulse Rate /min	Skin-fold cm.
						high	low		
Japan 40 Ager	n	38	38	38	30	34	34	24	26
	$\overline{x}$	44.03	168.0	68.8	92.4	134	86	59.0	2.50
	s	2.68	4.47	7.23	5.35	17.79	12.25	6.20	1.02
	M	44.0	162.8	59.8	88.4	132	83	71.8	
Japan 50 Ager	n	10	10	10	9	9	9	2	6
	$\overline{x}$	56.60	168.4	68.1	93.3	139	90	56.0	3.36
	s	2.01	4.45	9.35	9.30	13.47	11.19		0.51
	M	57.0	160.0	57.4	87.3	146	88	71.8	
Japan Over 60	n	7	7	7	6	5	5	4	4
	$\overline{x}$	65.26	167.6	67.6	90.3	161	99	62.5	3.50
	s	3.20	7.55	13.35	7.32	11.90	11.14	1.66	1.08
	M	65.0	158.0	55.9	86.5	155	89	72.0	
Canada 40 Ager	n	20	20	20	17				20
	$\overline{x}$	43.95	179.9	81.3	104.3				2.59
	s	3.22	4.91	8.57	6.38				0.81
Canada Over 50	n	5	5	5	5				5
	$\overline{x}$	56.6	179.6	86.7	112.0				2.98
	s	3.93	3.70	14.02	5.27				0.43

Table II. Average Scores of Canada and Japan Performance Test

		50 m Dash sec.	Standing L. Jump cm.	Grip Strength kg.	Side-Step Test times	One Foot Balance sec.	Bar Grip Test cm.
Japan 40 Ager	n	27	31	32	21	20	28
	x̄	7.56	227.3	48.8	44.8	17.0	20.1
	s	0.34	12.97	6.71	3.14	13.51	4.85
	M	8.00	204.0	44.1	39.5	46.0	22.6
Japan 50 Ager	n	4	10	10	2	2	10
	x̄	8.53	18.81	44.8	41.5	6.2	22.2
	s	0.56	12.10	7.74	4.50	1.50	5.96
	M		177.0	39.9	34.8	29.0	
Japan 60 Ager	n	5	7	6	4	3	5
	x̄	10.60	165.0	39.2	29.4	3.8	25.4
	s	1.31	23.77	4.64	2.29	1.69	
	M		157.0	36.7	31.1	21.0	
Canada 40 Ager	n	20	20	20	18	20	20
	x̄	7.74	207.9	54.2	37.2	12.7	20.5
	s	0.43	14.04	4.49	6.30	8.49	3.02
Canada Over 50	n	5	5	5	5	5	5
	x̄	8.52	171.0	44.6	31.8	6.0	19.2
	s	1.12	21.25	5.35	2.48	4.65	2.79

and with the progress of the game, they were handicapped in breaking up the scrimmage, following and backing up. In ruck and mole of scrimmage, because of the Canadian human wall of big bodies and the strength of their grip and arm power, the Japanese couldn't do anything at all. We didn't analyze it in detail, but we felt

Table III. Differences Between 40 and 50 Agers Physical Check

		Age	Height	Weight	Chest Girth	Blood Pressure		Arterial Pulse Rate	Skin-fold
Japan	x̄1	44.03	168.0	68.8	92.4	134	86	59.0	2.50
	x̄2	56.60	168.4	68.1	93.3	139	90	56.0	3.35
	x̄1-x̄2	-12.57	-0.4	0.7	-1.1	-5	-4	3.0	-0.85
	t								
Canada	x̄1	43.95	179.9	81.3	·104.3				2.95
	x̄2	56.60	176.9	86.7	112.0				2.98
	x̄1-x̄2	-12.65	3.0	-5.4					-0.39
	t								

Table IV. Differences Between 40 and 50 Agers
Performance Test

		50 m Dash	Standing Long Jump	Grip Strength	Side-Step Test	Closed Eyes Balance	Bar Gripping Test
Japan	$\bar{x}1$	7.56	227.3	48.8	44.8	17.0	20.1
	$\bar{x}2$	8.53	188.1	44.8	41.5	6.2	22.2
	$\bar{x}1-\bar{x}2$	-0.97	39.2	4.0	3.3	10.8	-2.1
	t	**	**				
Canada	$\bar{x}1$	7.54	207.9	54.2	37.2	12.7	20.5
	$\bar{x}2$	8.52	171.0	44.6	31.8	6.0	19.2
	$\bar{x}1-\bar{x}2$	-0.98	36.9	9.6	5.4	6.7	1.3
	t	**		**	*		

Table V. Differences Between Canada and Japan
Physical Check

	Age	Height	Weight	Chest Girth	Blood Pressure		Pulse Rate	Skin-fold
n1	38	38	38	30	34	34	24	26
n2	20	20	20	17			20	
$\bar{x}1$	44.03	168.0	68.8	92.4	134	86	69.0	2.50
$\bar{x}2$	43.95	179.9	81.3	114.3				2.95
$\bar{x}1-\bar{x}2$	0.08	-11.9	-12.5	-11.9				-0.09
t		**	**	**				
M	44.0	162.8	59.8	88.4	132	83	71.8	
$\bar{x}1-M$	0.03	5.2	9.0	4.0	2	3	-12.8	
t		**	**	**			**	

that holding time of the ball was a 70% to 30% advantage to Canadians. We could say the same thing in line out. Canadian average height was 179.9 cm and Japanese was 168.0 cm. Even if the Japanese were superior to Canadians in jumping power, the 11.9 cm difference in height is a great handicap.

Next, we would like to discuss physical power. In the 50-meter dash, there is only a 0.02 second difference between Japanese players and Canadians in average score (Table VI), although the Japanese players are 0.56 second faster than the average Japanese. In the standing long jump which is a barometer of jumping power, there is a 19.4 cm difference between the two countries and Japan has an advantage over Canada. The score of Japanese players compares to the 26- to 27-year-old normal score of Japan. Concerning muscle

Table VI. Differences Between Canada and Japan
Performance Test

	50 m Dash	Standing Long Jump	Grip Strength	Side-Step Test	Closed Eyes Balance	Bar Gripping Test
n1	27	31	32	21	20	28
n2	20	20	20	18	20	20
$\bar{x}1$	7.56	227.3	48.8	44.8	17.0	20.1
$\bar{x}2$	7.54	207.9	54.2	37.2	12.7	20.5
$\bar{x}1-\bar{x}2$	0.02	19.4	-5.4	7.6	4.3	-0.4
t		**	**	**		
M	8.00	204.0	44.1	39.5	46.0	21.0
$\bar{x}1$-M	-0.56	23.3	4.7	5.3	-29.0	-0.6
t	**	**	**	**	**	

power, we considered the pack in scrimmage or snap power of fingers in passing and we selected grip strength. Canadians were much stronger than Japanese and there is a 5.4 kg difference in the average score between the two. Japanese players showed 48.8 kg and this score is similar to the 24 to 25 year normal score of Japan. Rapid judgment and swift movement are required during rugby, so speed and agility are necessary. In side-step test, Japan is 7.6 times faster and in bar gripping reaction time, 0.4 cm superior to Canada. But we can't believe this score because Canadians had never tried this test before, so they didn't have any knowledge about this test and it was quite difficult for them to understand. The average score of side-step test, 44.8 cm, is similar to the 23 year normal score and bar gripping reaction time, 20.1 cm, matches the 23- to 24 year normal score. According to these results, we can say that the 40-year-old Japanese rugby players are far superior to the general Japanese public and they have almost a 20- to 30-year-old's physical power and fitness. We suppose that the reason why they have such youthful power is that they exercise daily and participate in rugby games almost every week regularly. Canadians are much superior to Japanese in physical characteristics, such as height, weight, chest girth and muscle power, but Japanese are superior to Canadians in power, agility and speed as shown in the standing long jump and side-step tests. For example, about pass work, cut in play and effective tackling skills which need speed and agility, Japanese have better sense than Canadians. But in scrimmage, mole, ruck and line out play which need big physiques and muscle power, Canadians were much stronger than Japanese. We couldn't gather many samples, but we tried to compare the

Table VII. Self-Diagnosis

			Japan		Canada	
			n	%	n	%
1. Do you have any trouble with your health now?		a) yes.	5	9.4	1	3.9
		b) no	48	90.6	25	96.1
2. Have you ever been told by a doctor that you have chest trouble or high blood pressure?		a) yes.	7	13.5	2	7.7
		b) no	45	68.3	24	92.3
3. Did you have any symptoms during the past year?		a) yes.	5	10.2	0	0
		b) no	44	89.8	26	100
4. Have you ever had a serious illness since you were born?		a) yes.	15	27.8	12	46.8
		b) no	39	72.2	14	53.8
5. Do you exercise regularly to keep your health in good condition?		a) yes.	29	54.8	26	100
		b) no	24	45.2	0	0
*kind of exercise.	a) running		15	51.7	10	38.5
	b) skiing		5	17.2	2	7.7
	c) swimming.		4	13.8	2	7.7
	d) golfing.		3	10.3	0	0
	e) gymnastics		3	10.3	2	7.7
	f) tennis		3	10.3	6	23.1
	g) squash		0	0	4	15.4
	h) others		6	20.7	4	15.4
*how often do you exercise?	a) every day		20	37.1	3	11.5
	b) 2 or 3 times a week		19	35.2	17	65.4
	c) once a week.		7	13.0	3	11.5
	d) 1 or 2 times a month		9	16.7	3	11.5
6. How many cigarettes do you smoke a day?	a) none.		22	40.7	21	80.8
	b) less than ten		2	4.7	2	7.7
	c) 10 to 20.		19	35.2	1	3.9
	d) more than 20.		11	20.4	1	3.9
	e) pipe		0	0	1	3.9
7. How much alcohol do you consume?	a) none.		4	7.5	4	15.4
	b) very little		4	7.5	3	11.5
	c) about average.		18	34.0	17	65.4
	d) more than average		21	39.3	7	7.7
	e) heavy drinker.		6	11.3	0	0

differences between those 40 and 50 years of age of each country (Tables III and IV). The 40-year-olds of Japan were superior to 50-year-olds in all six items we measured. There are obvious differences between 40- and 50-year-olds in 50-meter dash and side-step test in Canadians.

Finally, we would like to report about "self-diagnosis" (Table VII). We found many interesting results. Generally speaking, people over 40 become ill very easily, and most of them suffer from various kinds of illnesses such as headache, stomach ache, muscle and joint pain, high blood pressure, etc., but the rugby players we measured this time have few illnesses. They continue to play diverse sports as a daily habit. Over 50% of Japanese players do some exercise besides rugby regularly to keep in good condition and all of the Canadians exercise in addition to rugby. The kinds of sports they do are running, skiing, climbing and swimming, etc., in Japan and running, skiing, swimming and tennis in Canada.

It is widely said that athletes seldom smoke, and according to this study 40.7% of Japanese rugby players and 80.8% of Canadians don't smoke. Japanese players drink more alcohol than Canadians. We asked them how often they exercise including rugby in their daily life and 37.1% of Japanese and 11.5% of Canadians answered "almost every day"; 35.2% of Japanese and 65.4% of Canadians responded 2 to 3 times a week"; and 13.0% of Japanese and 11.5% of Canadians responded "once a week." As a result of this question we can say they do much more exercise than the general public.

The Relationship of Maximum Oxygen Intake to Gross Body Mass and Somatotype

N. B. Strydom, W. H. van der Walt, G. G. Rogers
and P. L. Jooste

Introduction

Submaximal oxygen consumption can be predicted with a fair degree of accuracy from gross body weight and work rate [2, 4]. Unfortunately, this is not true for $\dot{V}O_2$ max. Buskirk and Taylor [1] conducted a study on 59 men with a relatively wide weight range (coefficient of variation 20%) and found that only about 40% of the total variance in $\dot{V}O_2$ max could be accounted for by differences in gross body mass. Seventy percent of this variance could be accounted for by differences in fat-free mass. This observation is not substantiated by the work of other investigators [5, 6, 9] who found no improvement in the proportion of variance in $\dot{V}O_2$ max accounted for if lean body mass and/or fat-free mass is substituted for gross body mass. Furthermore, the proportion of variance in $\dot{V}O_2$ max accounted for by gross body mass has been shown to vary from 18% to 70% depending upon differences between samples with respect to gross body mass range and ethnic groups involved [6]. Differences between individuals with respect to body height have been shown to play only a marginal role independent of body mass in improving the prediction of $\dot{V}O_2$ max [6, 9]. In view of the above findings it is the purpose of this study to investigate the influence of somatotype on $\dot{V}O_2$ max and its influence on the $\dot{V}O_2$ max to gross body mass relationship.

Method

Fifteen untrained male subjects aged 20 to 25 were selected from a group of medical students classified as follows: five typical

N. B. Strydom, W. H. van der Walt, G. G. Rogers and P. L. Jooste, Industrial Hygiene Division, Chamber of Mines of South Africa, Johannesburg, Republic of South Africa.

ectomorphs, five typical mesomorphs and the remainder typical endomorphs by the method described by Sheldon et al [3]. Measurements of body mass and height were obtained on these subjects and each individual's $\dot{V}O_2$ max was determined while running on a treadmill [7].

Results

The subjects' physical characteristics are summarized in Table I. Student t-tests were used to determine whether the three groups differed significantly with respect to body mass, height, mass/height

Table I. Table of Physical Characteristics of Subjects

*	Parameter	Ectomorphs	Mesomorphs	Endomorphs	Total
			Group		
M	Mean	61.97	71.60	93.50	75.69
	S.D.	5.86	8.00	14.99	16.70
	Range	55.5–71.05	65.80–85.20	77.55–111.20	55.50–111.20
H	Mean	1.837	1.734	1.773	1.78
	S.D.	0.0599	0.0723	0.1079	0.0880
	Range	1.78–1.91	1.65–1.80	1.68–1.90	1.65–1.91
M/H	Mean	33.7	41.1	52.5	42.5
	S.D.	2.35	3.62	5.40	8.81
En	Mean	1.2	1.6	6.0	2.9
	S.D.	0.5	0.6	0.7	2.3
	Range	1–2	1–2	5–7	1–7
Me	Mean	2.4	6.0	2.4	3.6
	S.D.	0.6	0.7	0.6	1.8
	Range	2–3	5–7	2–3	2–7
Ec	Mean	6.0	1.8	1	2.9
	S.D.	1.0	0.5	0	2.3
	Range	5–7	1–2	1–1	1–7
$\dot{V}O_2$ (1)	Mean	2.72	3.75	3.57	3.35
	S.D.	0.507	0.608	0.218	0.640
	Range	2.09–3.46	3.13–4.75	3.27–3.85	2.09–4.75
$\dot{V}O_2$ (2)	Mean	43.6	52.2	38.8	44.9
	S.D.	4.5	2.9	5.1	6.9
	Range	37.7–48.7	47.6–55.8	31.5–43.7	31.5–55.8

*Definitions of variables:

M = Body Mass (kg)
H = Body Height (m)
M/H = Mass/Height (kg·m⁻¹)
En = Degree of Endomorphism

Me = Degree of Mesomorphism
Ec = Degree of Ectomorphism
$\dot{V}O_2$ (1) = Max O_2 Intake (l/min)
$\dot{V}O_2$ (2) = Max O_2 Intake (ml/kg/min)

ratio and $\dot{V}O_2$ max (l/min and l/kg/min). Mann Whitney tests were used to compare the groups' respective degrees of endo-, meso- and ectomorphism. The following significant differences could be shown to exist at the 5% level:

1. *Body mass:* The endomorphs had a significantly higher mean body mass than either of the other two somatotype groups.

2. *Height:* The mean height of the ectomorphs was significantly higher than that of the mesomorphs.

3. *Mass/height ratio:* All three somatotype groups could be shown to differ significantly from each other in this respect.

4. *Degree of endomorphism:* Significantly higher for endo-morphs than for the other groups.

5. *Degree of mesomorphism:* Significantly higher for meso-morphs than for the other groups.

6. *Degree of ectomorphism:* Significantly higher for both ecto-morphs and mesomorphs than for endomorphs and significantly higher for ectomorphs than for mesomorphs.

7. *$\dot{V}O_2$ max (l/min):* The mean $\dot{V}O_2$ max of the ectomorphs could be shown to be significantly lower than that for mesomorphs and endomorphs.

8. *$\dot{V}O_2$ max (ml/kg/min):* The mean $\dot{V}O_2$ max (ml/kg/min) was significantly higher for mesomorphs than for either ectomorphs or endomorphs.

9. *Relationship of $\dot{V}O_2$ max (l/min) to body mass for each of the three somatotypes.*

Linear regression lines of $\dot{V}O_2$ max against gross body mass were fitted on the data obtained for each of the three somatotypes. The correlation coefficients between $\dot{V}O_2$ max and body mass for ecto-, meso- and endomorphs, respectively, amounted to 0.95, 0.98 and 0.50, respectively. With 3 degrees of freedom only the correlation coefficients obtained for the ecto- and mesomorphs are significant at the 5% level.

The regression equations obtained were

(a) Ectomorphs: $\dot{V}O_2$ max = 0.0819 M − 2.354; RSD = 0.191 l/min
(b) Mesomorphs: $\dot{V}O_2$ max = 0.0744 M − 1.579; RSD = 0.141 l/min
(c) Endomorphs: $\dot{V}O_2$ max = 0.0072 M + 2.901; RSD = 0.219 l/min

where M = mass in kg and RSD = residual standard deviation in liters per minute.

The hypothesis that the three regression equations are identical in terms of the parameters of these equations (i.e., slope and intercept) was tested. Equations (a) and (b) could be shown to differ significantly from equation (c) at the 5% level of significance but equations (a) and (b) could not be shown to differ significantly in this respect. A similar linear regression equation of $\dot{V}O_2$ max against body mass was then fitted to data contained in the combined sample of ecto- and mesomorphs.

The equation obtained was

(d) $\dot{V}O_2$ max $= 0.0881$ M $- 2.650$; RSD $= 0.195$; r $= 0.97$
where M and RSD have the same meaning as before and r denotes the correlation between $\dot{V}O_2$ max and gross body mass.

The corresponding regression lines with 95% confidence limits for the combined group of ecto- and mesomorphs (equation (d)) and the endomorphs are given in Figure 1. Individual points are also plotted on this figure and dashed lines indicate extrapolation outside the observed range. From this figure it is clear that an ecto- or a mesomorph with a body mass in excess of 77.6 kg will always have a significantly higher $\dot{V}O_2$ max than an endomorph with the same body mass. Furthermore it should be clear that whereas a strong linear relationship exists between $\dot{V}O_2$ max (l/min) and body mass for ectomorphs and mesomorphs (94% of variance in $\dot{V}O_2$ max accounted for by differences in body mass) there is nearly no relationship between these two variables for endomorphs. (Only 25% of variance in $\dot{V}O_2$ max accounted for.)

10. *$\dot{V}O_2$ max (ml/kg/min) as a function of body mass and somatotype.*

The corresponding linear regression lines of $\dot{V}O_2$ max (ml/kg/min) against body mass for the combined group of ecto- and mesomorphs and the group of endomorphs with 95% confidence limits are given in Figure 2. The correlation between $\dot{V}O_2$ max (ml/kg/min) and gross body mass amounted to 0.84 (combined group of mesomorphs and ectomorphs) and -0.94 (endomorphs). Both these correlations are significant at the 5% level and one may therefore conclude that $\dot{V}O_2$ max expressed as ml/kg/min will always be dependent upon body mass (70% and 88% of the variance in $\dot{V}O_2$ max accounted for by variations in gross body mass, respectively).

From Figure 2 it follows that an ectomorph or mesomorph will have a significantly higher $\dot{V}O_2$ max (ml/kg/min) than an endomorph if gross body mass is in excess of 76 kg. The regression equations obtained were

(e) Ecto- and mesomorphs: $\dot{V}O_2$ max (ml/kg/min) $= 0.5755$ M $+ 9.45$
RSD $= 3.35$ ml/kg/min, degrees of freedom $= 8$.
(f) Endomorphs: $\dot{V}O_2$ max (ml/kg/min) $= -0.3192$ M $+ 68.69$
RSD $= 2.02$ ml/kg/min, degrees of freedom $= 3$.

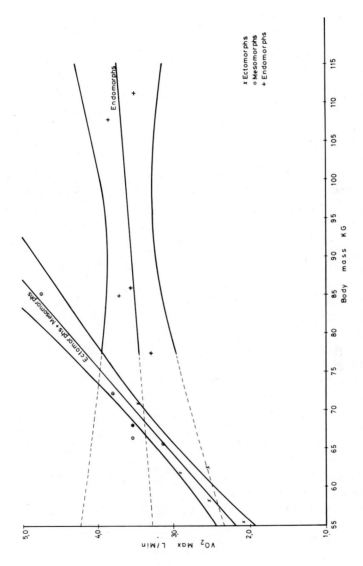

FIG. 1. Linear regression lines of $\dot{V}O_2$ max (1/min) against body mass with 95% confidence limits for different somatotypes.

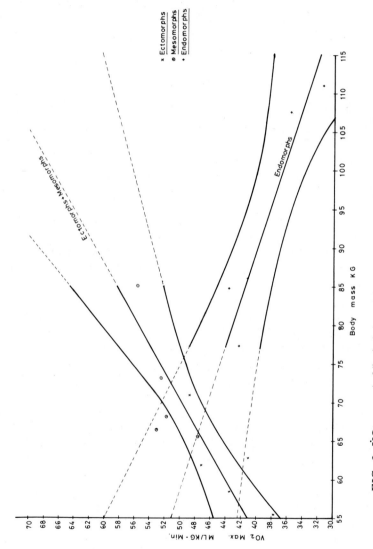

FIG. 2. V̇O₂ max (ml/kg/min) as a function of body mass and somatotype with 95% confidence limits.

The accuracy to which $\dot{V}O_2$ max can be predicted is not improved significantly if either of the variables H, En, Me or Ec is added to equations (c), (d), (e) or (f). If an individual's ecto- or mesomorphic characteristics dominate, his $\dot{V}O_2$ max (L/min) can be estimated with a fair degree of accuracy from equation (d) (coefficient of variation = 6%) and if his endomorphic characteristics dominate, his $\dot{V}O_2$ max (ml/kg/min) can be estimated from equation (f) (coefficient of variation = 5.2%).

Discussion

The three somatotypes differ significantly with respect to mass/height relationships. Tables of the average body mass of South African males in the age group of 20 to 29 years of a given height [8] suggest that all the ectomorphs are grossly underweight for their height while the exact opposite is true for the endomorphs.

From each of the endomorph's height a rough estimate of his gross body mass minus excess fat can be obtained from these tables. If the values thus obtained are substituted for their measured gross body mass, then the correlations between $\dot{V}O_2$ max (l/min) and body mass for the whole sample will amount to 0.86 (73% of variance accounted for) as against 0.614 (38% of variance accounted for) if gross body mass is used throughout.

It is interesting to note that the coefficient of variation of $\dot{V}O_2$ max (l/min) for the endomorphs amounted to only 6.1% despite a weight range of 77.6 to 111.2 kg. This figure is probably only slightly larger than what one would expect to be due to errors of measurement. One can therefore safely assume that the increase in gross body mass in these individuals is associated mainly with an increase in excess fat which does not consume much oxygen.

This finding has important implications for the lean body mass/gross body mass controversy. Buskirk and Taylor [1] dealt with subjects over a wide range of body composition (up to 37% fat). The mean body mass of their sample ± 2 standard deviations produces a range of 46 to 109 kg. The corresponding body mass range for Wyndham and Heyns' [6] samples amounts to 52 to 81 (Caucasians) and 47 to 71 kg (Bantu). Furthermore, the mean body mass/mean height ratios of these samples amounted to 44 kg/m (Buskirk), 38 kg/m (Wyndham and Heyns — Caucasians) and 35 kg/m (Wyndham and Heyns — Bantus). These figures are to be compared with those contained in Table I (34 kg/m for ectomorphs; 41 kg/m for mesomorphs; 53 kg/m for endomorphs and 42.5 kg/m for the combined sample). From these figures it would appear that

Buskirk and Taylor were dealing with a representative sample containing approximately equal proportions of all three somatotypes while it appears to be highly unlikely that Wyndham and Heyns' samples included anything but ectomorphs and mesomorphs. This fact explains why Wyndham and Heyns found correlations as high as 0.93 to 0.97 between fat free mass and gross body mass (the fat mass being proportional to total body mass in their subjects) and hence their conclusion that fat-free mass cannot play any significant role toward explaining the variation in $\dot{V}O_2$ max independent of gross body mass. Buskirk and Taylor, however, did deal with subjects in which the fat mass increased out of proportion to the increase in gross body mass and hence their finding that the proportion of variance in $\dot{V}O_2$ max accounted for is increased 40% to 70% if fat-free mass is substituted for gross body mass. Welch et al [5] found that $\dot{V}O_2$ max expressed as ml/min/kg gross body mass decreased significantly with an increase in percent fat and this observation is in line with what we found for endomorphs (−0.94 correlation between $\dot{V}O_2$ max (ml/kg/min) and gross body mass) (Fig. 2). Nevertheless, it would appear to be much simpler to use separate prediction equations for endomorphs, and ecto- and mesomorphs (as we have already suggested) than to go to the trouble of obtaining fat-free mass on all subjects, since this variable is at any rate highly correlated to gross body mass if one is dealing with ecto- and mesomorphs.

The dependency of $\dot{V}O_2$ max (ml/kg/min) on body mass has important implications for its use as an index of athletic performance. Ectomorphs will generally have lower $\dot{V}O_2$ max's than mesomorphs (Table I; Fig. 1) because of their lower body mass. However, there is evidence in the literature that for a given body mass increased body height is associated with an increased leg length which is in turn associated with an increased mechanical efficiency and consequently a decreased submaximal oxygen consumption in exercises such as running or walking [2, 4]. Linear regression equations of height against body mass fitted for each of the three somatotype groups differ significantly to the extent that if we wished to draw a 70 kg man from each of these groups, then the ectomorph will have to have a height of about 1.9 m, the mesomorph's height will be 1.7 m and the endomorph will have a height of 1.6 m. This observation implies that the ectomorph will have the lowest submaximal $\dot{V}O_2$ when running at a given speed followed by the mesomorph and endomorph in that order. Since the data contained in Figure 1 suggest that the $\dot{V}O_2$ max of both ectomorphs and mesomorphs of a given body mass will be very similar, it is possible that the ectomorph will in fact be working at a lower percent of his $\dot{V}O_2$ max than is the case for the mesomorph. There is evidence in the literature [6, 9] that an increased body height, independent of body mass, is also associated with a decrease in $\dot{V}O_2$ max. This may not apply for ectomorphs. In the present sample of 15 men the partial correlation between $\dot{V}O_2$ max (l/min) and height for a constant body mass amounts to −0.22. The mass/height relationships of the three somatotypes are, however, totally different and therefore the corresponding correlations for the groups of ectomorphs, mesomorphs and endomorphs amounted to 0.87, 0.57 and −0.57, respectively. Due to the small sample size neither of these correlations is significant but they are nevertheless indicative.

Summary

The maximal oxygen intake capacities of three groups of subjects, grouped according to the Sheldon somatotype rating, were measured by the intermittent treadmill technique in an effort to determine the influence of somatotype and body mass on $\dot{V}O_2$ max. Only typical samples of endo-, meso- and ectomorphism were used and the following conclusions were made:

1. Somatotype plays an important role in the prediction of $\dot{V}O_2$ max in the sense that it nearly uniquely determines both an individual's mass, height, mass/height relationship, aerobic capacity and aerobic capacity/mass relationship.

2. A strong linear relationship exists between $\dot{V}O_2$ max (l/min) and gross body mass for ectomorphs and mesomorphs while these two variables are unrelated in the endomorphs.

3. $\dot{V}O_2$ max (ml/kg/min) is dependent upon gross body mass and increases with increasing body mass for ectomorphs and mesomorphs. The opposite is true for endomorphs in which group a strong linear decrease in $\dot{V}O_2$ max expressed as ml/kg/min is observed with an increase in body mass.

4. The discrepancies that exist in the literature on the relative importance of fat-free mass and gross body mass in the prediction of $\dot{V}O_2$ max (l/min) are due mainly to differences in somatotype included in the various authors' samples.

References

1. Buskirk, E. and Taylor, H.L.: Maximal oxygen intake and its relation to body composition with special reference to chronic physical activity and obesity. J. Appl. Physiol. 11(1):72-78, 1957.

2. Cotes, J.E. and Meade, F.: The energy expenditure and mechanical energy demand in walking. Ergonomics 3:97-119, 1960.
3. Sheldon, W.H., Dupertuis, C.W. and McDermott, E.: Atlas of Men. New York and London:Harper Brothers, 1954.
4. van der Walt, W.H. and Wyndham, C.H.: An equation for the prediction of energy expenditure of walking and running. J. Appl. Physiol. 34(5):559-563, 1973.
5. Welch, B.E., Riendeau, R.P., Crisp, C.E. and Isenstein, R.S.: Relationship of maximal oxygen consumption to various components of body composition. J. Appl. Physiol. 12(3):395-398, 1958.
6. Wyndham, C.H. and Heyns, A.J.: Determinants of oxygen consumption and maximum oxygen intake of Bantu and Caucasian males. Int. Z. Angew. Physiol. 27:51-75, 1969.
7. Wyndham, C.H., Strydom, N.B., Leary, W.P. and Williams, C.G.: Studies of the maximum capacity of men for physical effort. I: A comparison of methods of assessing the maximum oxygen intake. Int. Z. Angew. Physiol. 22:285-295, 1966.
8. Wyndham, C.H., Watson, M. and Sluis-Cremer, G.K.: The relationship between weight and height of South African males of European descent between the ages of 20 and 60 years. S.A. Med. J. 44:406-409, 1970.
9. Wyndham, C.H., Williams, C.G., Watson, M.I. and Munro, A.H.: Improving the accuracy of prediction of an individual's maximum oxygen intake. Int. Z. Angew. Physiol. 23:354-366, 1967.

Age and Sex Trends in Aerobic Capacity Related to Lean Body Mass of Japanese From Childhood to Maturity

Sadayoshi Taguchi, Yuko Hata, Komei Ikuta
and Mitsumasa Miyashita

Introduction

Few studies have been designed to investigate aerobic capacity and body composition at various developmental ages [1, 5]. Therefore, it was decided to study aerobic capacity and its relationship to body composition in relation to developmental age in Japanese males and females.

Methods

The subjects were 100 ordinary males and 104 females who lived in Tokyo, aged 12 to 19 years, as well as a 20- to 28-year-old group.

Maximal Oxygen Uptake

Maximal oxygen uptake was measured by using a bicycle ergometer with a progressive load method as described by Ikai and Kitagawa [7]. Expired air was collected into Douglas bags and analyzed for CO_2 and O_2 by micro-Scholander analyzer.

Body Composition

Body composition was evaluated in terms of lean body mass (LBM) and body fat. Body density was determined by weighing the subjects under water with simultaneous determination of residual volume [11]. Estimation of body fat (%) from body density was made employing the formula of Brozek et al [3].

Sadayoshi Taguchi, Laboratory of Physiology, College of General Education, Kyoto University, Kyoto, Japan; Yuko Hata and Mitsumasa Miyashita, Laboratory for Exercise Physiology and Biomechanics, Faculty of Education, University of Tokyo, Japan; and Komei Ikuta, College of General Education, University of Tokyo, Japan.

Results

Table I represents the means and standard errors of height, weight, Rohrer's index, body density and percent body fat. In males body density increased from 1.063 at 12 years to 1.071 at 16 years and remained at the upper level thereafter. In females density was around 1.044 for all ages except 13 years. Consequently, the mean body fat for males fell from 16% at 12 years to about 12.5% at 16 years and remained constant thereafter. Females showed a small variation within 1% of body fat for all ages except 13 years, being about 23% to 24%.

LBM, body fat and total body weight according to age is shown in Figure 1. LBM for males increased during adolescence and the increment continued to 19 years. Females increased similarly up to 14 years leveling off thereafter.

The relationships between body weight and LBM for both sexes are illustrated in Figure 2. The regression equations of body weight vs. LBM were $Y = 0.901X - 1.639$ for males, and $Y = 0.629X + 6.710$ for females, where X is body weight and Y is LBM. The crosspoint of the regression lines between body weight and LBM in males and females was 30.7 kg in body weight or 26.0 kg in LBM.

Table I. Some Physical Characteristics of Subjects

	Age (years)	N	Height (cm)	Weight (kg)	Rohrer's Index	Body density (g/ml)	Fat (%)
Male	12	7	148.2±1.4	39.21±0.89	120.8±3.7	1.0627±.0053	15.9±2.2
Male	13	12	153.5±0.8	43.35±0.88	120.0±2.5	1.0625±.0034	16.0±1.4
Male	14	10	161.7±0.8	50.86±1.17	120.3±2.4	1.0646±.0025	15.1±1.0
Male	15	10	163.6±0.9	52.60±0.83	120.3±2.9	1.0672±.0034	14.1±1.4
Male	16	10	162.7±1.4	52.51±1.93	122.1±4.4	1.0716±.0035	12.3±1.4
Male	17	7	167.9±1.5	57.42±2.02	119.3±4.5	1.0761±.0031	10.5±1.2
Male	18	9	167.9±1.3	58.78±2.50	124.2±5.2	1.0690±.0030	13.3±1.2
Male	19	10	169.3±3.2	60.83±2.47	125.0±3.7	1.0710±.0020	12.5±0.8
Male	20-28	25	166.7±1.0	59.71±1.48	126.9±2.0	1.0714±.0017	12.4±0.7
Female	12	9	148.6±0.7	40.35±0.98	122.0±2.7	1.0455±.0023	22.9±1.0
Female	13	12	151.6±1.0	43.91±0.86	125.1±2.0	1.0521±.0024	20.1±1.0
Female	14	12	154.5±0.6	48.31±0.82	131.8±2.4	1.0472±.0028	22.4±1.1
Female	15	10	154.5±0.9	49.47±0.86	134.3±3.2	1.0418±.0025	24.5±1.0
Female	16	7	154.9±0.5	52.15±1.49	140.0±2.3	1.0409±.0032	24.8±1.3
Female	17	10	158.8±0.7	49.62±1.32	126.2±1.9	1.0433±.0026	23.9±1.1
Female	18	11	156.8±1.5	51.04±1.04	133.4±4.0	1.0433±.0024	24.1±1.1
Female	19	17	156.0±0.8	52.10±1.22	138.1±3.2	1.0443±.0017	23.4±0.7
Female	20-28	16	157.3±1.3	51.35±1.79	139.4±5.1	1.0438±.0028	23.7±1.2

*Values indicate means and standard errors.

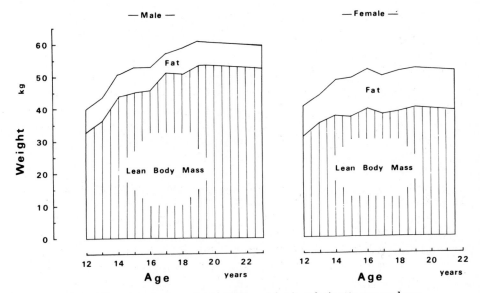

FIG. 1. The mean body weight, LBM and fat in relation to age and sex.

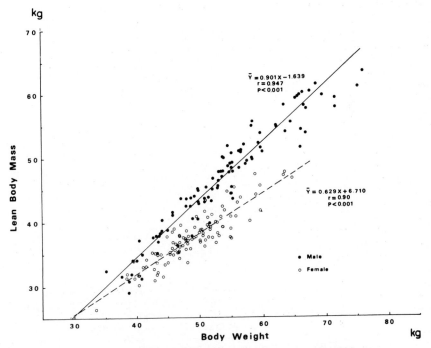

FIG. 2. Relationships between body weight and LBM.

Age trends for the maximal oxygen uptake (l/min) are presented in Figure 3. The maximal oxygen uptake for males had a tendency to increase with age, reaching a maximum of 2.81 l/min or 54 ml/kg LBM/min at 19 years. Similarly, the $\dot{V}O_2$ max for females showed a tendency to increase with age up to 16 years, reaching 1.90 l/min or 48.8 ml/kg LBM/min at that age. After 16 years of age, the level in the females was maintained up to the twenties. However, $\dot{V}O_2$ max decreased by 0.27 l/min from 16 to 17 years in these females. The mean maximal oxygen uptake when expressed in terms of ml/kg LBM/min is lower at all ages in females compared to males (Fig. 4). Differences between the means are statistically significant at all ages except 16 years. The age trend for males is somewhat irregular. Both sexes showed a gradual and slight decrease of the mean $\dot{V}O_2$ max (ml/kg LBM/min) after 12 years. The relationships between LBM (kg) and $\dot{V}O_2$ max (l/min) are illustrated in Figure 5. The regression equations were $Y = 0.042X + 0.579$ with a correlation coefficient of 0.815 ($P < 0.001$) for males and $Y = 0.030X + 0.586$ with a correlation coefficient of 0.493 ($P < 0.001$) for females, where X is LBM(kg) and Y is $\dot{V}O_2$ max (l/min). The sexual differences in mean

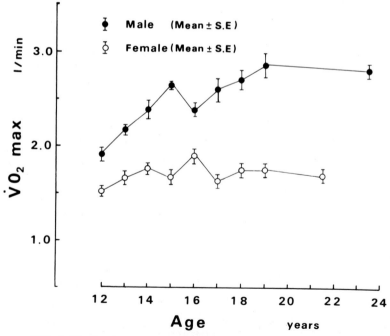

FIG. 3. Maximal oxygen uptake(l/min) in relation to age and sex.

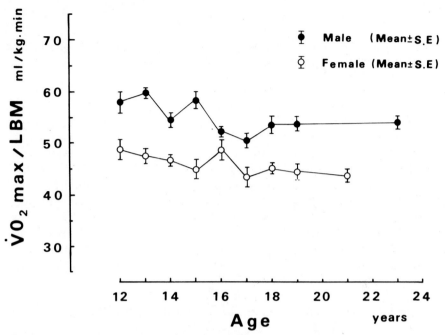

FIG. 4. Maximal oxygen uptake per unit LBM(ml/kg LBM/min) in relation to age and sex.

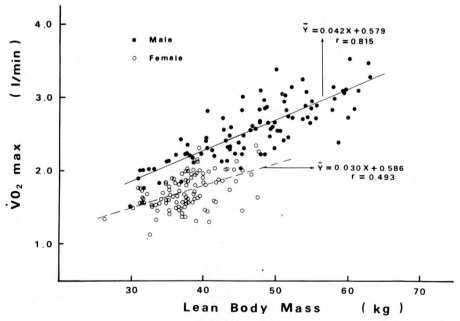

FIG. 5. Relationships between maximal oxygen uptake and LBM.

$\dot{V}O_2$ max (l/min) amounted to 20% at age 12 which is increased to 40% at age 19 years although it was different in general trend only at 16 years.

Discussion

Mean values of height and weight of this sample were found to be within the 95% confidence limit of the mean value of previously reported data on the Japanese population [12], indicating that the subjects studied were representative of the Japanese population. On the other hand, females at 16 years had a higher aerobic capacity than at any other age. It became apparent by the recall interview that this could be related to level of activity, since most of them participated in physical conditioning programs. Nevertheless, the results provide age trends for aerobic capacity and body composition.

Age trends for maximal oxygen uptake (l/min) of Japanese children in this study are in close agreement with those reported earlier by Ikai and Kitagawa [7], and Matsui et al [10]. Also, our data of males at 12 years(1.91 l/min) are almost equivalent to those at the same age reported for Norwegians [1] and British [5] and, in turn, substantially lower than the value at 12 to 13 years reported by Astrand [2]. However, the greater differences between our males and British, Norwegians and Americans [8] were found after 14 years of age. Our female subjects had lower levels of $\dot{V}O_2$ max(l/min) at 12 years than those of the British and Norwegians, and the differences continued thereafter. But, our females at 15 to 18 years had the same levels of $\dot{V}O_2$ max(l/min) as seen in American females [8].

Considerable discussion has arisen regarding the best parameter of body size that should be utilized in comparisons of individuals from different populations. Von Döbeln [14] recommended the use of $\dot{V}O_2$ max value per unit LBM, since fat is metabolically inactive. When $\dot{V}O_2$ max is expressed in terms of ml/kg LBM/min, our male subjects at 12 years had 7% to 8% lower values compared to the British [6] or Norwegians [1] at the same age. Although data for comparable ages of both sexes are limited in those countries cited above, the differences in mean values for males comparing Japanese and Norwegians at 14 years and/or British at 15 years became much greater. Similarly, the $\dot{V}O_2$ max for our females of comparable ages was consistently lower, 13.6% for 12 years and 9.2% for 14 years than those of the Norwegians [1], and 9.4% for 13 years and 13.8% for 15 years than those of the British [5].

It was found that Japanese adolescents had lower mean values of $\dot{V}O_2$ max per unit LBM compared to foreign children in general. However, it is not possible to draw a definite conclusion about a population baseline because the number of children investigated at each age class is small. Another possible reason includes the finding, in Japanese adult males studied, that the attained mean values of $\dot{V}O_2$ max(ml/kg LBM/min) are in agreement with those reported by MacNab et al [9], Buskirk and Taylor [4], Davies et al [6] and Sloan et al [13].

On the other hand, in the present study the sexual difference in $\dot{V}O_2$ max still remained on the basis of LBM unit (Fig. 5). This finding is in agreement with previous reports [1, 9]. There are apparently additional factors to be considered as pointed out by MacNab et al [9]. Further, Andersen et al [1] suggested that quality of muscle mass must deteriorate with age in girls, while it is unchanged in boys. The LBM for males in kilograms increased after 12 years while the absolute body fat was almost constant. However, females showed a gradual increase in absolute body fat between 12 and 15 years of age.

The most important finding of this study is the onset of sexual differences in body composition in terms of kilogram in body weight and LBM. The crosspoint of two regression lines between body weight and LBM indicates them to occur when body weight was 30.7 kg and LBM 26.0 kg (Fig. 2). On the average, these weights occurred between 8 and 9 years of age in the Japanese population [12].

References

1. Andersen, K.L., Seliger, V., Rutenfranz, J. and Mocellin, R.: Physical performance capacity of children in Norway. Europ. J. Appl. Physiol. 33:177-195, 1974.
2. Astrand, P.O.: Experimental studies of physical working capacity in relation to sex and age. Copenhagen:Munksgaard, 1952.
3. Brozek, J., Grande, F., Anderson, J.T. and Keys, A.: Densitometric analysis of body composition: Revision of some quantitative assumptions. Ann. N.Y. Acad. Sci. 110:113-140, 1963.
4. Buskirk, E. and Taylor, H.L.: Maximal oxygen intake and its relation to body composition, with special reference to chronic physical activity and obesity. J. Appl. Physiol. 11:72-78, 1957.
5. Davies, C.T.M., Barnes, C.A. and Godfrey, S.: Body composition and maximal exercise performance in children. Hum. Biol. 44:195-214, 1972.
6. Davies, C.T.M., Mbelwa, D., Crockford, G. and Weiner, J.S.: Exercise tolerance and body composition of male and female Africans aged 18-30 years. Hum. Biol. 45:31-40, 1973.
7. Ikai, M. and Kitagawa, K.: Maximum oxygen uptake of Japanese related to sex and age. Med. Sci. Sports 4:127-131, 1972.

8. Knuttgen, H.G.: Aerobic capacity of adolescents. J. Appl. Physiol. 22:655-658, 1967.
9. MacNab, R.B.J., Conger, P.R. and Taylor, P.S.: Differences in maximal and submaximal work capacity in men and women. J. Appl. Physiol. 27:644-648, 1969.
10. Matsui, H., Miyashita, M., Miura, M., Kobayashi, K. et al: Maximum oxygen intake and its relationship to body weight of Japanese adolescents. Med. Sci. Sports 4:29-32, 1972.
11. Rahn, H., Fenn, W.O. and Otis, A.B.: Daily variations of vital capacity, residual air, expiratory reserve including a study of the residual air method. J. Appl. Physiol. 1:725-736, 1949.
12. Shibuya, K. (ed.): Annual Report of Japanese Physical Fitness. Division of Physical Education, Ministry of Education, Tokyo, Japan, 1972.
13. Sloan, A.W., Koeslag, J.H. and Bredell, G.A.D.: Body composition, work capacity, and work efficiency of active and inactive young men. Europ. J. Appl. Physiol. 32:17-24, 1973.
14. Von Döbeln, W.: Human standard and maximal metabolic rate in relation to fat-free body mass. Acta Physiol. Scand. Suppl. 126:1-79, 1956.

Relationship Between Physique and Physical Fitness

Kyutoku Tomonari

Introduction

After World War II, growth of the school pupils was very accelerated in many countries. In Japan, too, we observe this phenomenon of growth as well as in Western nations [1, 7].

In contrast to the rapid growth, it is believed that there is a marked decline in student physical fitness. To cope with this situation, in primary and secondary schools throughout the country, attempts at physical fitness promotion are very popular. In this study, Hirata's evaluating method of physique and physical fitness is used. This method started from the study of the Stout/lean index (F—index) and developed to the synthetic evaluating chart of physique and physical fitness, and the polar coordinate diagram [3].

Particularly, the Stout/lean index (similar to Livi's Index, 1886) is most suitable to indicate the degree of stoutness and leanness, not only qualitatively but also quantitatively. This index was adopted as Ponderal Index by the International Conference on Standardization of Physical Fitness Test at Oxford University in 1970 [2].

Using the polar coordinate method we can represent very vividly the transition of physique of Japanese school children from 1900 to date. We can observe two opposite tendencies of becoming slender and becoming obese as a special feature of recent growth in school children.

Using Hirata's method, moderate stout physique proved to be more favorable for both phases of physical fitness.

Material and Method

Physique and Fitness for Protection

Physique during school age and differential of survival. The physiques of 4,374 pupils age 11 years around 1905 in Hamamatsu, a

---

Kyutoku Tomonari, Hirata Institute of Health, Mino City, Gifu Prefecture, Japan.

city of 470,000, located on the Pacific Coast just between Tokyo and Kyoto, and their survival after 50 years were investigated. It was found that 2870 were alive, 1021 deceased and 483 unknown.

The cause of death of the deceased group was investigated from medical certificates in the village and town offices. The mean physiques of the survivors and the deceased were evaluated by means of Hirata's method.

Physique and health of residents of senior citizens' homes. Among residents of 134 senior citizens' homes throughout the country, 2,983 were investigated about their level of health and physique.

The grade of health was classified into three groups: excellent (○), moderate (△) and bad (X).

Also, one year later, their survival was checked.

Physique and Fitness for Performance

Motor fitness tests* of 632 pupils of the Ose Primary School in Hamamatsu were investigated including 50 meter running, standing broad-jumping, and softball throwing ability.

Physiques were related to the scores of motor fitness tests.

Results

Physique and Fitness for Protection

Physique during school age and differential of survival. The mean physique of the survivors and deceased is listed in Table I and is presented by polar coordinate diagram in Figure 1.

The deceased are found among the tall-lean-narrow type. In contrast, the physiques of the survivors are the stout type. Except for death due to accident and heart and kidney diseases, the causes of death were diversified among the lean persons [5].

Physique and health of elderly persons. Table II and Figure 2 show the physique of old men and women according to their level of health.

In the order of excellent (○), moderate (△), bad (X) and dead (‡), physiques became leaner and smaller.

Physique and Fitness for Performance

Correlation between total scores of physique and scores of motor fitness test. Table III shows the correlation between the total scores

---

*Motor fitness test is used as fitness for performance.

Table I. Physique During School Age and Differential of Survival

	Number (N)	Height (H)	Weight (W)	Chest Circumference (B)	F-index (F)	σF (σF)	G-index (G)	σG (σG)	Relative Chest Circumference (b)	σb (σb)	γ-index (γ)	σγ (σγ)
Mean of the total	4374	129.3	27.1	63.9	23.20	0.59	26.68	0.90	49.30	2.21	144.2	5.98
Mean of the survived	2870	129.2	27.1	63.9	23.22	0.60	26.66	0.87	49.34	2.16	144.1	5.80
Mean of the deceased (except deaths from accident and battle)	930	130.1	27.3	63.8	23.12	0.60	26.78	0.96	49.06	2.34	145.0	5.45
Mean of the deceased confirmed by medical certificate	423	130.3	27.2	63.8	23.08	0.60	26.81	0.98	48.96	2.26	145.1	6.54
Arteriosclerosis	34	130.5	27.4	63.4	23.12	0.45	26.85	0.89	48.76	2.28	144.6	6.17
Tuberculosis	209	130.4	27.3	63.9	23.09	0.55	26.83	0.82	49.01	2.30	145.2	6.35
Digestive disease	42	130.7	27.3	64.0	23.05	0.63	26.86	1.20	48.93	2.48	145.5	8.25
Kidney and heart disease	34	127.8	26.5	63.5	23.24	0.63	26.47	0.97	49.65	1.96	143.1	6.75
Respiratory disease	24	130.6	27.1	64.5	23.00	0.57	26.83	0.85	49.23	1.70	146.0	5.05
Mental and nervous disease	43	129.8	26.5	63.3	22.99	0.55	26.71	1.09	48.44	2.52	145.2	7.04
Others	37	131.5	27.7	63.9	23.01	0.51	26.99	0.73	48.67	1.66	146.1	4.95
War deaths	58	131.2	28.2	65.0	23.16	0.38	26.98	0.90	49.41	2.06	146.5	5.65
Accidents	33	129.6	28.0	64.3	23.41	0.49	26.77	0.77	49.36	1.76	145.2	5.30

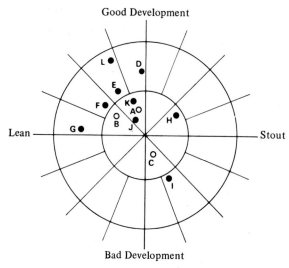

A: All deaths   G: Mental and nervous disease
B: Cause of death certified   H: Accidents
C: Survivors   I: Kidney and heart disease
D: War deaths   J: Tuberculosis
E: Digestive disease   K: Arteriosclerosis
F: Respiratory disease   L: Others

FIG. 1. Relationship between cause of death and physique by polar diagram.

of physique and the total scores of motor fitness test. There is no clear correlation between the two.

Correlation between factors of physique and scores of motor fitness test. It is possible to divide the growth into two factors, i.e., the growth of length (stature) and the growth of width (weight or chest circumference).

Table IV and Figure 3 show the correlation between the scores of stature and the scores of motor fitness test. There is no correlation between them, either. Table V and Figure 4 show the correlation between the scores of weight and the scores of motor fitness test. There is a definite correlation between them.

Body type in polar coordinate diagram and the scores of motor fitness test. Figure 5 shows polar coordination diagram. We classify the physique into lean, obese, large, small and standard. Moreover, the large and small are divided into lean and stout.

We compare the scores of motor fitness test by body type, i.e., lean with stout, small and lean with small and stout. In any case,

Table II. Physique and Health of Old Men

	Grade of Health	Number	Height	Weight	Chest Circum-ference	F-index	σF	G-index	σG	Relative Chest Circum-ference	σb	γ-index	σγ
Male	o	415	154.3	48.1	82.5	23.58	0.93	31.32	1.15	53.57	3.32	174.69	6.70
	△	488	153.5	46.4	81.5	23.44	0.99	31.09	1.05	53.10	3.21	173.75	6.15
	×	298	153.8	45.8	81.3	23.28	1.03	31.05	1.18	53.03	3.36	173.70	6.65
	‡	168	152.4	45.3	81.2	23.43	1.13	30.88	1.31	53.52	3.60	172.47	7.55
Female	o	432	141.5	41.3	78.8	24.42	1.24	29.29	1.05	54.82	4.50	163.83	6.13
	△	871	140.0	39.3	76.2	24.28	1.28	28.94	1.10	54.45	4.63	159.48	6.50
	×	466	139.5	38.0	75.8	24.11	1.30	28.75	1.02	54.43	4.40	158.48	6.33
	‡	221	139.6	37.5	75.1	24.01	1.36	28.74	1.04	53.49	4.66	158.55	6.05

o : excellent   △ : moderate   × : bad   ‡ : dead

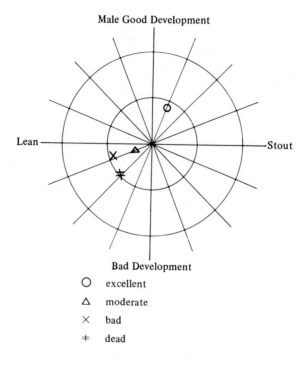

O   excellent

△   moderate

×   bad

+   dead

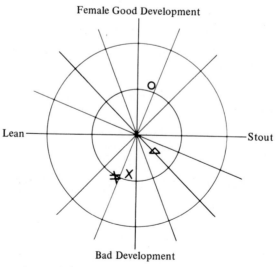

FIG. 2. Physique and health of old men by polar diagram.

Table III. Correlation Between Total Scores of Physique and
Scores of Motor Fitness Test

Scores of Physique	Scores of Motor Fitness Test													
	-6	-5	-4	-3	-2	-1	0	1	2	3	4	5	6	
6				1							1	1		3
5	2			1	2	1		1	1					8
4	1		1	2	1			3	1	1	1			11
3	2	1	2	3	1	4	2	2	1	3		1		22
2	2	1	2	3			2	3	6	5	3		4	32
1	3	2	1		6	5	4	5	11	4	5	8	2	56
	1	4	7	6	6	5	10	9	9	5	3	7	3	75
-1	5	2	1	5	2	8	10	5	8	8	8	2	3	67
-2	1			2		3	4	2	5	2		2	1	22
-3	1		1		2	1	2	1	2	3	1	1		15
-4		1		1		1	1				1			5
-5			2			1								3
-6										1				1
	18	11	17	24	20	30	35	31	44	32	23	22	13	320

Table IV. Correlations Between Stature and
Motor Fitness Test

	Scores of Height	-2	-1	0	1	2	3
♂	Number	4	24	57	56	12	
	Mean of scores of motor fitness test	-0.25	0.75	1.38	-0.11	1.0	
♀	Number	1	23	53	47	16	2
	Mean of scores of motor fitness test	-4.0	0.52	-0.75	-1.40	-1.31	-2.5

stout is better than the lean in scores of motor fitness test (Figs. 6 and 7).

Discussion

In Japanese schools, obese children are kept under the guidance and care of the school nurse and doctor. On the other hand, lean children are paid less attention of their health. It is obvious that the lean type is poor in the fitness for protection.

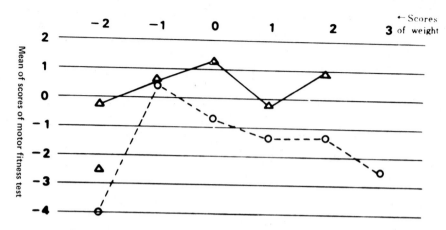

FIG. 3. Correlation between stature and motor fitness test.

Table V. Correlation Between Weight and Motor Fitness Test (Except Obese Children)

	Scores of Weight	−2	−1	0	1	2
	Number	11	102	158	40	11
♂	Mean of scores of motor fitness test	−1.45	0.44	0.58	−0.41	2.27
	Number	33	98	116	41	4
♀	Mean of scores of motor fitness test	−0.81	0.11	−0.11	0.14	2.50

Fitness for performance is composed of many factors: muscular strength, muscular endurance, agility, flexibility, body balance, coordination, circular endurance, etc. [4, 6].

But there is no motor fitness test which shows all these factors in one test. So we evaluate the fitness for performance by putting all kinds of tests together.

Hirata's method employs three tests: 50 meter running, standing broad-jumping and soft-ball throwing.

As concerns a practical motor fitness test, Hirata suggests that it should meet the following criteria: (1) be easy to perform and to measure; (2) be as free of errors of measurement as possible; (3) be adaptable to subjects of all ages; (4) require little space and time.

Although the three performance items suggested do not measure muscular endurance and circular endurance, Hirata's method is

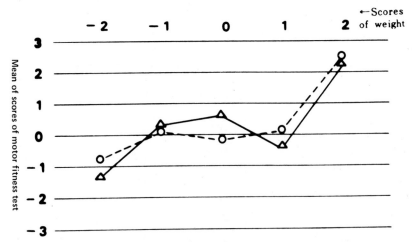

FIG. 4. Correlation between weight and motor fitness test (except obese children).

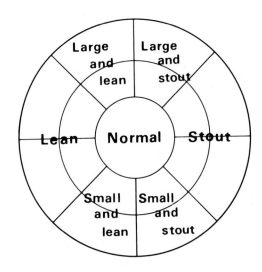

FIG. 5. The classification of physique by polar coordinates diagram.

believed to be the most feasible way for school children, because of the above-mentioned conditions.

Generally speaking, the physique in childhood continues to build up to adult ages: 79.8% in degree of growth, 74.9% in degree of stoutness and leanness [5].

male

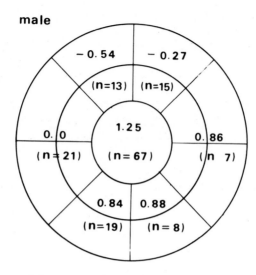

FIG. 6. The mean of the scores of motor fitness test in each body type (male).

female

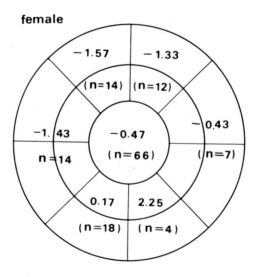

FIG. 7. The mean of the scores of motor fitness test in each body type (female).

As a conclusion, it can be said that special attention should be given to the physique of children through physical activity in the schools.

Summary

Generally speaking, physical fitness includes two phases of fitness, one for protection and the other for performance [4].

The relationship between physique and physical fitness in these two ways was studied.

Fitness for protection and physique. Longevity was used as one of the indicators of fitness for protection. Therefore, the relation between longevity and physique of 1,905 primary school graduates and residents of senior citizens' dormitories was investigated. The conclusion was that the mean physique of those who were alive at the time of the study was stouter than those who were dead.

Fitness for performance and physique. The relation between the scores of motor fitness test and physique was studied. The total of fitness test scores of stouter persons was larger than the total of scores of leaner individuals.

References

1. Hibino, Y.: Studies on the acceleration of Japanese student. Educ. Med. Vol. 11, 1966.
2. Hirata, K.: Ponderal Index, 1972.
3. Hirata, K. and Kaku, K.: The Evaluating Method of Physique and Physical Fitness and Its Practical Application, 1964.
4. Ikai, M.: Sport and physical fitness. Handbook of Sports Medicine, 1965.
5. Tomonari, K.: The Relation Between Longevity and Physique, 1959.
6. Wolanski, N.: Motorics of the Child as a Subject of Research and Educational Activity, 1974.
7. Wolanski, N.: Basic problems in physical development in man in relation to the evaluation of development of children and youth. Curr. Anthropol. 8, No. 1-2, 1967.

Modification du test PWC_{170}

Krastiu Krastev

Le test PWC_{170} (Sjostrand, Wahlund, Karpman, etc.), recommandé par l'Organisation mondiale de la santé (1958), trouve une application de plus en plus large tant par la facilité qu'il présente pour être effectué que par sa valeur pour juger du niveau des possibilités fonctionnelles de l'organisme. Comme on le sait, ce test repose sur la dépendance linéaire qui existe entre la fréquence du pouls dans le diapason de 120 à 180 pulsations par minute et la grandeur de l'effort physique. Grâce à cette dépendance, il est suffisant — selon les auteurs du test — de déterminer la fréquence du pouls pour deux efforts dans le diapason susmentionné afin d'obtenir par voie d'extrapolation ou par la formule (celle de Karpman, par exemple)

$$PWC_{170} = N_1 + (N_2 - N_1)\left(\frac{170 - f_1}{f_2 - f_1}\right)$$

la valeur du PWC_{170} (en kilogrammètres ou en watts), où N_1 et N_2 désignent chacun les deux efforts, tandis que f_1 et f_2 — les fréquences respectives du pouls lors de ces efforts.

Ce test, pour être fait suivant la méthode adoptée, demande 13 minutes de temps "pur", notamment pour deux efforts chacun de 5 minutes et une pause entre eux de 3 minutes.

D'après cette méthode, environ 200 examens portant sur des sportifs (hommes et femmes) à divers niveaux d'entraînement, ainsi que sur des étudiants et des étudiantes non entraînés ont été effectués dans notre laboratoire. Il a été constaté que plus le degré d'entraînement est élevé, surtout dans les disciplines où prédomine l'endurance, d'autant plus lentement s'accélère la fréquence du pouls pour un accroissement égal de l'effort physique. Les courbes pour les divers sports et pour des sportifs à divers niveaux d'entraînement se présentent sous forme d'éventail (Fig. 1).

Compe tenu de cette régularité, on peut admettre la possibilité — rien que sur la base d'un effort pour une fréquence du pouls d'environ 150 à 170 pulsations — d'obtenir par extrapolation la

Krastiu Krastev, Institut supérieur de culture physique et des sports, Sofia, Bulgarie.

valeur du PWC_{170}. La pente de la droite du pouls est dans ces cas déterminée par l'emplacement du point obtenu des valeurs de la fréquence du pouls et de l'effort dans le système des ordonnées (Fig. 1, a, b, c).

Admettant ce qui vient d'être énoncé comme une régularité objective, nous avons élaboré un tableau où, en fonction des valeurs de l'effort (en watts) et de la fréquence du pouls mesurée, on peut trouver sans des calculs complémentaires la valeur du PWC_{170} en kilogrammètres (Tableau I). Le traitement mathématique des données obtenues des mêmes tests, mais évaluées suivant le procédé courant et notre procédé (celui à l'aide du Tableau I), a montré que l'erreur d'après le deuxième procédé est minimale (0.62%).

Les avantages de procéder au test suivant la manière proposée sont évidents:

1. Sans que l'exactitude du test en soit diminuée, celui-ci est ramené à un effort de 5 minutes avec environ 50% de la capacité d'effort maximale de l'organisme. D'après la méthode pratiquée jusqu'alors, on effectuait au maximum 4 tests par heure. Suivant la méthode proposée, leur nombre est monté à 10 par heure.

2. La détermination des valeurs du PWC_{170} suivant le tableau proposé se fait en quelques secondes. Tout travail de calcul est évité et, de ce fait, les erreurs y relatives.

Le test PWC_{170} sert, en réalité, à juger de l'adaptation du système cardiocirculatoire à l'effort physique. Afin de pouvoir se faire une idée plus complète de l'état des sportifs examinés, de grande importance sont aussi les données de l'adaptation de l'appareil respiratoire. A cet effet, nous ajoutâmes à ce test également l'élément respiratoire.

A la fin de l'effort de 5 minutes, parallèlement à la mesure du pouls on recueille l'air expiré dans un sac de Douglas à volume déterminé: environ 50 litres. Lors du gonflage du sac, on détermine le volume respiratoire par minute. En cas où on recourt à un manomètre pour mieux fixer le moment où le sac est rempli d'air, l'erreur suivant cette méthode est inférieure à 2%. Les valeurs STPD du volume respiratoire par minute sont ramenées à 50 watts de travail d'après la formule courante:

$$V_e = \frac{\text{Volume respiratoire par minute}}{\text{Effort-watts}} \times 50$$

La valeur obtenue de l'équivalent de ventilation (V_e), qui est de l'ordre de 10 à 20 litres, est en rapport inverse avec l'adaptation de l'appareil respiratoire à l'effort physique. Considérable est la dépend-

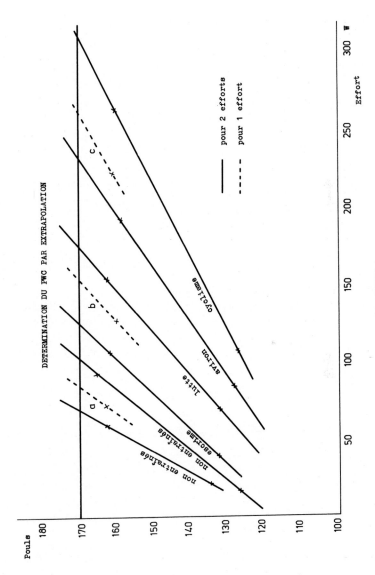

FIGURE 1.

Tableau I. Estimation de la capacité d'effort physique (PWC$_{170}$) d'après la frequence du pouls et l'effort

Watts Pouls	30	45	60	75	90	105	120	135	150	165	180	195	210	225	240	255	270	285	300	315	330	345
141	432	528	627	726	846	969	1092	1215	1320	1431	1536	1644	1752	1854	1956	2058	2160	2241	2325	2406	2490	2574
144	406	502	600	698	815	935	1055	1174	1278	1386	1490	1596	1702	1802	1903	2004	2105	2187	2272	2353	2438	2522
147	381	476	573	670	784	901	1017	1134	1235	1342	1443	1547	1651	1750	1850	1951	2051	2133	2218	2301	2386	2471
150	356	450	546	642	753	867	980	1094	1193	1298	1397	1499	1601	1698	1798	1897	1996	2080	2165	2248	2334	2419
153	330	424	519	614	723	833	943	1053	1151	1253	1351	1451	1551	1647	1745	1843	1942	2026	2112	2195	2282	2367
156	305	398	492	586	692	799	906	1013	1109	1209	1305	1402	1500	1595	1692	1790	1887	1972	2058	2142	2229	2316
159	279	371	465	558	661	764	869	973	1067	1164	1259	1354	1450	1543	1639	1736	1833	1918	2005	2090	2177	2264
162	254	345	438	530	630	730	831	932	1024	1120	1212	1306	1400	1491	1587	1683	1778	1865	1952	2038	2125	2213
165	229	319	411	503	599	696	794	892	982	1075	1166	1257	1349	1439	1534	1629	1724	1811	1898	1985	2073	2161
168	203	293	384	475	568	662	757	851	940	1031	1120	1209	1299	1381	1481	1575	1669	1757	1845	1932	2021	2109
171	178	267	357	447	538	628	720	811	898	986	1074	1161	1249	1335	1428	1522	1615	1703	1792	1880	1969	2058
174	153	241	330	419	507	594	682	771	855	942	1027	1113	1199	1283	1376	1468	1560	1649	1739	1827	1917	2006
177	127	215	303	391	476	560	645	730	813	897	981	1064	1148	1232	1322	1415	1505	1596	1685	1775	1865	1955
180	102	189	276	363	445	526	608	690	771	853	935	1016	1098	1180	1270	1361	1451	1542	1632	1722	1813	1903

NOTE: Les valeurs sont données en kilogrammètres

ance de cet équivalent avec le taux d'assimilation de l'oxygène de l'air inspiré.

Par le precédé énoncé ci-haut, sans compliquer les examens avec des efforts complémentaires et diverses manipulations, nous obtenons un test cardio-respiratoire PWC_{170} qui en dit beaucoup.

Il existe une forte dépendence corrélative entre les parties cardiaque et respiratoire du test ($r = 0.74$). Dans beaucoup de cas, pourtant, il se manifeste une hétérogénéité dans l'adaptation des sportifs de haute classe. Certains de nos meilleurs sportifs ayant à leur actif nombre de compétitions internationales (courses, aviron, cyclisme, etc.) se distinguent par example de leurs collègues moins remarquables non pas tant par l'adaptation cardiaque que respiratoire (ils ont un équivalent de ventilation très bas).

Suivant le test ainsi modifié, nous avons procédé à plus de 1000 examens sur des sportifs et des personnes non entraînées. Pour juger de la capacité d'effort, nous utilisons divers tableaux d'estimation, compte tenu du sport dont il s'agit et du niveau d'entraînement. Le Tableau II est utilisé par nous pour juger de compétiteurs d'élite (hommes) pratiquant des sports d'endurance, tels que aviron, cyclisme, courses sur moyens et longs parcours, etc. Les tableaux d'estimation comportent 7 degrés et sont élaborés d'après la méthode des écarts-types.

Le test PWC_{170}, sous sa forme modifiée, donne la possibilité de résoudre d'une manière plus complexe certaines tâches de caractère scientifique ou scientifico-pratique. Ainsi, par exemple, au mois de juillet 1975, lors du séjour de nos compétiteurs d'athlétisme à Montréal, nous avions procédé à des examens complexes — physiologiques et biochimiques, ainsi que portant sur la technique sportive

Tableau II. Estimation de l'adaptation cardio-respiratoire chez des sportifs d'élite d'après le test PWC_{170} modifié

PWC_{170} Kilogrammètres par Kg/Poids	Equivalent de Ventilation – Litres pour 50 Watts	Estimation	
Au-dessus de 30,0	Au-dessous de 9,6	Très haute	7
de 23,6 à 30,0	de 10,9 à 8,6	Haute	6
de 21,0 à 23,5	de 12,6 à 11,0	Au-dessus de la moyenne	5
de 18,3 à 20,9	de 14,0 à 12,5	Moyenne	4
de 15,8 à 18,2	de 15,5 à 14,1	Sous la moyenne	3
de 13,0 à 15,7	de 17,0 à 15,6	Basse	2
Au dessous de 13,0	Au-dessus de 17,0	Très basse	1

— en vue d'élucider le caractère de l'adaptation des sportifs au décalage de 6 heures dans le cycle journalier et aux particularités du climat chaud et humide de Montréal à cette époque de l'année. Les données du test PWC_{170} nous permettent de distinguer nettement deux phases dans l'adaptation: la phase aiguë, d'une durée de 5 à 6 jours, et celle de stabilisation allant jusqu'au 10e—12e jour (Fig. 2). Il est intéressant de noter que l'adaptation du système cardio-vasculaire devance l'adaptation de l'appareil respiratoire. L'équivalent de ventilation se rapproche de ses valeurs initiales le dixième jour seulement après l'arrivée à Montréal. La courbe d'adaptation obtenue par ce test coïncide dans une grande mesure également avec les données des autres examens.

Caractéristiques sont aussi les changements dans les deux parties de ce test en cas de surcharge hypoxique. Lors de la respiration de mélanges de gaz avec baisse graduelle de la pression partielle d'oxygène (celle-ci correspondant à l'altitude respective), on observe des changements symétriques dans les deux parties du test (Fig. 3). Jusqu'à une altitude de 4.5 km, on constate une baisse graduelle presque linéaire des valeurs du PWC_{170} et une hausse de l'équivalent de ventilation. Une réaction adéquate du système cardio-pulmonaire est en présence. L'hypoxie plus poussée encore a pour effet, pourtant, de susciter une décompensation hypoxique de l'organisme liée au changement (baisse) brusque et non adéquat des valeurs du PWC_{170} et celles de l'équivalent de ventilation (hausse). Chez les alpinistes ayant un plus grand stage dans les conditions de haute altitude, la partie "cardiaque" du test montre une baisse adéquate jusqu'à 6,000 m d'altitude, tandis que l'équivalent de ventilation ne se distingue pas dans son "comportement" de celui chez les autres sportifs.

Ce test peut être utilisé avec succès aussi pour contrôler le niveau de fatigue et de récupération après des efforts d'entraînement. Nos recherches nous ont permis de mettre en évidence, après de rudes entraînements, une baisse des valeurs du PWC allant jusqu'à environ 30%. Ce qu'il importe de signaler est que les deux parties du test varient différemment en fonction du caractère de l'entraînement effectué.

Comme on le voit, la modification du test PWC_{170} permet de procéder à une estimation plus intégrale de l'adaptation cardio-respiratoire de l'organisme et à une prise en considération plus différentiée des divers autres facteurs du milieu interne et externe de l'organisme (hypoxie, climat, fatigue, etc.). Pour cette raison, nous nous permettons de recommander cette modification à un usage plus généralisé dans le contrôle scientifique de l'état d'entraînement.

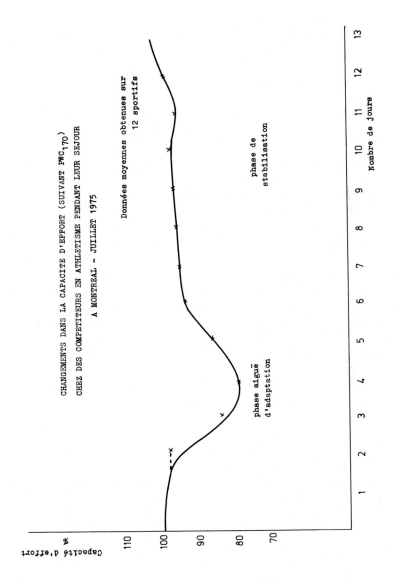

CHANGEMENTS DANS LA CAPACITE D'EFFORT (SUIVANT PWC_{170})
CHEZ DES COMPETITEURS EN ATHLETISME PENDANT LEUR SEJOUR
A MONTREAL – JUILLET 1975

Données moyennes obtenues sur
12 sportifs

FIGURE 2.

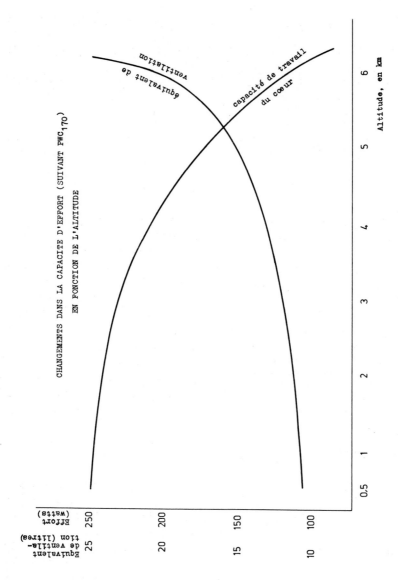

FIGURE 3.

Endurance Training and the $\dot{V}O_2$ Max With Special Reference to Validity of the Astrand-Ryhming Nomogram and the Cooper 12-Minute Run as Indirect Tests for Maximal Oxygen Uptake

B. F. Thiart, J. H. Blaauw and J. P. van Rensburg

Introduction

Although the maximal oxygen consumption ($\dot{V}O_2$ max) of a person is a highly reproducible characteristic, several studies have emphasized the importance of the active muscle mass [9, 11], the physical condition [8], the working posture [1, 10] and the type of apparatus used [3, 5] in determining the maximal oxygen uptake.

Divergent correlations have also been reported between the directly determined and the predicted values based on the Cooper test [2, 12] and the A.-R. nomogram [6, 13]. The validity of these two indirect methods is often disputed. The main objectives of this study were to (1) establish whether the specific trained condition of a subject might influence the maximal oxygen uptake when assessed on the bicycle and the treadmill, respectively, and (2) investigate the validity of the indirect tests as a means of assessing maximal oxygen uptake.

Materials and Methods

One hundred and sixteen young men were classified according to their physical condition into four groups: (A) 33 regular cyclists; (B) 33 active sportsmen taking part in activities such as rugby and track and field; (C) 31 untrained men not taking part in any organized endurance sport; and (D) 19 trained runners (middle- and long-distance athletes).

B. F. Thiart, J. H. Blaauw and J. P. van Rensburg, Exercise Physiology Laboratory, Department of Physical Education, University of Stellenbosch, Republic of South Africa.

In the direct assessment of the $\dot{V}O_2$ max on the bicycle and the treadmill, respectively, the workloads were increased stepwise with resting periods between successive loads. On the treadmill the inclination was held constant at 5%. Groups A and B were tested on both the bicycle and the treadmill, each subject working five minutes per session except for the "supramaximal" loads when the subject indicated an inability to complete the work session. The tests were conducted on separate days until there was no further increase in the oxygen uptake despite a further increase in workload. This "leveling off" of the oxygen consumption was accepted as the only criterion that the "maximal" value was reached.

In the A.-R. nomogram test the subjects performed two submaximal work sessions on the bicycle. The average of the two predicted values was calculated for each subject and compared with the directly determined values.

Groups C and D performed a maximal test on the treadmill as well as the Cooper 12-minute run on a 400 meter track. Approximately one week prior to the Cooper test each subject had a trial run to accustom himself to the test procedure. During the final test the accumulative time was announced every minute.

Twelve subjects of group C were subjected to a training program consisting of 12 minutes of jogging per day, five days per week. The program lasted for 12 weeks after which the subjects were retested to determine the predicted and the directly determined values. The Pearson product-moment coefficient was used to establish the correlation between the treadmill and the Cooper test values.

Results and Discussion

The average physical characteristics of the four groups are summarized in Table I and in Table II the average maximal heart rate, oxygen uptake and pulmonary ventilation (BTPS) of groups A and B are tabulated.

Table I. Average Age, Height and Mass of the Four Groups

	A (Cyclists) 33	B (Sportsmen) 33	C (Untrained Men) 31	D (Runners) 19
Age (years)	22.42	21.57	20.30	20.40
Height (cm)	176.22	178.18	177.20	177.16
Mass (kg)	73.33	72.69	72.90	70.80

Table II. Average Maximal Heart Rate, Oxygen Uptake and
Pulmonary Ventilation (BTPS) of Groups A and B

	A (Cyclists)		B (Sportsmen)			
	Bicycle	Treadmill	Bicycle			Treadmill
Heart rate/min	192.18	194.03	179.48	†		190.27
$\dot{V}O_2$ max l/min	4.44	4.38	4.20	‡		4.58
ml/kg/min	60.74	59.89	58.05	‡		63.46
$\dot{V}E$ (BTPS) l/min	157.90	†	144.98	159.77	*	153.62

*Significant difference at 10% level
†Significant difference at 2.5% level
‡Significant difference at 0.1% level

From the results summarized in Table II it is clear that the average maximal heart rate and the oxygen uptake of group B (noncyclists) were significantly higher on the treadmill than on the bicycle ergometer. The average higher treadmill value (9%) obtained in the present study compares favorably with the values reported by Glassford [4] 8%; McArdle [7] 9.9% and Faulkner [3] 11%. In group A (cyclists), however, no significant difference was found between the treadmill and bicycle values for the same variables. Consequently, the application of either the treadmill or the bicycle ergometer is justified in determining the "true" $\dot{V}O_2$ max of trained cyclists. When testing noncyclists, the treadmill value tends to be significantly higher than the bicycle value. It appears that noncyclists do not command the trained local muscle mass and specific stamina to exert themselves truly maximally on the bicycle ergometer. When maximal oxygen consumption is assessed on the bicycle the value is therefore decidedly influenced by the specifically trained condition of the subject.

It is interesting to note that in both groups, the maximal pulmonary ventilation was on average higher on the bicycle than on the treadmill. In the cycling group this difference was even more pronounced. On the bicycle the pedaling rate was held constant (60 rpm) and only the resistance was increased at each workload. It would appear that the higher exertion demanded on the bicycle during maximal work could contribute to this difference. Neurogenic factors such as stimulatory impulses from the motor cortex and proprioceptive reflexes from joint receptors might be involved.

Table III shows that in group B the average predicted values based on the A.-R. nomogram were significantly higher than both the treadmill (P <0.05) and bicycle values (P <0.001). With regard to

B. F. THIART ET AL

Table III. Comparison Between Directly Determined and Predicted
A.-R. Nomogram Values

| | A (Cyclists) | | | B (Sportsmen) | | | |
	Bicycle	Nomogram	Treadmill	Bicycle		Nomogram	Treadmill
$\dot{V}O_2$ max							
l/min	4.43	4.27	4.37	4.20	†	4.83	* 4.58
ml/kg/min	60.74	57.70	59.89	58.05		66.50	63.46

*Significant at 5% level
†Significant at 0.1% level

group A (cyclists) the corresponding average results did not yield a statistically significant difference.

In the case of highly trained subjects the nomogram consistently recorded an overestimation of their "true" maximal values. This overestimation was especially noticeable in conditioned long-distance athletes and individual overestimations > 25% with regard to their maximal treadmill values and > 35% in respect to the corresponding bicycle values were registered. Although the individual over-estimations were not as pronounced as in the case of long-distance athletes, a few highly trained cyclists showed the same tendency. Unfit persons, on the other hand, recorded an underestimation of the "true" $\dot{V}O_2$ max. The major defect in the nomogram lies in its failure to take account of changes in stroke volume and in the economy of labor performance which accompany prolonged inten-sive endurance training.

Several workers have already investigated the validity and reliability of the Cooper test and have reported variable correlations ranging from 0.22 to 0.90 between the directly determined and the predicted values [2, 12]. In this study the subjects in group C showed a correlation of 0.67 between the predicted and the "true" values while 0.85 was registered in group D (Table IV).

Twelve subjects of group C were tested before and after a 12-week training program. The results are summarized in Table V.

Table IV. Comparison Between Directly Determined and
Predicted Cooper Test Values

| | C (Untrained Men) (31) | | | D (Trained Athletes) (19) | | |
	Treadmill	Cooper Test	r	Treadmill	Cooper Test	r
$\dot{V}O_2$ max						
l/min	4.12	3.84	0.67	4.70	4.81	0.85
ml/kg/min	56.71	52.68		66.71	68.38	

Table V. Average $\dot{V}O_2$ Max (l/min) Before and After Training

| | Before N = 12 | | | After N = 12 | | |
	Treadmill	Cooper Test	r	Treadmill	Cooper Test	r
$\dot{V}O_2$ max						
l/min	4.12	3.54	0.48	4.14	4.15	0.77
ml/kg/min	55.10	49.60		55.00	55.10	

The correlation between the actual and predicted values before the start of the training program was 0.48 compared to 0.77 after training.

The maximal distance a person is able to cover in 12 minutes may increase considerably as a result of regular exercise. This increase is not necessarily reflected in a similar increase in the "true" $\dot{V}O_2$ max. In the present experiment there was no significant difference between the directly determined average values before and after the jogging program. The explanation for this is that specific training improves the stamina and economy of running which enables the person to run farther with the same consumption of oxygen. For obvious reasons highly trained runners tend to be overestimated, while the opposite tendency is true of very unfit persons. As an indirect test the "accuracy" of the Cooper test compares favorably with that of the A.-R. nomogram and especially in medium to fairly well-trained runners the distance covered in 12 minutes enabled us to calculate the $\dot{V}O_2$ max with a considerable degree of accuracy. Motivation as well as the training condition, however, are two important factors affecting the validity of the Cooper test, and differences in these factors have undoubtedly contributed to the highly divergent correlations reported in the literature.

For the accurate determination of an individual's VO_2 max both the A.-R. nomogram and the Cooper test are unsuitable. However, insofar as these indirect methods are used as a so-called screening method to classify subjects as good or bad with regard to the $\dot{V}O_2$ max, their application is justified.

References

1. Astrand, P.-O and Saltin, B.: Maximal oxygen uptake and heart rate in various types of muscular activity. J. Appl. Physiol. 16:977-981, 1961.
2. Doolittle, T.L. and Bigbee, R.: The twelve-minute run-walk. A test of cardiorespiratory fitness of adolescent boys. Res. Q. 39:491-495, 1968.
3. Faulkner, J.A., Roberts, D.E., Elk, R.L. and Conway, J.F.: Cardiovascular responses to submaximum and maximum effort in cycling and running. J. Appl. Physiol. 30:457-461, 1971.

4. Glassford, R.G., Baycraft, G.H., Sedgwick, A.W. and Macnab, R.B.J.: Comparison of maximal oxygen uptake by predicted and actual methods. J. Appl. Physiol. 20:509-513, 1965.

5. Hermansen, L., Ekblom, B. and Saltin, B.: Cardiac output during submaximal and maximal treadmill and bicycle exercise. J. Appl. Physiol. 29:82-86, 1970.

6. Maksud, M.G. and Coutts, K.D.: Application of the Cooper twelve-minute Run-walk test to young males. Res. Q. 42:54-59, 1971.

7. McArdle, W.D. and Magel, J.R.: Physical work capacity and maximum oxygen uptake in treadmill and bicycle exercise. Med. Sci. Sports 2:118-123, 1970.

8. Saltin, B., Blomquist, G., Mitchell, J.A. et al: Response to exercise after bed rest and after training. A longitudinal study of adaptive changes in oxygen transport and body composition. Circulation 38 (suppl. VII):1-78, 1968.

9. Simmons, R. and Shephard, R.J.: Measurements of cardiac output in maximum exercise. Application of an acetylene rebreathing method to arm and leg exercise. Intern. Z. Angew. Physiol. 219:1386-1392, 1970.

10. Stenberg, J.: The significance of the central circulation for the aerobic work capacity under various conditions in young healthy persons. Acta Physiol. Scand. 68 (suppl. 273):1-26, 1966.

11. Stenberg, J.P., Astrand, P.-O., E᭞ᵐ, B. et al: Hemodynamic response to work with different muscle groups, sitting and supine. J. Appl. Physiol. 22:61-70, 1967.

12. Wanamaker, G.S.: A study of the validity and reliability of the twelve-minute run under selected motivational conditions. Paper presented at the Research Section N.A.A.H.P.E.R., 1970, Seattle, Washington.

13. Wyndham, C.H., Strydom, N.B., Maritz, J.S. et al: Maximum oxygen intake and maximum heart rate during strenuous work. J. Appl. Physiol. 14:927-936, 1959.

Specificity of Aerobic Testing in Competitive Cyclists Compared With Runners

H. Hartung and J. McMillen

Introduction

Previous studies have shown a specificity of physiological adaptation to training including arm vs. leg work, lactate accumulation, swimming and heart rate response [2, 3, 10, 17]. Studies have also indicated that there is a strong specificity of training effects resulting from bicycle training [21-23]. These authors and others [8, 12, 18] have concluded that the specific muscular adaptations to training relate to the mode of testing and favor the cycle-trained individual on a maximal bicycle test and the subject trained by running on a running test. Studies have also shown that maximal oxygen uptake ($\dot{V}O_2$ max) during uphill running is 5% to 15% greater than during cycling in subjects not trained for cycling [1, 7, 8, 13, 17, 21].

The maximal aerobic capacity of well-trained competitive cyclists has not received much attention in the exercise physiology literature. Di Prampero and others [6] reported a mean $\dot{V}O_2$ max of only about 50 ml/kg/min for seven Cuban and Guatemalan cyclists at the 1968 Olympic Games. The test used, however, was an indirect step-test method and $\dot{V}O_2$ was estimated from submaximal heart rates. Saltin and Astrand [24] found a mean $\dot{V}O_2$ max of 75 ml/kg/min for six Swedish competitive cyclists tested on a bicycle ergometer. This aerobic power compares closely with that found for runners which they tested in the same study. Hagberg [9] measured the $\dot{V}O_2$ max of seven U.S. competitive cyclists riding their bikes on a treadmill. Mean $\dot{V}O_2$ max was found to be 66.8 ml/kg/min.

The purpose of this investigation was to determine if specificity of training vs. testing methods was evident in the maximal cardiorespiratory responses of competitive cyclists and distance

H. Hartung and J. McMillen, Human Performance Laboratory, Central Missouri State University, Warrensburg, Missouri, U.S.A.

runners tested on the bicycle ergometer (BE) and treadmill (TM). A secondary purpose was to add to the small amount of data currently available concerning the aerobic fitness levels of trained cyclists.

Methods

Eight competitive cyclists of varying levels of ability and nine collegiate distance and middle-distance runners of varying ability served as subjects for the study. Testing took place in the late spring in the early part of the competitive cycling season and during the track season.

Each subject was tested for maximum oxygen uptake during a continuous treadmill running test and a continuous cycling test. Previous studies have shown that continuous tests produce results much the same as discontinuous TM and BE tests [16, 17]. An initial orientation session was held at which each subject was acquainted with the test procedures and ran and cycled at test speeds and workloads. The two maximum tests were conducted at least three days apart. The order of test administration was randomly selected to attempt to preclude any systematic effect due to testing order.

Testing was done in an air-conditioned laboratory with a temperature range of 20 to 24 C and moderate humidity; an electric fan was used to circulate air to cool the subject on each test. Each subject was tested at the same time of day on each test at least two hours following the last meal.

For the TM test, the subject warmed up by running three minutes at 6.0 mph (161 m/min), 0% grade. Following a two-minute seated rest, during which the headband and breathing valve were attached, the subject ran at 7.0 mph (188 m/min), 0% grade for two minutes. The treadmill grade was then increased 2.5% each two minutes continuously until the subject could not continue.

Preliminary studies of trained cyclists had indicated that the usual pedal speeds of 50 to 70 rpm [12] for BE tests were too slow and caused leg tightness and discomfort at increased workloads compared with their training speeds of 80 to 100 rpm. Maximum O_2 was also greater at higher crank speeds and the cycling test was therefore modified for the cyclists. Following a three-minute warm-up on the ergometer at 60 rpm and workload of 630 kpm/min, the subject pedaled at 60 rpm, 840 kpm/min for two minutes. The resistance was then increased by .5 kg each two minutes continuously, with the pedaling speed increasing to 80 rpm after four minutes. The test procedure for the runners was the same, except that the pedal speed remained at 60 rpm throughout the test.

Oxygen uptake was determined using an oxygen consumption computer (OCC-1000, Technology Inc.) which had been validated using known gas samples and gas chromatography [14]. Expired air was routed via a Daniels valve [5] through a 5-liter mixing chamber to the oxygen transducer. Samples were read every other minute until it was apparent that the subject could only continue a short time, at which time 30-second readings were made each minute. Ventilation volume was determined from readings taken each minute from a high velocity dry gas meter (CD-4, Parkinson-Cowan).

A two-way analysis of variance was used to determine if there were statistically significant differences between the groups for each variable measured. Where a significant interaction was found, the Tukey post hoc comparison method was applied to determine specifically where the difference was located. Product-moment correlations were also computed between test types for the physiological variables.

Results

The groups could not easily be equated on the basis of physical characteristics, since they were composed of a few highly select subjects rather than a random sample. The cyclists were significantly taller and heavier than the runners (Table I), but the range and variability of weight was much greater for the cyclists. The mean age of the cyclists was almost two years greater than that of the runners, also a significant difference.

The cyclists had a higher mean maximum heart rate ($P < .05$) when both tests were considered together. Heart rates on the TM were significantly ($P < .01$) higher than on the BE when both groups were considered. The mean heart rate for the cyclists on the TM was 197.5 which was significantly greater than for either the cyclists or

Table I. Physical Characteristics of Subjects

| Variable | Test | Runners (N = 9) | | | Cyclists (N = 8) | | | P* |
		Mean S.D.		Range	Mean S.D.		Range	
Age (yr)		20.37 ± 0.91		(18.8–22.1)	22.23 ±	2.09	(19.2–24.8)	<.01
Ht. (cm)		173.28 ± 6.82		(162–185)	180.96 ±	6.93	(170–188)	<.01
Wt. (kg)	TM[a]	61.76 ± 4.59		(56.2–70.1)	70.39 ±	11.42	(50.4–90.3)	<.01
Wt. (kg)	BE[b]	62.32 ± 5.14		(55.8–71.2)	70.93 ±	11.31	(51.0–90.3)	<.01

*Statistical probability level based on analysis of variance
[a]TM = Treadmill
[b]BE = Bicycle ergometer

the runners tested on the BE. Table II presents the mean, range, standard deviation and statistical probability level for each variable by test and by group.

No significant difference was found between the runners tested on the TM and cyclists tested on the BE except for maximum ventilation volume ($\dot{V}E$) in which the cyclists were 13% (P < .05) higher than the runners. The cyclists attained a higher $\dot{V}O_2$ max when tested on the BE than on the TM by 8.8% (l/min) and 8.3% (ml/kg/min). Neither of these differences was significant, however. The runners achieved a greater $\dot{V}O_2$ max on the TM than the BE by 10.4% (ml/kg/min) and 9.9% (l/min), with the former reaching significance at P < .05.

In terms of absolute $\dot{V}O_2$ max (l/min) there were no runners who attained a higher value on the BE test than on the TM. There was one cyclist, however, who reached a higher, and one an equal, absolute $\dot{V}O_2$ max on the TM test. Practically the same results were obtained when relative $\dot{V}O_2$ max (ml/kg/min) was considered; one cyclist was higher on the TM than on the BE and no runners higher on the BE than on the TM (Fig. 1).

Oxygen pulse was significantly higher (P < .05) for the cyclists (24.4 ml/beat) on the BE test than for the same group on the TM and for the runners on the BE test. The mean values of $\dot{V}E$ for the cyclists on the TM (153.4 l/min) and the BE (158.8 l/min) were both significantly higher (P < .01) than the runners on the BE (119.0

Table II. Maximum Test Variables For Runners and Cyclists

Variable	Test	Runners (N = 9)			Cyclists (N = 8)			P*
		Mean	S.D.	Range	Mean	S.D.	Range	
$\dot{V}O_2$	TM[a]	4.25 ±	0.51	(3.72-5.15)	4.13 ±	0.53	(3.50-5.25)	NS
(l/min)	BE[b]	3.83 ±	0.39	(3.15-4.63)	4.53 ±	0.50	(3.65-5.17	<.05
$\dot{V}O_2$	TM	68.73 ±	4.08	(63.4-74.9)	59.23 ±	5.08	(53.0-69.6)	<.01
(ml/kg/min)	BE	61.57 ±	4.08	(52.7-66.9)	64.57 ±	6.62	(56.0-71.6)	NS
HR	TM	187.44 ±	3.27	(183-195)	197.50 ±	8.11	(188-214)	NS
(bpm)	BE	181.67 ±	6.60	(167-188)	185.63 ±	10.69	(167-207)	NS
$\dot{V}E$	TM	138.17 ±	13.57	(125-157)	153.36 ±	13.14	(135-176)	NS
(l/min)	BE	119.02 ±	18.13	(86-153)	158.82 ±	11.85	(140-173)	<.01
O_2 Pulse	TM	22.68 ±	2.60	(19.8-27.4)	20.89 ±	2.42	(17.4-26.1)	NS
(ml/beat)	BE	21.07 ±	1.67	(18.9-24.6)	24.39 ±	2.51	(19.4-27.5)	<.05

*Statistical probability level based on analysis of variance
[a]TM = Treadmill
[b]BE = Bicycle ergometer

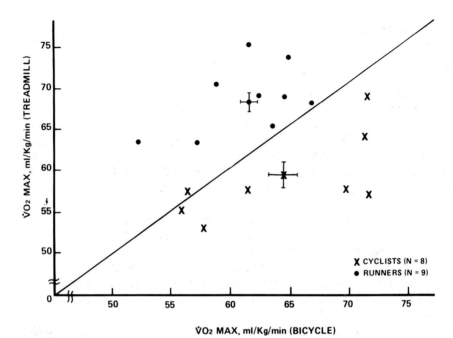

FIG. 1. Individual values for max oxygen uptake (ml/kg/min) on the treadmill and bicycle ergometer tests. Means ± S.E.M. are also shown.

l/min). The cyclists on the BE also had significantly (P < .05) greater V̇E than the runners on the TM (138.2 l/min).

Discussion

Although the total group of cyclists tested did not have a V̇O₂ max which approached the 75 ml/kg/min of the Swedish cyclists [24], the mean of the four highest subjects was 71 ml/kg/min on the BE test. These subjects were clearly in better condition and were more experienced than the others in the group. The V̇O₂ max of the runners, on the other hand, compares favorably with that of eight university track athletes [20] and for ten marathon runners [4] previously studied.

The two cyclists who had V̇O₂ max on the TM equal to or greater than on the BE were the two who were the least experienced and in poorest condition at the time of testing. One of these subjects has also trained some by running as well as cycling during the preceding several months.

The relative V̇O₂ max for the runners was 10.4% greater on the TM test than the BE which approximates the difference noted in several other studies [17, 18]. The higher $\dot{V}O_2$ max for the cyclists on a BE test has been reported previously for individual subjects [12, 18, 19], but not for the mean value of an entire group of subjects.

Studies of untrained college-age [21] and middle-aged subjects [22, 23] in which one group trained by cycling and another by running or walking have indicated that the effects of cycle training are more specific than those of running. The cyclists in the present study were not able to achieve a TM relative $\dot{V}O_2$ max a great deal higher than young untrained subjects in several other studies [15, 21] even though they were highly trained in endurance cycle work. A significantly higher max heart rate and lower O_2 pulse for the cyclists on the TM compared with the BE test indicate a greater cardiovascular stress during the unaccustomed type of work.

The lower $\dot{V}O_2$ max normally found in BE compared with TM testing has been explained in previous reports [7, 11] as resulting from a lower cardiac output ($\dot{Q}$) due to a lower stroke volume (SV), with heart rate and arteriovenous O_2 difference (a-v O_2 diff.) remaining the same in both tests. This would not explain the $\dot{V}O_2$ max differences found in the present study, since the heart rate was lower on the BE test for both groups. The lower BE $\dot{V}O_2$ max of the runners could be explained by the finding of Miyamura and Honda [19] that this difference results from both a decreased $\dot{Q}$ due to a lower heart rate and a lower a-v O_2 diff. with no difference in SV. Neither of these studies explain the increased $\dot{V}O_2$ max of the cyclists on the BE despite a lower heart rate. It is possible that a slight increase in a-v O_2 diff. might explain part of the increase, but an increase in SV would have to occur to keep the $\dot{Q}$ from decreasing. The trained cyclists lean forward on the cycle handlebars so that the upper body is nearly horizontal and this posture may facilitate venous return and possibly increase end-diastolic volume allowing an increased SV.

The results of this study indicate that higher $\dot{V}O_2$ max results may be obtained on a continuous BE test in highly trained cyclists using higher pedal speeds than previous studies have shown [12]. Recent work [9] showing improved efficiency at 90 to 100 rpm by competitive cyclists tends to substantiate our use of a higher crank speed (80 rpm) in the present study.

References

1. Astrand, P.-O. and Saltin, B.: Maximal oxygen uptake and heart rate in various types of muscular activity. J. Appl. Physiol. 16:977-981, 1961.
2. Brouha, L.: Spécificité de l'entraînement au travail musculaire. Rev. Can. Biol. 4:144-148, 1945.

3. Clausen, J.P., Trap-Jensen, J. and Lassen, N.A.: The effects of training on the heart rate during arm and leg exercise. Scand. J. Clin. Lab. Invest. 26:296-301, 1970.

4. Costill, D.L. and Winrow, E.: Maximal oxygen intake among marathon runners. Arch. Phys. Med. Rehabil. 51:317-320, 1970.

5. Daniels, J.: Portable respiratory gas collection equipment. J. Appl. Physiol. 31:164-167, 1971.

6. Di Prampero, P.E., Limas, F.P. and Sassi, G.: Maximal muscular power, aerobic and anaerobic, in 116 athletes performing at the XIXth Olympic Games in Mexico. Ergonomics 13:665-674, 1970.

7. Faulkner, J.A., Roberts, D.E., Elk, R.L. and Conway, J.: Cardiovascular responses to submaximum and maximum effort cycling and running. J. Appl. Physiol. 30:457-461, 1971.

8. Glassford, R.G., Baycroft, G.H.Y., Sedwick, A.W. and Macnab, R.B.J.: Comparison of maximal oxygen uptake values determined by predicted and actual methods. J. Appl. Physiol. 20:509-513, 1965.

9. Hagberg, J.M.: Effects of different gear ratios on the metabolic responses of competitive cyclists to constant load steady state work. Med. Sci. Sports 7:74, 1975 (Abst.).

10. Hartung, G.H.: Specificity of training as indicated by heart rate response to exercise. Percept. Mot. Skills 36:639-645, 1973.

11. Hermansen, L., Ekblom, B. and Saltin, B.: Cardiac output during submaximal and maximal treadmill and bicycle exercise. J. Appl. Physiol. 29:82-86, 1970.

12. Hermansen, L. and Saltin, B.: Oxygen uptake during maximal treadmill and bicycle exercise. J. Appl. Physiol. 26:31-37, 1969.

13. Kamon, E. and Pandolf, K.B.: Maximal aerobic power during laddermill climbing, uphill running, and cycling. J. Appl. Physiol. 32:467-473, 1972.

14. Londeree, B.R.: Validation of the oxygen consumption computer. Med. Sci. Sports 5:187-190, 1973.

15. Magel, J.R., Foglia, G.F., McArdle, W.D. et al: Specificity of swim training on maximum oxygen uptake. J. Appl. Physiol. 38:151-155, 1975.

16. Maksud, M.G. and Coutts, K.D.: Comparison of a continuous and discontinuous graded treadmill test for maximal oxygen uptake. Med. Sci. Sports 3:63-65, 1971.

17. McArdle, W.D., Katch, F.I. and Pechar, G.S.: Comparison of continuous and discontinuous treadmill and bicycle tests for max VO_2. Med. Sci. Sports 5:156-160, 1973.

18. McArdle, W.D. and Magel, J.R.: Physical work capacity and maximum oxygen uptake in treadmill and bicycle exercise. Med. Sci. Sports 2:118-123, 1970.

19. Miyamura, M. and Honda, Y.: Oxygen intake and cardiac output during maximal treadmill and bicycle exercise. J. Appl. Physiol. 32:185-188, 1972.

20. Novak, L.P., Hyatt, R.E. and Alexander, J.F.: Body composition and physiologic function of athletes. JAMA 205:764-770, 1968.

21. Pechar, G.S., McArdle, W.D., Katch, F.I. et al: Specificity of cardiorespiratory adaptation to bicycle and treadmill training. J. Appl. Physiol. 36:753-756, 1974.

22. Pollock, M.L., Dimmick, J., Miller, H.S. Jr. et al: Effects of mode of training on cardiovascular function and body composition of adult men. Med. Sci. Sports 7:139-145, 1975.

23. Roberts, J.A. and Alspaugh, J.W.: Specificity of training effects resulting from programs of treadmill running and bicycle ergometer riding. Med. Sci. Sports 4:6-10, 1972.
24. Saltin, B. and Astrand, P.-O.: Maximal oxygen intake in athletes. J. Appl. Physiol. 23:353-358, 1967.

Physique, Performance and Oxygen Intake Capacity

Thomas K. Cureton, Jr.

Introduction

It is the purpose of this presentation to view the relative contributions of physique and oxygen intake to performance as a multivariate problem. Wyndham [34], for instance, has done this in analyzing the *net* effect of height, weight and fat on oxygen intake (l/min). He used partial correlations and concluded that 70% of oxygen intake (l/min) was due to weight, height and fat. In this study the usual method of analysis by the multivariate "Path Coefficient" System, based on the square of the Beta weights in the prediction equation, is used.

Accounting for performance of any kind involves many unique factors which are usually not correlated with each other. One rotational factor analysis [16] demonstrated that among 102 variables, including items of physique, cardiovascular-respiratory fitness, O_2 intake and O_2 debt, the percent contribution to the total variance was as follows: *Factor I*: Stroke Volume from the Brachial Pulse Wave (29.04%); *Factor II*: Hill's Oxygen Requirement (14.04%); *Factor III*: Pulse Pressure at end of an All-out Treadmill Run, 8.6% grade, 10 mph (10.93%); *Factor IV*: Body Weight (7.22%); *Factor V*: Progressive Pulse Ratio, Adjustment to Physical Work (5.14%); *Factor VI*: Endurance Run Time (5.08%); *Factor VII*: Pulse Rate (3.41%); *Factor VIII*: Oxygen Intake in the All-out Run, l/min (3.54%). The low relative proportionate part of the total variance led us to pursue the problem further to determine the relative value of physique, performance and oxygen intake by multivariate analysis.

A factor analysis of 22 tests made on 110 young men [11] revealed that the most important item is the 18-Item Motor Test, followed by the Sum of Four Dynamometer Strength Test, the

Thomas K. Cureton, Jr., Physical Fitness Institute, University of Illinois, Urbana, Ill., U.S.A.

623

Somatotype Rating (Physique), Pulse Rate Recovery from the Harvard 5-Min Step Test, Thinness by Calipered Fat, Pulse Wave and Schneider Index, Mile Run for Time, Vital Capacity Residual, Calf Girth (physique) in that order. This last item has been shown to correlate highly with $\dot{V}O_2$ max in more recent studies.

Physique Studies on Young Men and Relationship to Performance

An early study of somatotyping was carried out on 585 young men at Springfield College [11]. There was a significant difference between the mesomorph and ecto-mesomorph classes as compared to endomorphs and ectomorphs in *motor performance*. The mean overall performance score on the Cozens All-Around Athletic Performance Test was 334.4 points. Mesomorphs and ecto-mesomorphs were significantly above this mean while endomorphs and ectomorphs were significantly below it. However, the endomorphs and ecto-mesomorphs excelled on the McCurdy-Larson Organic Efficiency Test. Later these findings were verified on another group of 110 medical students tested in Chicago.

An early study to separate the bone, muscle bulk and fat components by anthropometrical techniques on a class of graduate students in physical education is shown in Table I. Oxygen intake (l/min) correlates (0.40) with the bone component and moderately correlates (0.48) with muscular bulk but *not* with fat, Larson Chinning-Vertical Jump-Dipping Test or the 18-Item Motor Test. When weight was divided into the $\dot{V}O_2$, the correlations were negative and low. Schvartz et al [26] found a low correlation between predicted $\dot{V}O_2$ max and the time of a 1-km run; also Gitin et al found $\dot{V}O_2$ max as determined by laboratory procedures on 18 U. S. Marines to correlate 0.16 with the U. S. Marine Fitness Test Score and -0.48 with the 3-mile run time.

A study of endurance running in college age men [10] revealed that the ectomorphs' prediction score for endurance running on the basis of a *4-Item CV* (cardiovascular) equation was better than endo- or mesomorphs. The criterion endurance measure was the composite standard score from four endurance events: mile run, 2 mile run, 3½ mile steeplechase run, and the 1000/100 yard drop-off test. Since the cardiovascular items did not correlate with age, the body build was the dominant influence on endurance running. Other studies have confirmed this influence originally reported in 1945 [1, 4, 5, 20, 24, 33]. More recent studies have shown that $\dot{V}O_2$ max is related to weight and even somewhat more with lean body mass (LBM). Running is likewise affected by body build, or weight and lean body

Table I. Separation of Bone Muscle Fat Proportions (Athletic Subjects)
(Male and Female 20-29 Yr.)

Subjects Identity	Predicted RB-WT	Sex	Height (in)	Weight (lbs.)	Percent Weight of Bones	Percent of Muscle	Percent of Fat	Density of Body
1. M.O.	+32.0	M	75	227	42.8	32.8	24.4	1.039
2. B.F.	+28.0	M	72	194	43.3	40.7	16.0	1.058
3. R.T.	+20.8	M	73.5	155	44.4	32.4	23.2	1.042
4. L.S.	+20.37	M	68	155	41.8	46.2	22.0	1.042
5. A.P.	+13.8	M	72	207	45.4	38.9	16.6	1.059
6. W.G.S.	+17.7	M	71	160	44.7	43.2	16.6	1.076
7. G.K.	+17.4	M	71	184	43.8	49.9	12.3	1.070
8. G.F.	+13.87	M	68	148	45.7	44.7	9.65	1.078
9. G.E.O.	+13.7	M	70.5	178	50.0	36.7	13.3	1.067
10. N.K.	+13.4	M	66	138	43.3	47.7	10.0	1.075
11. S.A.M.	+10.5	F	68	140	42.7	47.3	11.0	1.076
12. J.O.H.	+ 9.58	M	72	193	42.4	36.3	21.3	1.046
13. G.K.	+ 3.4	F	67	132	38.9	48.6	12.6	1.069
14. D.B.	+ 1.7	F	62	105	38.1	54.5	7.4	1.082
15. J.S.	+ 1.0	M	71	192	42.2	45.8	12.0	1.070
16. P.C.	- 1.0	F	64	155	38.6	45.4	16.0	1.060
17. N.A.	- 2.0	M	68	165	42.8	41.2	16.0	1.059
18. M.A.B.	- 3.0	M	68	180	39.8	40.8	19.4	1.053
19. D.B.	+30.0	M	72	204	52.6	32.9	14.5	1.061

mass. High correlations are reported in the literature between $\dot{V}O_2$ max (ml/min/kg) and time, or distance, but it has been shown that body build affects both. Endurance running is moderately (0.48) correlated with cardiovascular fitness, pulse rate, pulse pressure, brachial pulse wave as reflected by formulas related to heart minute volume. Still, these do not account for more than one third of the total variance in careful work. If lean body mass, or weight, is partialed out of the $\dot{V}O_2$ max (either ml/min/kg or l/min) the relationship is poor between running endurance and the residual $\dot{V}O_2$ max. A correlation of 0.46 between the Astrand-Ryhming "predicted" $\dot{V}O_2$ max and 12-minute running distance decreasing to 0.33 with weight partialed out has been shown. Weight correlated -0.42 with the running distance. The data on 14 male subjects showed a low relationship between $\dot{V}O_2$ max and running performance, due to the overshadowing effects of weight, or body build (somatotype) and LBM [21-23].

Experiments conducted in the water with swimmers have shown that up to 1500 meters fat has very little effect on performance, but is generally considered helpful to performance in long-distance swimming. It is well known that body fat in runners is a handicap. It was found [28] that the mechanical efficiency of leg kicking, arm stroking and gliding speed could be combined to predict time of 60 or 100 yard sprints, and that a drop-off type of endurance test was more valuable in combination with the mechanical velocity tests to predict 100 or 440 yard swimming times than combinations of oxygen intake and oxygen debt.

Cardiovascular-respiratory fitness seems to be more reliable in predicting swimming 440 yards or longer racing distances, with the O_2 *net debt* more significant than O_2 intake [28]. Furthermore, the breath holding time (after a two-minute step test) is helpful and is moderately correlated with O_2 debt. A test for swimming time prediction of 440 yards correlates 0.83 with swimming time based on a modification of the McCurdy-Larson Organic Efficiency Test [11] and a land exercise test of ten items. This test is only slightly dependent upon the body shape and fat ranges found in young men and women on swimming teams.

Other studies have shown that physical aptitude is highly specific to the sport. A test made to predict "general fitness" is not apt to work very well in sports highly dependent upon specific skill, size, endurance and experience [12]. Furthermore, a test like $\dot{V}O_2$ max is of very little interest to coaches or competitors in the sports. Its validity can be challenged. The interest is, of course, in the direct performance. For instance, to examine the efficiency of kicking, stroking, gliding and endurance (as in the drop-off type test) in the pool is more valuable to swimmers and coaches than the more "nonrelated" type tests. However, it is not suggested that purely "physiological" exploration is futile, or that the more "generalized" parameters have no value. Excellence in sports is related very closely to body type and body build [12]. More specifically, certain specific anthropometric measurements are related to athletic performances: the Davenport Index (the Crural Ratio: Length of Forelegs to Length of Thigh), the Vertical Jump, Standing Broad Jump, the Bone-Muscle-Fat Proportions, the Omomorphy Index (Width of Shoulders to Width of Hips), the Heel Length to Foot Length. We have shown that measurements of the feet and forelegs and thighs are significantly related to jumping using multivariate procedures.

The body build and anthropometric ratios of swimmers do relate to their swimming ability but not as much as their dynamic stroke characteristics, or their smooth gliding ability through the water. The relative weight of their legs in the water (density) is related negatively to performance but good flotation which helps to ride naturally high with better breathing is an asset.

How the body proportion ratios relate to performance has been frequently studied but how density relates to the body ratios is yet to be analyzed.

Difficulties With The Ratio: $\dot{V}O_2$/Body Weight

The oxygen intake (ml/min/kg) causes great confusion when used with full-normal distributions, or random samples from a full-normal sample. The heavier an individual is, the more energy is expended but increased lean body mass will increase the $\dot{V}O_2$ intake and total energy expended proportionately. But less lean body mass will cause the $\dot{V}O_2$ to decrease. Changing the ventilation volume from one test to another in an individual will change the $\dot{V}O_2$ or $\dot{V}O_2$ max. Changing the stride length or manner of using the arms or lifting the knees will change the $\dot{V}O_2$ or $\dot{V}O_2$ max. Slight to moderate changes (improvements) are related to improved economy (mechanical), improved skill (elimination of awkwardness) and breathing changes. To attribute such changes to "oxygen transport" from lungs to muscles is most certainly not the whole story, but added capillarization and increased number and size of mitochondria within the muscles being used are probable factors of importance. But when weight (the whole body weight) is divided into the $\dot{V}O_2$, confusion may occur because the changing fat content or lean body mass, the changing mechanics of performance, and the changing state of relaxation (minimal tension) in the muscles all effect it. There is no guarantee that the improvements in $\dot{V}O_2$ or $\dot{V}O_2$ max mean more than changes in some of these variables. The meaning of the changes associated with progressive stages of longitudinal training is badly clouded as was demonstrated by a study of Orban on six boys who trained in ice race-skating. Three of the boys deteriorated over approximately 90 consecutive days of training (workouts), but their skating times improved as O_2 intake measured in l/min/kg did not improve. Three other boys improved with two of these never plateauing, but the third did after about 100 days of training. It demonstrates that boys respond differently to training. By following the body fat changes it was deduced that those who gained lean body mass improved, and those who did not remained almost the same. Many things are unknown, such as the blood volume changes, the actual density and the influence of the strongest boy with the greatest ability getting a cold. Unfortunately, such oxygen intake measures are affected by several influences, some opposite to others, and neither in l/min nor in l/min/kg could the O_2 intake measures be interpreted.

Another study by Stanley Brown in 1960 found that boys who lost fat and weight improved their $\dot{V}O_2$ max but those who made insignificant changes in fat but gained in muscle bulk and strength improved in $\dot{V}O_2$ max (l/min/kg). Similar conclusions now appear in several papers now published by Jack Daniels, Victor Katch and S. Brown. At the U. S. Marine Physiological Center, LeJeune, N. C. it was found that the $\dot{V}O_2$ max test was insignificantly related to the mile run time and the Marine Circuit Test given to high school boys in various high schools in the United States. The situation has been the same in relating the $\dot{V}O_2$ max test to endurance runs in the schools by physical educators [7, 32]. It was also shown that in long-distance running, by correcting the statistics or by equalizing the weight, $\dot{V}O_2$ max and/or body type was related poorly to endurance running [4-6, 14, 15, 17-19, 33]. The better runners know how to economize by using relatively less oxygen per minute.

Various experiments have been done to clarify the meaning of size, density and body mass in longer runs.

Critical Experiments to Clarify the Meaning of $\dot{V}O_2$ max

The early experiment of Seltzer at Harvard [25] in 1940 should be mentioned because he demonstrated that chest measurements, the width of the shoulders (Omomorphy Index) to width of the hips, and weight were highly related to oxygen intake, which was confirmed with respect to weight by Buskirk [2] and Cotes [3].

More recently, the demonstrations made by Cotes, Davies, Shephard and Cummings that simple external measurements of the body, such as width or circumference of the calf, the volume of the legs up to the crotch and body density, correlate highly with the $\dot{V}O_2$ max test (l/min or ml/min/kg) suggest that size, structural proportions and body build influence greatly the $\dot{V}O_2$ max as well as performance. By statistical analyses it is seen that the *net* (Beta square) contribution of O_2 intake ($\dot{V}O_2$) or $\dot{V}O_2$ max (ml/min/kg) is very small compared to the structural variables and to the "ability to run fast."

Comparison of Density, Speed of Running and $\dot{V}O_2$ to Predict Running Time in the 600-yard and Mile Runs

In the last three years, experiments at the University of Illinois, Urbana, by Kirk J. Cureton et al [8, 9] related three runs for time to the density (^{40}K), speed of running and $\dot{V}O_2$ using the "Path Analysis" multivariate system. The relative value of the parameters mentioned in the *net* (direct) contribution to the runs (time) revealed that the strongest relationship was just ability to run (speed, 50 yds), next density. Last and poorest was $\dot{V}O_2$. That same type of result has been shown in studies with young men [13, 14, 16]. In a study of young middle-aged men the data were computed to permit the *net* causal percent (Beta square) contributions to be calculated, using as dependent variables age, weight, two-mile running time to predict $\dot{V}O_2$ max (the criterion). The results have been shown to be age = 19%; weight = 80%; and two-mile run time = 1%, rounding off to whole numbers.

It is clear that $\dot{V}O_2$ max and $\dot{V}O_2$ have gotten credit for much that belongs to the body type and structural and mechanical efficiency of the individual.

In the perusal of the literature of the past 15 years, there are many examples of "biased samples" (highly trained individuals very much alike), or small, platykurtic distribution samples which give the highest (inflated) raw correlations, due to the cluster of poor performers at one end and good performers at the other end, but with too few cases in the middle of the distribution. Correlations as high as 0.90 drop to as low as 0.22 when treated with nonparametric statistics or when similar, larger and well-distributed samples are obtained.

The "predicted $\dot{V}O_2$ max" means that subjects on the regression line can be *predicted* quite well as to running performance but the situation reduces to correlating body build (as a component within $\dot{V}O_2$ max) with body build (influence in performance). Actually then, in such a case, the two variables being correlated are almost one and the same. If anyone doubts this, one can line up a well-distributed sample of all types, conforming approximately to a random sample of body types, and run them through a 1½ mile for time or distance, and the results will show the great *bias* of body type in affecting endurance running.

The overemphasis on $\dot{V}O_2$ max has only diverted the search for the most critical variables which explain performance. The relative value of pH of the blood is a critical variable indicating the ability of the body in action to keep the levels of lactate down but more importantly indicates the ability of the subjects relatively to stand high levels of lactate and extremely low pH. The build-up of CO_2 in the blood *can be felt*, and this stress effect of exertion is what a runner, or swimmer, or any athlete reacts to rather than restriction of lowering of O_2 intake. The human is built with the unique feature of a relatively large "reserve capacity," usually called O_2 debt capacity, but in holding the breath it is the CO_2 build-up and inability to get rid of it that is the critical problem.

It is the mistaken belief that O_2 intake or $\dot{V}O_2$ max is some type of miracle test. Other than structural size, the test has very little value after weight is partialed out [27, 29]. It might be helpful to look at some of the results of studies which have put the relative contribution of the several competing variables on a *net* (Beta square) computing basis to show the relative value which they have to affect the endurance performances [13, 16, 24]. Both the factor analysis and the *net Beta square* analysis show that $\dot{V}O_2$ max is a dubious and quite uninterpretable measure to the coach or practical physical educator who may wish to test pupils and tell them of their cardiovascular status. Of course, differences between individuals can be identified on standardized workloads and with measures of pulse rate, blood pressures and stroke volume. The $\dot{V}O_2$ max test is so complicated by the fat, density variations and speed variations that its practical use is uninterpretable and should not be used to rate circulatory-respiratory fitness from either time or distance runs on a track [3, 7, 13-15, 26, 28, 29, 34]. The interest is now focused on determining reliable fat and density measures and in actual interpretable cardiovascular measures [8, 9, 23, 31].

To conclude, I must call your attention to the very high correlations obtained by Kjellberg, Rude and Sjostrand [21] between heart size and total hemoglobin and oxygen intake, correlations as high as 0.95. Applying this principle it follows that if body weight is purged from this apparent relationship, then the relationship is quite largely destroyed. It is the same with vital capacity [11] that by holding the body size constant, it eliminated 85% of the variability in the measurement, and age variation accounted for 7% more. The residual was a poor index to work with. Fantastic claims were made for gross vital capacity in the past and history has repeated itself with respect to the same kind of claims for $\dot{V}O_2$ max. The same univariate way of thinking can set off waves of "temporary delusion" with respect to strength, or enzymes, or muscle fiber counts, thus neglecting the capacity of man to react as a *total mind-body* integrated organism with great endurance, nervous capacity and drive.

References

1. Brown, W.C. and Wilmore, J.W.: Physical and physiological profiles of champion long distance runners. Med. Sci. Sports 6:71, 1971.
2. Buskirk, E.R. and Taylor, H.L.: Maximal oxygen intake and its relations to body composition with special reference to chronic physical activity and obesity. J. Appl. Physiol. 11:72-78, 1957.
3. Cotes, J.E., Davies, C.M.T., Edholm, C.G. et al: Factors relating to the aerobic capacity of 45 healthy British males and females, ages 18-28 years. Proc. R. Soc. Lond. [Biol.] 174:91-114, 1969.
4. Costill, D.L.: The relationship between selected physiological variables and distance running performance. J. Sports Med. Phys. Fitness 7:61-66, 1967.
5. Costill, D.L., Bowers, A. and Kramer, W.F.: Skinfold estimates of body fat among marathon runners. Med. Sci. Sports 2:93-99, 1970.
6. Costill, D.L., Thomason, H. and Roberts, H.: Fractional utilization of the aerobic capacity during distance running. Med. Sci. Sports 5:248-257, 1973.
7. Corbin, C.B.: Relations between physical working capacity and running performance in young boys. Res. Q. (AAHPER), 43:235-238, 1972.
8. Cureton, K.J., Boileau, R.A. and Lohman, T.G.: Relationship between the body composition measures and the AAHPER test performance in young boys. Res. Q. (AAHPER), 46:218-229, 1975.
9. Cureton, K.J., Boileau, R.A., Meisner, J.E. et al: Distance running times in the AAHPER youth fitness test as measures of circulatory-respiratory fitness in children 7 through 12 years of age. Milwaukee, Wisconsin: Report to the Research Council of AAHPER, April 6, 1976.
10. Cureton, T.K. Jr., Huffman, W.J., Welser, L. et al: Endurance of Young Men. Washington, D. C.: Society for Research in Child Development, Vol. X., Volume No. 40, No. 1, 1945.
11. Cureton, T.K. Jr.: Physical Fitness Appraisal and Guidance. St. Louis: C. V. Mosby Co., 1947.
12. Cureton, T.K. Jr.: Physical Fitness of Champion Athletes. Urbana, Ill.:University of Illinois Press, 1951.

13. Cureton, T.K. Jr.: The relative value of stress indicators, related to prediction of strenuous (athletic) treadmill performance. Medicine and Sport. New York and Basel:S. Karger, 1969, Vol. III, pp. 73-80.

14. Cureton, T.K. Jr.: What is oxygen intake (the $\dot{V}O_2$ max) measure? Am. Corr. Ther. J. 27:17-23, 1973.

15. Cureton, T.K. Jr.: In Enc. of the Sc. and Med. of Sport. New York: MacMillan, 1971, pp. 222-226.

16. Cureton, T.K. Jr. and Sterling, L.F.: Factor analysis of cardiovascular variables. J. Sports Med. Phys. Fitness 4:124-227, 1963.

17. Katch, V.L.: The role of maximal oxygen intake in endurance performance. Research Abstracts (AAHPER), p. 11, April 3, 1970.

18. Katch, V. and Henry, F.M.: Prediction of running performance from maximal oxygen debt and intake. Med. Sci. Sports 4:187-191, 1972.

19. Kearney, J.T. and Byrnes, W.G.: Measures of $\dot{V}O_2$ max and their relationship to running performance among three subject groups. Am. Corr. Ther. J. 28:145-150, 1974.

20. Kireilis, R.W. and Cureton, T.K. Jr.: The relationship of external fat to physical education activities and fitness tests. Res. Q. (AAHPER) 18:123-134, 1947.

21. Kjellberg, S.R., Rudhe, U. and Sjostrand, T.: The relation of cardiac volume tò the weight and surface area of the body, the blood volume and the physical capacity for work. Acta Radiologica 31:113-122, 1949.

22. Laubach, L.L.: Body composition in relationship to muscle strength and range of joint movement. J. Sports Med. Phys. Fitness 9:89-97, 1969.

23. Novak, L.P., Hyatt, R.E. and Alexander, J.F.: Body composition and physiologic function of athletes. JAMA 295:764-770, 1968.

24. Porbix, J.A.: A study of the relationship between the somatotype and motor fitness. Res. Q. (AAHPER) 25:84-90, 1954.

25. Seltzer, C.C.: Body build and oxygen metabolism at rest and during exercise. Am. J. Physiol. 129:1-13, 1940.

26. Shvartz, E., Shapiro, Y., Vurtzel, E. and Shapiro, A.: Relationship of a kilometer run to aerobic capacity. J. Sports Med. Phys. Fitness 13:180-182, 1973.

27. Thompson, J.M., Dempsey, J.A., Crosby, L.W. et al: Oxygen transport and oxyhemoglobin dissociation during prolonged muscular work on the ergometer bicycle. J. Appl. Physiol. 37:653-654, 1974.

28. Van Huss, W.D. and Cureton, T.K. Jr.: Relationship of selected tests with energy metabolism and swimming performance (25, 100 and 440 yards). Res. Q. (AAHPER) 26:205-221, 1955.

29. Welch, B.E., Riendieu, R.F., Crisp, G.R. and Eisenstein, R.S.: Relationship of maximal oxygen consumption to various components of body composition. J. Appl. Physiol. 12:395-402, 1958.

30. White, R.I. Jr. and Alexander, J.K.: Body oxygen consumption and pulmonary ventilation in obese subjects. J. Appl. Physiol. 20:197-201, 1965.

31. Wilmore, J.H. and Behnke, A.H.: Anthropometric estimation of body density and lean body weight in young men. J. Appl. Physiol. 27:25-31, 1969.

32. Wiley, J.F. and Shaver, L.G.: Prediction of maximal oxygen intake from running performance of untrained young men. Res. Q. (AAHPER) 43:89-93, 1972.

33. Wyndham, C.H., Strydom, N.B., Van Rennburg, A.J. and Benade, A.J.N.: Requirements of world class performances in endurance running. S. Afr. Med. J. 41:992-1002, 1969.
34. Wyndham, C.H.: Influence of body size and composition on oxygen consumption during exercise and on maximal aerobic capacity of Bantu and Caucasian men. Arch. Phys. Med. Rehabil. pp. 539-554, 1971.

Author Index Auteurs

Subject Index ⊗ Sujets

SUBJECT INDEX / SUJETS

NOTICE

By decision of the Scientific Commission, *French* and *English* were adopted as the two official languages of the International Congress of Physical Activity Sciences – 1976.

In these Proceedings, the communications appear *in the language in which they were presented* for French and English and *in English* as concerns the papers which were delivered in either German, Russian or Spanish. Abstracts in the two official languages accompany each paper included in Books 1 and 2 and the seminar presentations in the other books of the series.

AVERTISSEMENT

Les langues *anglaise* et *française* furent adoptées par la Commission scientifique comme langues officielles du Congrès international des sciences de l'activité physique – 1976. De ce fait, les communications apparaissent au présent rapport officiel *dans la langue où elles ont été présentées* pour ce qui est de l'anglais et du français, et dans la langue *anglaise* pour ce qui est des communications qui furent faites dans les langues allemande, russe et espagnole.

Des résumés dans chacune des deux langues officielles accompagnent chacune des communications qui paraissent aux Volumes 1 et 2 ainsi que les présentations faites par les conférenciers invités dans les autres volumes de la série.